Advanced Nutrition and Dietetics in Diabetes

Editors

Louise Goff PhD RD

Pamela Dyson PhD RD

Series Editor

Kevin Whelan PhD RD

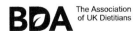

BDA The Association of UK Dietitians

WILEY Blackwell

Registered Office
John Wiley & Sons, Ltd, The Atrium, Southern Gate, Chichester, West Sussex, PO19 8SQ, UK

Editorial Offices
9600 Garsington Road, Oxford, OX4 2DQ, UK
The Atrium, Southern Gate, Chichester, West Sussex, PO19 8SQ, UK
1606 Golden Aspen Drive, Suites 103 and 104, Ames, Iowa 50010, USA

For details of our global editorial offices, for customer services and for information about how to apply for permission to reuse the copyright material in this book please see our website at www.wiley.com/wiley-blackwell.

The right of Louise Goff and Pamela Dyson to be identified as the authors of this work has been asserted in accordance with the UK Copyright, Designs and Patents Act 1988.

Library of Congress Cataloging-in-Publication Data

Advanced nutrition and dietetics in diabetes / edited by Louise Goff & Pamela Dyson.
    p. ; cm. – (Advanced nutrition and dietetics (BDA))
  Includes bibliographical references and index.
  ISBN 978-0-470-67092-7 (pbk.)
I. Goff, Louise, editor. II. Dyson, Pamela, editor. III. Series: Advanced nutrition and dietetics (BDA)
[DNLM: 1. Diabetes Mellitus–diet therapy. 2. Diabetic Diet. 3. Health Behavior. 4. Life Style.
5. Nutrition Therapy. WK 818]j
  RC662
  616.4′620654–dc23
                              2015022542

A catalogue record for this book is available from the British Library.

Set in 9.5/12pt Times by SPi Global, Pondicherry, India

Printed in the UK

ADVANCED NUTRITION AND DIETETICS BOOK SERIES

Dietary recommendations need to be based on solid evidence, but where can you find this information? The British Dietetic Association and the publishers of the *Manual of Dietetic Practice* present an essential and authoritative reference series on the evidence base relating to advanced aspects of nutrition and dietetics in selected clinical specialties. Each book provides a comprehensive and critical review of key literature in the area. Each covers established areas of understanding, current controversies and areas of future development and investigation, and is oriented around six key themes:

- Disease processes, including metabolism, physiology and genetics
- Disease consequences, including morbidity, mortality and patient perspectives
- Clinical investigation and management
- Nutritional consequences of disease
- Nutritional assessment, including anthropometric, biochemical, clinical, dietary, economic and social approaches
- Nutritional and dietary management of disease

Trustworthy, international in scope, and accessible, *Advanced Nutrition and Dietetics* is a vital resource for a range of practitioners, researchers and educators in nutrition and dietetics, including dietitians, nutritionists, doctors and specialist nurses.

Contents

Preface

Diabetes has been with us since ancient times, and the first mention of an illness that could be diabetes was recorded in an Egyptian papyrus of 1500 BC. A simplistic definition of diabetes is that of a disease typified by excessively high blood glucose concentrations, but this conceals the true nature of diabetes as a complex biochemical disorder affecting carbohydrate, fat and protein metabolism. Treatment of diabetes is multifactorial and aims to reduce both short- and long-term complications of the disease while maintaining quality of life. Diabetes belongs to the group of diseases that cannot be managed by medication alone, and lifestyle factors, including diet and physical activity, are fundamental to successful management. Dietary advice has been subject to various fashions over the years from low to high carbohydrate (and back) and each new approach has been greeted with almost equal amounts of enthusiasm and criticism. The fundamental question for all health professionals concerned with the management of diabetes is – what is the best diet for diabetes?

Evidence-based medicine (and lifestyle advice) is the cornerstone of successful management, and although there are numerous randomised controlled trials indicating the efficacy and safety of most medications used to treat diabetes, this is not always true of lifestyle interventions. Many studies designed to investigate the effects of lifestyle and dietary interventions are not well-designed and there are issues with small numbers of subjects, lack of comparison or control groups, study design and intervention, data quality, data reporting and target populations. It is impossible to conduct randomised, controlled trials in free-living populations over the periods of time required for unambiguous results, and in many cases short-term trials using surrogate end-points are the only evidence available. Despite this, many national and international diabetes associations now publish evidence-based guidelines and recommendations for the dietary management of diabetes, although most of these guidelines identify areas where there is little evidence and recommendations are made based on consensus opinion.

This book is designed to offer both evidence for and the practical aspects of the nutritional management of diabetes, and offers a global view of the lifestyle interventions for the prevention and management of diabetes, including management of complications and special groups. Recognised authorities from around the world have shared their expertise in areas such as the management of diabetes in older people, the glycaemic index, public health and prevention and formulating nutritional guidelines. The book is divided into nine different sections, each addressing a particular aspect of diabetes and each providing a critical review of key literature in the area with an emphasis on translating evidence into practice. The epidemiology, aetiology and clinical management of diabetes are addressed, with an emphasis on lifestyle management, and specifically diet and nutrition, in all areas of the treatment and prevention of diabetes.

This book is aimed at those who work at an advanced level in diabetes, including clinicians, researchers and educators, and is intended for the multi-disciplinary team, including specialist dietitians, diabetes specialist nurses, physicians and psychologists. It will also appeal to general dietitians who wish to learn more about diabetes, and to those undertaking Masters degrees in dietetics, nutrition, medicine or nursing with a specific diabetes component. It is a useful reference and resource for those teaching diabetes at any level.

Louise Goff PhD RD
Senior Lecturer in Nutritional Sciences
King's College London

Pamela Dyson PhD RD
Research Dietitian
University of Oxford
Editors
Advanced Nutrition and Dietetics in Diabetes

This book is the second title in a series commissioned as part of a major initiative between the British Dietetic Association and the publishers Wiley. Each book in the series provides a comprehensive and critical review of the key literature in a clinical area. Each book is edited by one or more experts who have themselves undertaken extensive research and published widely in the relevant topic area. Each book chapter is written by experts drawn from an international audience and from a variety of disciplines as required of the relevant chapter (e.g. dietetics, medicine, public health, basic sciences). Future titles in the series will cover areas including obesity and nutritional support.

The book editors and I are proud to present the second title in the series: Advanced Nutrition and Dietetics in Diabetes. We hope that it impacts on health professionals' understanding and application of nutrition and dietetics in the prevention and management of diabetes and improves outcomes and reduces complications for such patients.

Kevin Whelan PhD RD
Professor of Dietetics
King's College London
Series Editor
Advanced Nutrition and Dietetics Book Series

Foreword

Diabetes management is complex and requires a multidisciplinary team approach, including a wide range of healthcare professionals as well as people with diabetes and their carers. Diet and lifestyle advice form the cornerstone of diabetes self-management, education and counselling, and for most patients with diabetes, this is one of their main concerns. It is therefore crucial that all healthcare professionals, not just dietitians, involved in diabetes care have a good knowledge of the role of diet and skills in advising patients about their lifestyle.

This book is a comprehensive text and reviews concisely and succinctly the literature relating to diabetes pathophysiology and aetiology and the latest evidence on the role of diet in the prevention and management of the many different types and presentations of diabetes.

This book has contributions from leading clinicians, dietitians and researchers in the field of diabetes and covers diabetes in more depth and breadth than other diet-oriented texts; included are sections on diabetes in older adults, diabetes in ethnic minority groups, diabetes in pregnancy, diabetes and coeliac disease, cystic fibrosis-related diabetes and gastroparesis as well, focusing clearly on both type 1 and type 2 diabetes.

I would recommend *Advanced Nutrition and Dietetics in Diabetes* as essential reading for not only dietitians but also physicians, nurses and scientists who want to – and indeed need to – know about the role of diet in diabetes management.

Professor Sir George Alberti
Emeritus Professor of Medicine,
University of Newcastle
Senior Research Investigator,
Endocrinology & Metabolism Group,
Imperial College London
Visiting Professor, Division of Diabetes &
Nutritional Sciences, King's College London

Editor biographies

Louise Goff

Louise Goff is a Senior Lecturer in Nutritional Sciences in the Division of Diabetes and Nutritional Sciences at King's College London. Her research interest is diabetes in African and Caribbean populations. Dr Goff leads a programme of research focused on prediabetes and the development of type 2 diabetes in people of African and Caribbean ancestry funded by Diabetes UK. Dr Goff is on the editorial board of *Ethnicity and Health*.

Pamela Dyson

Pamela Dyson is a Research Dietitian in the Oxford Centre for Diabetes, Endocrinology and Metabolism at Oxford University. Her clinical speciality includes nutritional management of both type 1 and type 2 diabetes in adults. Dr Dyson's research interests include weight management in type 2 diabetes, delivery of dietary education and community approaches to diabetes prevention. Dr Dyson led the writing of the Diabetes UK guidelines for the nutritional management of diabetes and was invited to write the diabetes chapter for the 5th edition of the *Manual of Dietetic Practice*. She is on the editorial board of *Diabesity in Practice*.

Kevin Whelan

Kevin Whelan is the Professor of Dietetics in the Division of Diabetes and Nutritional Sciences at King's College London. He is a Principal Investigator leading a research programme exploring the interaction between the gastrointestinal microbiota, diet and health and disease. In 2012 he was awarded the Nutrition Society Cuthbertson Medal for research in clinical nutrition. Prof Whelan is the Series Editor for the *British Dietetic Association Advanced Nutrition and Dietetics* book series and is also on the editorial boards of *Alimentary Pharmacology and Therapeutics* and the *Journal of Human Nutrition and Dietetics*.

Contributors

Ahmed H Abdelhafiz MD FRCP
Consultant Physician, Honorary Senior Clinical Lecturer
Rotherham General Hospital
Rotherham, UK

Francesca Annan MSc RD
Paediatric Diabetes Dietitian
Alder Hey Children's NHS Foundation Trust
Liverpool, UK

Suzanne Barr PhD RD
Research Dietitian
Imperial College London
London, UK

Pratik Choudhary MD MRCP
Consultant Diabetologist and Senior Lecturer
King's College Hospital NHS Foundation Trust and
King's College London
London, UK

Thushara Dassanayake BSc RD
Specialist Renal Dietitian
Imperial College Healthcare NHS Foundation Trust
London, UK

Trudi Deakin PhD RD
Consultant Diabetes Dietitian
X-PERT Health Charity
Hebden Bridge, UK

Anne Dornhorst DM FRCP
Imperial College Healthcare NHS Foundation Trust
London, UK

Alastair Duncan MSc RD
Principal Dietitian
Guy's and St Thomas' NHS Foundation Trust
London, UK

Trisha Dunning AM
Professor of Nursing
Deakin University and Barwon Health
Victoria, Australia

Pamela Dyson PhD RD
Research Dietitian
University of Oxford, Oxford Centre for Diabetes
Endocrinology and Metabolism, Churchill Hospital
Oxford, UK

Marion J. Franz MS RD
Nutrition Concepts by Franz, Inc.
Minneapolis, USA

Maeve Gacquin BSc MINDI
Senior Dietitian
Galway Clinic
Doughiska, Ireland

Louise Goff PhD RD
Senior Lecturer in Nutritional Sciences
King's College London
London, UK

Simon Heller DM FRCP
Professor of Clinical Diabetes
University of Sheffield
Sheffield, UK

C. Jeya Henry PhD
Professor and Director of Clinical Nutritional Sciences
National University of Singapore
Singapore

Elaine Hibbert-Jones BSc RD
Chief Diabetes Dietitian
Royal Gwent Hospital
Newport, UK

Alyson Hill PhD RD
Lecturer in Dietetics
University of Ulster
Londonderry, UK

Mohammed S. B. Huda PhD MRCP
Consultant in Diabetes and Endocrinology
Barts Health NHS Trust
London, UK

Ahmed Iqbal MBBS MRCP
MRC Fellow in Diabetes and Endocrinology
University of Sheffield
Sheffield, UK

David R. Matthews DPhil FRCP
Professor in Diabetic Medicine and Emeritus
Founding Chairman of OCDEM
University of Oxford, Oxford Centre for Diabetes
Endocrinology and Metabolism
Oxford, UK

Hilary McCoubrey BSc RD
Paediatric Diabetes Dietitian
Birmingham Children's Hospital
Birmingham, UK

Shivani Misra MSc MRCP
Specialist Registrar in Diabetes and Endocrinology
Imperial College Healthcare NHS Foundation Trust
London, UK

Lindsay Oliver BSc RD
Consultant Dietitian in Diabetes
North Tyneside General Hospital
North Shields, UK

Sathish Parthasarathy MBBS MRCP
Specialist Registrar in Diabetes and Endocrinology
King's College Hospital NHS Foundation Trust
London, UK

Princy Paul
Consultant Paediatrician and Lead for Diabetes
Alder Hey Children's NHS Foundation Trust
Liverpool, UK

Baldeesh Rai BSc RD
Specialist Cardiac Dietitian
London North West Healthcare NHS Trust
London, UK

Alan J. Sinclair MD FRCP
Dean and Professor of Medicine
Bedfordshire & Hertfordshire PG Medical School
Luton, UK

Kimber L. Stanhope PhD RD
Associate Research Nutritional Biologist
University of California
Davis, USA

P. Sangeetha Thondre PhD
Post-Doctoral Research Fellow
Oxford Brookes University
Oxford, UK

Nicola Tufton MRCP
Specialist Registrar in Diabetes and Endocrinology
Barts Health NHS Trust
London, UK

Karen Walker PhD
Associate Professor of Nutrition
Monash University
Melbourne, Australia

Kerry-Lee Watson BSc RD
Specialist Cystic Fibrosis Dietitian
King's College Hospital NHS Foundation Trust
London, UK

Catherine Whitmore RN
Research Nurse in Diabetes and Endocrinology
University of Liverpool
Liverpool, UK

John Wilding DM FRCP
Professor of Medicine, Head of the Department of
Obesity and Endocrinology
University of Liverpool
Liverpool, UK

Katie Wynne PhD MRCP
Hunter New England Health and University of Newcastle
Newcastle, Australia

Abbreviations

AACE	American Association of Clinical Endocrinologists
ABCD	Association of British Clinical Diabetologists
ACCORD	Action to Control Cardiovascular Risk in Diabetes
ACE	Angiotensin converting enzyme inhibitor
ACSM	American College of Sports Medicine
ADA	American Diabetes Association
ADS	Australian Diabetes Society
ADP	Adenosine diphosphate
ADVANCE	Action in Diabetes and Vascular Disease: Preterax and Diamicron MR Controlled Evaluation
AGS	American Geriatrics Society
AKPD	Atypical ketosis prone diabetes
AMP	Adenosine monophosphate
AMPK	AMP-activated kinase
apoB	Apolipoprotein B100
ARB	Angiotensin receptor blockade
ASDIAB	Asian Young Diabetes Research Study
ATP	Adenosine triphosphate
AUC	Area under the curve
BG	Blood glucose
BMI	Body mass index
BP	Blood pressure
CAPD	Continuous ambulatory peritoneal dialysis
CARE	Cholesterol and Recurrent Events study
CD	Coeliac disease
CEMACH	Confidential enquiry into maternal and child health
CF	Cystic fibrosis
CFRD	Cystic fibrosis-related diabetes
CHD	Coronary heart disease
CI	Confidence interval
CKD	Chronic kidney disease
CMV	Cytomagelavirus
CSII	Continuous subcutaneous infusion of insulin
CVD	Cardiovascular disease
DAFNE	Dose adjusted for normal eating
DAG	Diacylglycerol
DASH	Dietary approaches to stop hypertension
DCCT	Diabetes Control and Complications Trial
DE-PLAN	Prevention using lifestyle, physical activity and nutrition intervention
DGP	Diabetic gastroparesis
DiaMond	Diabetes mondiale project group
DKA	Diabetic ketoacidosis
DMEG	Diabetes Management and Education Group
DNA	Deoxyribonucleic acid
DNL	*De novo* lipogenesis
DPP-4	Dipeptidyl peptidase 4
DPP	Diabetes prevention programme
DPS	Diabetes prevention study
DR	Diabetic retinopathy
DSME	Diabetes self-management education

Early ACTID	Activity early in diabetes	HHS	Hyperosmotic hyperglycaemic state
EASD	European Association for the Study of Diabetes	HIV	Human immunodeficiency virus
EDIC	Epidemiology of Diabetes Interventions and Complications trial	HLA	Human leucocyte antigen
		HOPE	Heart Outcomes Prevention Evaluation
EPBP	European Best Practice (Guidelines)	HOT	Hypertension optimal treatment
ESPEN	European Society for Clinical Nutrition and Metabolism	IBW	Ideal body weight
		IDF	International Diabetes Federation
EURODIAB	European type 1 diabetes study	IFCC	International Federation of Clinical Chemistry
FAI	Free androgen index	IFG	Impaired fasting glycaemia
FAO	Food and Agriculture Organisation	IGT	Impaired glucose tolerance
		ILI	Intensive lifestyle interventions
FEV1	Forced expiratory volume in 1 second	IOM	Institute of Medicine
FIN-D2	Finland type 2 diabetes prevention programme	IR	Insulin resistance
		IRS-1	Insulin receptor substrate-1
FPG	Fasting plasma glucose	ISPAD	International Society for Paediatric and Adolescent Diabetes
FSA	Food Standards Agency		
FSH	Follicle stimulating hormone		
FTO	Fat mass and obesity-associated protein		
		IV	Intravenous
GAD	Glutamic acid decarboxylase	JBDS	Joint British Diabetes Society
GDA	Guideline daily amount	JNK	c-jun NH_2-terminal kinase
GDM	Gestational diabetes mellitus	LADA	Latent autoimmune diabetes in adults
GORD	Gastro-oesophageal reflux		
GES	Gastric emptying scintigraphy	LDL	Low density lipoprotein
GF	Gluten-free	LH	Lutenising hormone
GFD	Gluten-free diet	LMIC	Low and middle-income countries
GFR	Glomerular filtration rate		
GI	Glycaemic index	LPL	Lipoprotein lipase
GIP	Gastric Inhibitory polypeptide	Look AHEAD	Action for health in diabetes
GL	Glycaemic load	MCP-1	Monocyte chemoattractant protein-1
GLP-1	Glucagon-like peptide-1		
GPEDM	Global Partnership for Effective Diabetes Management	MDI	Multiple daily injections
		MDT	Multidisciplinary team
GWAS	Genome-wide association studies	MICS	Malnutrition-inflammation complex syndrome
HAART	Highly active antiretroviral therapy	MODY	Maturity onset diabetes of the young
HbA1c	Glycated haemoglobin (haemoglobin A1c)	MRFIT	Multiple Risk Factor Intervention Trial
HD	Haemodialysis	MTP	Microsomal triglyceride-transfer protein
HDL	High density lipoprotein		
HFCS	High fructose corn syrup	MUFA	Monounsaturated fat

NaDIA	National diabetes inpatient audit	RNI	Reference nutrient intake
NAFLD	Non-alcoholic fatty liver disease	RR	Relative risk
NASH	Non-alcoholic steatohepatitis	RT-CGM	Real-time continuous glucose monitoring
NCD	Non-communicable disease	SABRE	Southall and Brent Revisited Study
NGT	Normal glucose tolerance		
NHS	National Health Service	SFA	Saturated fatty acid
NICE	National Institute of Health and Clinical Excellence	SGLT-2	Sodium glucose transporter 2
		SHBG	Sex hormone binding globulin
NODAT	New-onset diabetes after organ transplantation	4S	Scandinavian Simvastin Survival Study
NPH	Neutral protamine Hagedorn	4-T	Treating to Target in Type 2 diabetes Trial
nPKC	Novel-protein kinase C		
OGTT	Oral glucose tolerance test	TC	Total cholesterol
ONS	Oral nutritional supplements	TDD	Total daily dose
PAD	Peripheral arterial disease	TNDM	Transient neonatal diabetes
PAI-1	Plasminogen activator inhibitor-1	TODAY	Treatment options for type 2 diabetes in adolescents and youth
PCOS	Polycystic ovary syndrome		
PD	Peritoneal dialysis	TPN	Total parenteral nutrition
PEM	Protein energy malnutrition	TZD	Thiazolidinedione
PNDM	Permanent neonatal diabetes	UKPDS	UK Prospective Diabetes Study
PPARγ	Peroxisome proliferator-activated receptor gamma	VACSDM	Veterans Affairs Cooperative Study in Type 2 Diabetes Mellitus
PUFA	Polyunsaturated fat		
PVD	Peripheral vascular disease	VADT	Veteran Affairs Diabetes Trial
QUM	Quality use of medicines	VA-HIT	Veterans Affairs High Density Lipoprotein Cholesterol Intervention Trial
RACF	Residential aged care facility		
RACGP	Royal Australian College of General Practitioners		
		VLDL	Very low density lipoprotein
RAS	Renin-angiotensin-aldosterone system	VO_2max	Maximum capacity of an individual's body to transport and use oxygen
RCPCH	Royal College of Paediatrics and Child Health		
		VRIII	Variable rate intravenous insulin infusion
RCT	Randomised controlled trial		
RD	Registered dietitian	WC	Waist circumference
RDA	Recommended daily allowance	WHO	World Health Organisation

SECTION 1

Background

Chapter 1.1

Prevalence, public health aspects and prevention of diabetes

Pamela Dyson

University of Oxford, Oxford Centre for Diabetes, Endocrinology and Metabolism, Churchill Hospital, Oxford, UK

1.1.1 Prevalence

Globally, diabetes is one of the most common non-communicable diseases (NCD), affecting an estimated 371 million people (8.3% of the adult population) worldwide in 2012 [1]. Type 2 diabetes accounts for 85–90% of global diabetes, and conservative estimates by the International Diabetes Federation (IDF) predict that diabetes will increase to 776 million by 2035 (9% of the population), and that over 80% of those with diabetes will live in low and middle-income countries (LMIC) [2]. The predicted increase in diabetes is largely due to type 2 diabetes and is strongly associated with lifestyle factors, including obesity, physical inactivity and unhealthy diet. The rising incidence of diabetes is not confined to one part of the world and the IDF reports a wide geographic spread. Table 1.1.1 shows the rising pandemic, split by world region. It illustrates that the diabetes epidemic, although well established in high-income countries, will be much more prominent as an increasing problem in LMIC. For example, it is predicted that the number of people with diabetes will double in Africa and the Middle East and North Africa between 2010 and 2030.

Approximately 80–90% of those with diagnosed diabetes have type 2 diabetes and 10–20% have type 1 diabetes. Different countries exhibit different rates of diabetes with a range from <5% in parts of Africa to >30% amongst adults in Narau. In the United Kingdom (UK), prevalence rates were estimated at 4.26% (2.8 million adults) in 2010 based upon data from the Qualities and Outcomes Framework [3] although this may be an underestimate as a more recent study reported that the prevalence amongst adults in the UK was 3.1 million (7.4%) in 2011 [4].

The global statistics for the prevalence of diabetes refer only to those who have received a diagnosis but population-based studies have reported a high prevalence of undiagnosed diabetes. Globally, approximately 175 million people may be unaware of their diabetes [2] and in the UK, for example, it has been estimated that 850 000 people are living with undiagnosed diabetes [5]. There are large differences between countries for the prevalence of undiagnosed diabetes, with rates of 90% reported in some African countries and much lower rates in high-income countries. As with diagnosed diabetes, over 80% of people with undiagnosed diabetes live in LMIC.

1.1.2 Pre-diabetes

Pre-diabetes or impaired glucose tolerance (IGT) is characterized by elevated blood glucose levels, and is considered a risk factor for the development of type 2 diabetes and for cardiovascular disease. Approximately 316 million people in the world were estimated to have IGT in 2013, and 70% of these live in LMIC. By 2035, the numbers with IGT are projected to increase to 471 million, meaning that over one billion people, or approximately 20% of the

Advanced Nutrition and Dietetics in Diabetes, First Edition. Edited by Louise Goff and Pamela Dyson.
© 2016 John Wiley & Sons, Ltd. Published 2016 by John Wiley & Sons, Ltd.

Table 1.1.1 Regional estimates for diabetes (20–79 age group), 2010 and 2030

	2013			2035		
Region	Population (20–79 y) (millions)	No. of people with DM (millions)	Diabetes prevalence (%)	Population (20–79 y) (millions)	No. of people with DM (millions)	Diabetes prevalence (%)
NAC	325	36.7	9.6	405	50.4	9.9
MENA	375	34.6	10.9	584	67.9	11.3
SEA	883	72.1	8.7	1217	123.0	9.4
EUR	659	56.3	6.8	669	68.9	7.1
SACA	301	24.1	8.2	394	38.5	8.2
WP	1613	138.2	8.1	1818	201.8	8.4
AFR	408	19.8	5.7	776	41.5	5.3
Total	4564	381.7	8.3	5863	592.9	8.8

Source: *Diabetes Atlas* 6th edition.
Key: NAC North America and Caribbean, MENA Middle East and North Africa, SEA South East Asia, EUR Europe, SACA South and Central America, WP Western Pacific, AFR Africa

adult population, will be living with diabetes or pre-diabetes by 2035 [2].

1.1.3 Public health aspects

Diabetes, in common with other NCDs, is regarded as a clinical disease and is traditionally managed by application of the acute medical model to the individual with diabetes. As type 2 diabetes prevalence has increased, it has become a public health concern requiring a broad, multidisciplinary approach that targets individuals, families, communities and societies. Diabetes requires more than the traditional approach of medical management of each individual, and effective treatment and prevention will entail a population-based public health approach.

Public health includes the concepts of surveillance for assessment and monitoring, prevention strategies and policy implications. Surveillance can provide data about the prevalence of diabetes and associated risk factors, including health behaviour and obesity. These data can be used to define and ultimately reduce the burden of diabetes by targeting services and prevention strategies at relevant populations. Many countries do not maintain national diabetes registers

and do not have systems to assess risk factors, and uncertainties about prevalence in the general population and in high-risk groups prevent instigation of effective public heath strategies to prevent and manage diabetes.

Public policies for prevention and management of diabetes can be introduced at local, state and national levels. Management of diabetes can be improved by policies at a national level e.g. the UK retinal screening programme and at a local level e.g. school policies for the management of children with type 1 diabetes. Health care policies are an important factor for the management of diabetes, and integration of health care (whether provided by the state or through private insurance) with public policy is essential.

Economic impact of diabetes

Diabetes affects quality of life, general health and well-being and is responsible for the loss of healthy years of life (disability-adjusted life years or DALYs). The premature mortality associated with diabetes is preceded by years of disability. Apart from the human consequences of the morbidity and mortality associated with diabetes, the economic impact is enormous and is related to both the direct medical costs of treatment and the indirect costs of labour units lost. Type 2 diabetes in particular is now affecting people at a younger age during their prime economically productive years and it has been estimated that the global economic impact could total US $490 billion over the next 20 years [2]. The estimated global cost of diabetes alone was US $471 billion in 2012, accounting for 11–12% of total health-care expenditure in the world. Diabetes is forecast to have substantial negative effects on individual, national and international economic well-being over the next 20 years, and this will have particular effect in newly emerging economies.

1.1.4 Prevention

Type 1 diabetes

The aetiology of type 1 diabetes remains poorly understood and there is no evidence for effective prevention; studies in high-risk groups have used strategies including insulin therapy [6] and nicotinamide supplementation [7] without success. A more recent randomised controlled trial is investigating early exposure to complex dietary proteins in high-risk infants and has shown a reduction of approximately 50% in diabetes-associated antibodies in those weaned to a highly hydrolysed formula. Whether this translates to diabetes prevention will be clear at the study's end in 2017 [8].

Type 2 diabetes

Risk factors for type 2 diabetes include both non-modifiable (age, genetic predisposition, ethnicity) and modifiable (obesity, physical inactivity, diet) factors. There is strong evidence for type 2 diabetes prevention from studies in high-risk individuals from different ethnic groups, using both pharmacological and lifestyle interventions [9–13]. The most effective intervention is that of lifestyle change, incorporating weight loss, dietary modification and increased physical activity; this combination can reduce the risk of diabetes by 28–59% [14,15]. In addition, three studies have reported long-term reductions in progression to diabetes in lifestyle intervention groups at 7–20 years

after completion of the study – the so-called legacy effect [16–18].

Components of lifestyle interventions

The main components of lifestyle interventions for diabetes prevention were similar in all published studies. The Diabetes Prevention Programme (DPP) achieved 7% weight loss amongst participants by recommending an energy deficit of 500–1000 kcal/day, reduction of fat intake to 25% total energy intake and promoting 150 minutes of moderate activity per week [9]. The Finnish Diabetes Prevention Study (DPS) recommended ≥5% weight loss, a reduction in total fat intake to <30% and saturated fat to <10% total energy, an increase in fibre intake to ≥15 g/1000 kcal and 30 minutes of moderate physical activity daily [10]. The Indian diabetes prevention study included energy restriction, fat reduction, avoidance of sugar and increased dietary fibre. In addition, participants were asked to take ≥ 30 minutes of moderate exercise daily [11]. The Japanese prevention trial promoted weight loss by a 10% reduction in portion size for all foods except vegetables, low fat intake (<50 g/day) and low alcohol intake (<50 g/day) with 30–40 minutes of moderate exercise per day [12]. The Chinese study attempted to define the relative effects of physical activity, diet and a combination of the two by adopting block randomisation, although specific details of each intervention are not described [13].

Weight loss

The most dominant predictor for diabetes prevention is weight loss; every kilogram lost is associated with a 16% reduction in risk [14]. Although all the published data support the use of a low fat, increased fibre, moderate energy reduction diet, there are no head to head trials assessing the most effective strategy for weight loss and diabetes prevention [19]. There is limited evidence that alternative approaches, including the Mediterranean diet [20], meal replacements [21] and low carbohydrate diets [22] may be effective for weight loss and diabetes prevention in high-risk individuals.

Dietary components

Epidemiological studies have shown that specific foods may have a role in diabetes prevention, including higher intakes of low fat dairy products [23,24] dark yellow [25] and green leafy vegetables [26] and coffee [27]. Moderate intakes of alcohol also protect against diabetes [28]. Some foods are associated with a higher risk of diabetes and these include red and processed meat [29] and fried potato products [30].

In addition, there are also specific vitamins and minerals that have been associated with a lower incidence of diabetes, although these are usually taken as supplements rather than obtained from food. Epidemiological evidence suggests that high intakes of Vitamin D and calcium [31] and magnesium [32] may reduce risk, but the effect of chromium remains uncertain[33].

Physical activity

Increased physical activity reduces the risk of diabetes, and at least 30 minutes per day of moderate activity has been recommended by most studies.

Guidelines for diabetes prevention

European evidence-based guidelines for diabetes prevention have recently been published [34], and the American Diabetes Association and Diabetes UK have included lifestyle-specific guidelines in their latest recommendations for the prevention and management of diabetes [35,36]. These guidelines recommend:

- Intensive lifestyle interventions incorporating low fat, high fibre diets and increased physical activity should be used to prevent diabetes in adults.
- Weight reduction is an essential component of prevention, and long-term losses of 5–7% are effective.
- At least 30 minutes of moderate physical activity should be taken daily.

One of the most challenging aspects of diabetes prevention remains the application of positive results from clinical trials into routine clinical use. There are on-going studies investigating different strategies in the community [37–39] but at present these trials are aimed at high-risk individuals [40] and there is little evidence of translation of the success of randomised controlled trials to public health and, as a result, global diabetes prevalence continues to rise.

Key points

- Diabetes affected 8.3% of the global adult population in 2013, with 80% of those living in low / middle income countries.
- Significant numbers are either undiagnosed or have pre-diabetes.
- Prevalence of type 2 diabetes is increasing due to ageing, physical inactivity and increasing obesity.
- There is no evidence for prevention of type 1 diabetes.
- There is strong evidence for the role of lifestyle in the prevention of type 2 diabetes in high-risk individuals.
- A healthy lifestyle, including weight loss and increased physical activity, is the cornerstone of diabetes prevention.

References

1. WHO. *World Health Statistics 2012*. Geneva: World Health Organization, 2012.
2. International Diabetes Federation. *Diabetes Atlas*, 6th edn, Brusssels, Belgium: International Diabetes Federation, 2013.
3. NHS. *Quality and Outcomes Framework*. Online GP practice results database, 2010.
4. Holman N, Forouhi NG, Goyder E, Wild SH. The Association of Public Health Observatories (APHO) Diabetes Prevalence Model: estimates of total diabetes prevalence for England, 2010–2030. *Diabet Med* 2011; **28**(5): 575–82.
5. Diabetes UK. State of the Nation: England 2012. London: Diabetes UK, 2012.
6. Diabetes Prevention Trial - Type 1 Diabetes Study Group. Effects of insulin in relatives of people with type 1 diabetes mellitus. *N Eng J Med* 2002; **346**: 1685–1691.
7. Gale EA, Bingley PJ, Emmett CL, Collier T; European Nicotinamide Diabetes Intervention Trial (ENDIT) Group. European Nicotinamide Diabetes Intervention Trial (ENDIT): a randomised controlled trial of intervention before the onset of type 1 diabetes. *Lancet* 2004; **363**(9413): 925–931.

8. Knip M, Virtanen SM, Becker D, Dupré J, Krischer JP, Akerblom HK; for the TRIGR Study Group. Early feeding and risk of type 1 diabetes mellitus: experiences from the Trial to Reduce Insulin-dependent diabetes Mellitus in the Genetically at Risk (TRIGR). *Am J Clin Nutr* 2011: **94**(Suppl 6): 1814S–1820S.

9. Knowler WC, Barrett-Connor E, Fowler SE, Hamman RF, Lachin JM, Walker EA, et al.; Diabetes Prevention Program Research Group. Reduction in the incidence of type 2 diabetes with lifestyle intervention or metformin. *N Engl J Med* 2002; **346**(6): 393–403.

10. Tuomilehto J, Lindström J, Eriksson JG, Valle TT, Hämäläinen H, Ilanne-Parikka P, et al.; Finnish Diabetes Prevention Study Group. Prevention of type 2 diabetes mellitus by changes in lifestyle among subjects with impaired glucose tolerance. *N Engl J Med* 2001; **344**(18): 1343–1350.

11. Ramachandran A, Snehalatha C, Mary S, Mukesh B, Bhaskar AD, Vijay V; Indian Diabetes Prevention Programme (IDPP). The Indian Diabetes Prevention Programme shows that lifestyle modification and metformin prevent type 2 diabetes in Asian Indian subjects with impaired glucose tolerance (IDPP-1). *Diabetologia* 2006; **49**(2): 289–297.

12. Kosaka K, Noda M, Kuzuya T. Prevention of type 2 diabetes by lifestyle intervention: a Japanese trial in IGT males. *Diabetes Res Clin Pract* 2005; **67**: 152–162.

13. Pan XR, Li GW, Hu YH, Wang JX, Yang WY, An ZX, et al. Effects of diet and exercise in preventing NIDDM in people with impaired glucose tolerance. The Da Qing IGT and Diabetes Study. *Diabetes Care* 1997; **20**(4): 537–544.

14. Walker KZ, O'Dea K, Gomez M, Girgis S, Colagiuri R. Diet and exercise in the prevention of diabetes. *J Hum Nutr Diet* 2010; **23**(4): 344–352.

15. Knowler WC, Fowler SE, Hamman RF, Christophi CA, Hoffman HJ, Brenneman AT, et al.; Diabetes Prevention Programme Research Group. 10-year follow-up of diabetes incidence and weight loss in the Diabetes Prevention Program Outcomes Study. *Lancet* 2009; **374**(9702): 1677–1686.

16. Li G, Zhang P, Wang J, Gregg EW, Yang W, Gong Q, et al. The long-term effect of lifestyle interventions to prevent diabetes in the China Da Qing Diabetes Prevention Study: a 20-year follow-up study. *Lancet* 2008; **371**(9626): 1783–1789.

17. Lindström J, Ilanne-Parikka P, Peltonen M, Aunola S, Eriksson JG, Hemiö K, et al.; Finnish Diabetes Prevention Study Group. Sustained reduction in the incidence of type 2 diabetes by lifestyle intervention: follow-up of the Finnish Diabetes Prevention Study. *Lancet* 2006; **368**(9548): 1673–1679.

18. Diabetes Prevention Programme (DPP) research group. The Diabetes Prevention Program (DPP): description of lifestyle intervention. *Diabetes Care* 2002; **25**(12): 2165–2171.

19. Hamman RF, Wing RR, Edelstein SL, Lachin JM, Bray GA, Delahanty L, et al. Effect of weight loss with lifestyle intervention on risk of diabetes. *Diabetes Care* 2006; **29**(9): 2102–2107.

20. Salas-Salvadó J, Martinez-González MA, Bulló M, Ros E. The role of diet in the prevention of type 2 diabetes. *Nutr Metab Cardiovasc Dis* 2011; **21**(Suppl 2): B32–48.

21. Noakes M, Foster PR, Keogh JB, Clifton PM. Meal replacements are as effective as structured weight-loss diets for treating obesity in adults with features of metabolic syndrome. *J Nutr* 2004; **134**(8): 1894–1899.

22. Hession M, Rolland C, Kulkarni U, Wise A, Broom J. Systematic review of randomized controlled trials of low-carbohydrate vs. low-fat/low-calorie diets in the management of obesity and its comorbidities. *Obes Rev* 2009; **10**(1): 36–50.

23. Choi HK, Willett WC, Stampfer MJ, Rimm E, Hu FB. Dairy consumption and risk of type 2 diabetes mellitus in men: a prospective study. *Arch Intern Med* 2005; **165**(9): 997–1003.

24. Liu S, Choi HK, Ford E, Song Y, Klevak A, Buring JE, et al. A prospective study of dairy intake and the risk of type 2 diabetes in women. *Diabetes Care* 2006; **29**(7): 1579–1584.

25. Liu S, Serdula M, Janket SJ, Cook NR, Sesso HD, Willett WC, et al. A prospective study of fruit and vegetable intake and the risk of type 2 diabetes in women. *Diabetes Care* 2004; **27**(12): 2993–2996.

26. Carter P, Gray LJ, Troughton J, Khunti K, Davies MJ. Fruit and vegetable intake and incidence of type 2 diabetes mellitus: systematic review and meta-analysis. *BMJ* 2010; **341**: 4229.

27. van Dam RM, Willett WC, Manson JE, Hu FB. Coffee, caffeine, and risk of type 2 diabetes: a prospective cohort study in younger and middle-aged U.S. women. *Diabetes Care* 2006; **29**(2): 398–403.

28. Wannamethee SG, Camargo CA Jr, Manson JE, Willett WC, Rimm EB. Alcohol drinking patterns and risk of type 2 diabetes mellitus among younger women. *Arch Intern Med* 2003; **163**(11): 1329–1336.

29. van Dam RM, Willett WC, Rimm EB, Stampfer MJ, Hu FB. Dietary fat and meat intake in relation to risk of type 2 diabetes in men. *Diabetes Care* 2002; **25**(3): 417–424.

30. Halton TL, Willett WC, Liu S, Manson JE, Stampfer MJ, et al. Potato and french fry consumption and risk of type 2 diabetes in women. *Am J Clin Nutr* 2006; **83**(2): 284–290.

31. Pittas AG, Dawson-Hughes B, Li T, Van Dam RM, Willett WC, Manson JE, et al. Vitamin D and calcium

intake in relation to type 2 diabetes in women. *Diabetes Care* 2006; **29**(3): 650–656.

32. Larsson SC, Wolk A. Magnesium intake and risk of type 2 diabetes: a meta-analysis. *J Intern Med* 2007; **262**(2): 208–214.

33. Trumbo PR, Ellwood KC. Chromium picolinate intake and risk of type 2 diabetes: an evidence-based review by the United States Food and Drug Administration. *Nutr Rev* 2006; **64**(8): 357–363.

34. Paulweber B, Valensi P, Lindström J, Lalic NM, Greaves CJ, McKee M, et al. A European evidence-based guideline for the prevention of Type 2 diabetes. *Horm Metab Res* 2010; **41**(Suppl 1): S3–S36.

35. Evert AB, Boucher JL, Cypress M, Dunbar SA, Franz MJ, Mayer-Davis EJ, et al. Nutrition therapy recommendations for the management of adults with diabetes. *Diabetes Care* 2014 Jan; **37**(Suppl 1): S120–S143.

36. Dyson PA, Kelly T, Deakin T, Duncan A, Frost G, Harrison Z, et al.; Diabetes UK Nutrition Working Group. Diabetes UK evidence-based nutrition guidelines for the prevention and management of diabetes. *Diabet Med* 2011 Nov; **28**(11): 1282–1288.

37. Ackermann RT, Marrero DG. Adapting the Diabetes Prevention Program lifestyle intervention for delivery in the community: the YMCA model. *Diabetes Educ* 2007; **33**(1): 69, 74–75, 77–78.

38. Lakerveld J, Bot SD, Chinapaw MJ, van Tulder MW, van Oppen P, Dekker, JM, et al. Primary prevention of diabetes mellitus type 2 and cardiovascular diseases using a cognitive behavior program aimed at lifestyle changes in people at risk: Design of a randomized controlled trial. *BMC Endocr Disord* 2008; **8**: 6.

39. Williams K, Prevost, AT, Griffin S, Haredeman W, Hollingowrth W, Spiegelhalter D, et al. The ProActive trial protocol - a randomised controlled trial of the efficacy of a family-based, domiciliary intervention programme to increase physical activity among individuals at high risk of diabetes [ISRCTN61323766]. *BMC Public Health* 2004; **4**: 48.

40. Uusitupa M, TuomilehtoJ, Puska P. Are we really active in the prevention of obesity and type 2 diabetes at the community level? *Nutr Metab Cardiovasc Dis* 2011; **21**(5): 380–389.

Diagnostic criteria and classification of diabetes

Pamela Dyson

University of Oxford, Oxford Centre for Diabetes, Endocrinology and Metabolism, Churchill Hospital, Oxford, UK

1.2.1 Diagnostic criteria

Diabetes

The diagnostic criteria for diabetes have been developed and revised by the World Health Organisation (WHO) [1] and use the occurrence of diabetes-specific complications to derive diagnostic cut-points for diabetes. A diagnosis of diabetes can be made under the following circumstances:

- fasting plasma glucose ≥ 7.0 mmol/l (126 mg/dl)
- or 2-hour glucose ≥ 11.1 mmol/l (200 mg/dl) after ingestion of a 75 g oral glucose load (oral glucose tolerance test – OGTT)

Glycaemia is commonly assessed by a test known as HbA1c, a simple blood test measuring levels of glycated haemoglobin, and both the WHO and American Diabetes Association (ADA) now support its use as a suitable test for the diagnosis of diabetes [2,3]. HbA1c can be used for the diagnosis of diabetes, but only if the assays are standardised to international reference levels and if stringent quality assurance is in place. The cut-off point is 48 mmol/mol (6.5%), although a value <48 mmol/mol does not exclude diabetes if it has been previously diagnosed based upon blood glucose measurements. The advantage of using HbA1c as a diagnostic test is that it uses a non-fasting sample and does not require the dietary preparation necessary for an OGTT. The disadvantages of HbA1c are that it is relatively expensive, not widely available in low and middle-income countries (LMIC) and the result may be affected by a variety of factors including haemoglobinopathies. In addition, the WHO states that a diagnosis of diabetes should not be made based upon a single abnormal HbA1c value in the absence of symptoms, and that at least one additional test of HbA1c, or plasma glucose levels (fasting or 2-hour following OGTT) should be taken to confirm the diagnosis.

Impaired glucose tolerance and increased fasting glucose

Both impaired glucose tolerance (IGT) and increased fasting glucose (IFG) have been identified as risk factors for developing diabetes, and IGT as a risk factor for cardiovascular disease. The diagnostic criteria for IGT and IFG are:

- Impaired Glucose Tolerance: fasting plasma glucose <7.0 mmol/l (126 mg/dl) and 2-hour plasma glucose ≥ 7.8 and <11.1 mmol/l (140 and 200 mg/dl) after OGTT
- Increased Fasting Glucose: fasting plasma glucose 6.1 – 6.9 mmol/l (110 – 125 mg/dl) and (if measured) 2-hour glucose < 7.8 mmol/l (142 mg/dl)

Gestational diabetes

There is no agreed international standard for the screening and diagnosis of gestational diabetes (GDM), although there is consensus that the diagnosis of diabetes during pregnancy should use similar criteria to those for adults generally [4,5]. A more recent report has caused some controversy by recommending changes to the diagnosis of GDM and advocating screening for women with risk factors in early pregnancy, with screening for all other women at 24–28 weeks of pregnancy [6]. A 75 g OGTT is recommended as the test for GDM and a diagnosis should be made if any one glucose level reaches a specified level of:

- Fasting ≥ 5.1 mmol/l
- 1-hour ≥ 10.0 mmol/l
- 2-hour ≥ 8.5 mmol/l

There is concern that these new diagnostic criteria will increase the diagnosis of GDM and will have a large impact on resources without proven benefit [7].

1.2.2 Classification

There are two broad categories of diabetes: type 1 and type 2, although other rarer categories do exist.

Type 1 diabetes

Type 1 diabetes is an autoimmune condition characterised by pancreatic β-cell failure leading to complete insulin deficiency and susceptibility to ketoacidosis. It is usually characterised by the presence of anti-GAD, islet cell or insulin antibodies, although these may not be present in certain cases and this type of diabetes is referred to as 'idiopathic type 1'. The cause of type 1 diabetes remains unknown, although genetic factors and certain viruses may play a part. Type 1 diabetes usually presents in children and young adults, although it can be diagnosed at any age. Type 1 diabetes accounts for approximately 10–20% of diabetes and is treated by a combination of insulin replacement by injection or pump therapy and lifestyle modification.

Type 2 diabetes

Type 2 diabetes is characterised by defects in insulin secretion, usually accompanied by resistance to the action of insulin. Type 2 diabetes accounts for 80–90% of diabetes and has a strong genetic propensity to run in families, but is also associated with lifestyle factors and is more common in societies with high levels of obesity and low levels of physical activity. The risk factors for type 2 diabetes include non-modifiable (age, race and genetic predisposition) and modifiable (obesity, physical inactivity and unhealthy diet). Approximately 80–90% of people with type 2 diabetes are overweight or obese, and a recent European study has shown that nearly 50% of people with diabetes are obese (BMI ≥30 kg/m^2), twice the prevalence in the background population [8]. It is most frequently diagnosed in the middle-aged and elderly population, typically in people over the age of 40, although it is now increasingly diagnosed in obese children and adolescents. Traditionally, over 95% of diabetes in children is categorised as type 1, but in the United States (US), among older children, the proportion of type 2 diabetes ranges from 6% in non-hispanic white adolescents to 76% in American Indians [9]. Despite reports from around the world of an increase in the incidence of type 2 diabetes in children and adolescents, the true prevalence is largely unknown, although it is estimated that the prevalence in the United States (US) is approximately 12 per 100 000 [10]. The majority of type 2 diabetes is found in ethnic groups, including African-Americans, Hispanic, Pacific Islanders, with the highest prevalence reported in Pima Indian adolescents (22.3 per 1000) [11]. It has been estimated that as many as 1400 children in the United Kingdom (UK) had type 2 diabetes [12] in 2004, but recent evidence based on prescription of anti-diabetic medication suggests that the prevalence may be as high as 1.9 per 100 000 [13]. Type 2 diabetes is treated by a combination of diet, physical activity, oral medications and, increasingly, injectable therapies, including GLP-1 agonists and insulin.

Other types of diabetes

- Genetic defects in β-cell function (maturity onset diabetes in the young – MODY)
- Genetic defects in insulin action
- Diseases of the exocrine pancreas, including cancer, acute and chronic pancreatitis, cystic fibrosis
- Drug-induced diabetes e.g. glucocorticoids, thyroid hormone, thiazide diuretics.

Key points

- Diabetes can be diagnosed by three different means; fasting glucose, 2-hour glucose after an oral glucose tolerance test or HbA1c levels.
- IFG and IGT are risk factors for type 2 diabetes.
- There is no consensus for the diagnosis of gestational diabetes.
- There are two main types of diabetes; type 1 and type 2.

References

1. World Health Organization. Definition and diagnosis of diabetes mellitus and intermediate hyperglycaemia: Report of a WHO/IDF consultation. Geneva: World Health Organization, 2006.
2. International Expert Committee. International Expert Committee report on the role of A1c assay in the diagnosis of diabetes. *Diabetes Care* 2009; **32**: 1327–1334.
3. World Health Organization. Use of glycated haemoglobin (HbA1c) in the diagnosis of diabetes mellitus. Geneva: World Health Organization, 2011.
4. WHO Expert Committee on diabetes mellitus: Second report. Geneva: World Health Organization, 1980.
5. American Diabetes Association. Diagnosis and classification of diabetes mellitus. *Diabetes Care* 2009; **32**(Suppl 1): S62–S67.
6. Metzger BE, Gabbe SG, Persson B, Buchanan TA, Catalano PA, Damn P, et al. International association of diabetes and pregnancy study group recommendations on the diagnosis and classification of hyperglycaemia in pregnancy. *Diabetes Care* 2010; **33**(3): 676–682.
7. Cundy T. Proposed new diagnostic criteria for gestational diabetes – a pause for thought? *Diabet Med* 2011; **29**(2): 176–180.
8. Haslam DW. UK findings on overweight, obesity and weight gain from PANORAMA, a pan-European cross-sectional study of patients with Type 2 diabetes. *Diabet Med* 2011; **28**(Suppl 1): 264–265.
9. Liese AD, D'Agostino RB, Hamman RF, Filgo PD, Lawrence JM, Liu LI, et al. The burden of diabetes mellitus among US youth: prevalence estimates from the SEARCH for Diabetes in Youth Study. *Pediatrics* 2006; **118**(4): 1510–1518.
10. Reinehr T. Type 2 diabetes mellitus in children and adolescents. *World J Diabetes* 2013; **4**(6): 270–281.
11. Fagot-Campagna A, Pettitt DJ, Engelgau MM, Burrows NR, Geiss LS, Valdez R, et al. Type 2 diabetes among North American children and adolescents: an epidemiologic review and a public health perspective. *J Pediatr* 2000; **136**: 664–672.
12. Lobstein T, Leach R. Diabetes may be undetected in many children in the UK. *BMJ* 2004; **328**(7450): 1261–1262.
13. Hsia Y, Neubert AC, Rani F, Viner RM, Hindmarsh PC, Wong IC. An increase in the prevalence of type 1 and 2 diabetes in children and adolescents: results from prescription data from a UK general practice database. *Br J Clin Pharmacol* 2009; **67**(2): 242–249.

SECTION 2

Dietary principles of diabetes

Chapter 2.1

Historical perspectives of dietary recommendations for diabetes

Maeve Gacquin
Galway Clinic, Doughiska, Ireland

The nutritional management of diabetes has been subject to much change over the years due to factors such as economic forces, changes in staple foods and eating patterns, new medications and insulin formulations (Table 2.1.1). Since the first published guidelines by the British Diabetic Association in 1982 [1], the availability of evidence-based research and knowledge in science and medicine has improved greatly. This evolution is likely to continue and nutritional recommendations in the future may once again be substantially different from those of today.

2.1.1 From early times to the seventeenthth century

In 1000 BC traditional Indian medicine noted two types of diabetes. One that occurred in thin young individuals and one that was common in the overweight [2].

The earliest known record of diabetes was mentioned in a Third Dynasty Egyptian papyrus in 1552 BC by the physician Hesy-Ra and describes polyuria as a symptom [2,3].

The Greeks were the first to advocate diet and lifestyle management. In the first century AD, diabetes was described by Arateus as the 'melting down of flesh and limbs into urine'. He gave it the name diabetes which means 'siphon'. Aetius prescribed a 'cooling diet of diluted wine

and cooling applications to the loins'. Avicenna directed that all diuretic foods and drugs be avoided and that patients engage in exercise (preferably on horseback). In the later stages of diabetes he recommended 'tepid baths and fragrant wines' [2–4].

In the seventeenthth century a London Physician, Dr Thomas Willis, used urine sampling/tasting to diagnose diabetes 'mellitus' (Latin for honey). This method of monitoring remained unchanged till the twentieth century [2–4].

2.1.2 Eighteenth and nineteenth centuries

There were many significant developments in the nineteenth century with key individuals contributing to the understanding and management of diabetes, often with some unusual and unconventional diet and lifestyle measures.

John Rollo, an army surgeon, was interested in the physiology and source of glycosuria. He proposed that sugar may be formed in the stomach from fruit and vegetables and recommended that a diet consisting predominantly of animal foods was appropriate [2–4]. An example of a daily regimen from his 1797 book consisted of:

Breakfast: 1½ pints of milk and a half a pint of lime water mixed together, bread and butter.

Advanced Nutrition and Dietetics in Diabetes, First Edition. Edited by Louise Goff and Pamela Dyson.
© 2016 John Wiley & Sons, Ltd. Published 2016 by John Wiley & Sons, Ltd.

Table 2.1.1 Historical changes in the nutritional management of diabetes (Sanders, 2001 [4]; Canadian Diabetic Association, 2008 ADA, 2008 [16]; Diabetes UK, 2011 [18]; Tattersall, 2009 [2])

Date	Progress achieved
1000 BC	Traditional Indian medicine noted two types of diabetes: one that occurred in thin young individuals; one that was common in the overweight
150 BC	The Egyptians were writing about diabetes in the papyrus scrolls
45–117 AD	Ancient Greeks were the first to advocate diet and lifestyle management for individuals with diabetes
18th century	Mathew Dobson and John Rollo observed that there was sugar in the urine and blood of individuals with diabetes
1813	Claude Bernard linked diabetes with glycogen metabolism
1816	L. Taube related the intake of carbohydrate and its digestion to increased amounts of sugar in urine
1850	French physician, Priory, advised patients with diabetes to eat extra large quantities of sugar to treat their diabetes
1870	French physician, Bouchardat, noticed the disappearance of glycosuria in his diabetic patients during the rationing of food in Paris while under siege by Germany during the Franco-Prussian war
Late 19th century	Italian diabetes specialist, Catoni, isolated his patients under lock and key in order to get them to adhere to their diets
1900+	'Fad diets' included the 'oat cure' the 'milk diet', the 'rice cure', 'potato therapy' and even the use of opiates
1919	Frederick Allen (US diabetes specialist) published the 'Total Dietary Regulation in the Treatment of Diabetes'.
1920s	R.D. Lawrence empowers people with diabetes with education and dietary guidelines
1921	The discovery and isolation of insulin radically reduced death rates in type 1 diabetes
1940s	A link was made between diabetes and long-term complications (eye and kidney)
1940–1955	Oral medications were developed to help lower blood glucose levels
1959	Two major types of diabetes were recognised; 'type 1' – insulin-dependent diabetes – and 'type 2' – non-insulin-dependent diabetes
1970	Blood glucose meters and insulin pumps were developed
1993	The findings of the Diabetes Control and Complications Trial were published
1998	The findings of the UK Prospective Diabetes Study were published
2000	The Diabetes and Nutrition Study Group of the European Association for the Study of Diabetes (2000) published its recommendations for the nutritional management of people with diabetes mellitus
2002	The ADA (2002) published a position statement on evidence-based nutrition principles and recommendations for the treatment and prevention of diabetes and related complications
2003	The Nutrition Sub-Committee of the Diabetes Care Advisory Committee of Diabetes UK published a paper on 'The implementation of nutritional advice for individuals with diabetes'
2005	IDF published global guidelines for management of type 2 Diabetes
2008	The ADA produced a position statement, 'Nutrition Recommendations and Interventions for Diabetes'
2009	ISPAD published 3rd edition
2011	Diabetes UK published evidence-based nutrition guidelines for the prevention and management of diabetes

Lunch: Plain blood puddings, made of blood and suet only.

Dinner: Game or old meats which have been long kept, and as far as the stomach may bear, fat and rancid old meats.

This type of diet provides 600 kcal a day from carbohydrate and approximately 1200 kcal from fat.

The importance of Rollo's diet, although seemingly unfavourable for cardiovascular health, was that it was an attempt to treat diabetes rationally by preventing the formation of glucose.

When Dr John Camplin developed the symptoms of diabetes in 1844, he was advised by his colleagues William Prout (1785–1850) and Henry Bence Jones (1814–1873) to adopt a high protein and fat diet [2–4] and, on complaining of 'great biliary derangement' and irregular bowel function, Prout introduced him to bran cake. It was also common for physicians of that time to prescribe generous amounts of purgatives such as rhubarb, aloes, senna, magnesium sulfate and castor oil with these high protein, low carbohydrate diets.

One diet that was made popular for a short period by a French physician, Dr Pierre Priory (1794–1879) in the 1850s was sugar feeding [2–4]. His concern was for the amount of sugar lost through urine and he felt that replacing this sugar from dietary sources may restore strength.

In 1870, during the siege of Paris in the Franco-Prussian war, French physician Bourchardat (1806–1886) noticed that, as a result of starvation, the urine of some of his patients was sugar free. Furthermore, incidence rates and mortality rates of type 2 diabetes were shown to decrease during all wars. Bourcardat subsequently advised 'mangez le moins possible' (eat as little as possible). Italian Born physician Guelpa (1850–1930) showed that fasting and saline enemas made people with diabetes 'sugar free' in three days [2–4].

One feature that has changed very little over the years is that of dietary adherence. At this time many physicians complained of the lack of patient compliance with dietary advice stating that many patients either could not or would not follow the diet. Some ensured dietary compliance with extreme measures. The Italian physician,

Catoni kept his patients under lock and key to ensure adherence. Many with diabetes longed for a drug to replace restrictive diets [2].

2.1.3 Twentieth century

By the beginning of the twentieth century many physicians promoted 'dietary cures' based on specific foods. These included Donkins skim-milk (1784), Mosse's potato (1902) and Von Noordens oatmeal cure (1903). The oatmeal diet, for example, consisted of 8 oz of oatmeal and 8 oz of butter daily. These diets included periods of semi-starvation before the introduction of the specific 'curative' food [2–4].

During the twentieth century onwards, great emphasis was placed on patient education and diet as the key elements in controlling diabetes. Classes were popular in the United States (US) and Germany while one-to-one education was more common in the United Kingdom (UK). Although well meaning, the teachers had not been taught how to teach and many lesson plans were described as overly scientific and negative or dictatorial.

The author of a 1920 article about diabetes education commented: "there is no use talking in the language of the laboratory to a patient that understands only the language of the kitchen. We must either teach them the new language or translate our Greek into understandable English" [2]. Unfortunately, this advice was ignored in most diabetes units for the next 60 years and compliance and understanding of diet and lifestyle management of diabetes remained poor.

In 1919 Frederick Allen, a US diabetes physician, published 'The total regulation of diabetes'. This publication advised the combination of starvation diets with bed rest, often allowing only 450 kcal a day. Although he had some limited success with this approach, many people died of ketoacidosis or undernutrition related illnesses.

The discovery of insulin in 1921 extended the lives of those who were able to obtain a supply, but had little immediate effect on dietary prescriptions. In 1923, for example, the diet remained extremely restrictive; essentially a low carbohydrate intake meant a lower dose of insulin. At the end of the 1920s, some physicians in America and Canada introduced higher carbohydrate diets with the rationale that this type of diet was more palatable, less expensive, achieved greater compliance and, contrary to general expectations, led to a reduction in insulin requirements in many with diabetes. However, many physicians continued to advise low carbohydrate diets due to an ingrained belief that carbohydrate was bad for those with diabetes [2,4].

In 1923, R.D. Lawrence was appointed chief biochemist in King's College Hospital London. He had been diagnosed with diabetes in 1920 at the age of 28 and developed a strong interest in the management of diabetes. He set up a 'diet kitchen' where patients could be taught as outpatients about management of diabetes, including diet and insulin injections. He believed ardently that people with diabetes should be given the opportunity to take control of their own treatment and that this would also improve their quality of life. This was predominantly focused at managing type 1 diabetes.

To aid this he devised several influential diet schemes, such as the Line-Ration Diet, now called the Lawrence Weighed diet, and the Lawrence Unweighed Diabetic Diet, providing simple, accurate methods of measuring and regulating dietary intake.

In deriving his diet schemes he aimed to fulfil three main criteria; that each diet should:

- Contain sufficient carbohydrate to prevent ketosis.
- Satisfy the patient in quantity and quality as far as possible.
- Be accurate, simple to calculate, and varied.

In 1925 he published the first edition of 'The Diabetic Life' and in 1929 he published the first edition of 'The Diabetic ABC', which he described as a "short practical book for patients and nurses". The Lawrence line diet of 1929 aimed to restrict carbohydrate and provide similar amounts of protein, fat and carbohydrate from day to day to ensure consistency. Carbohydrates were labelled as 'black lines' and protein and fat were labelled as 'red lines'. Each black line provided 10g carbohydrate and 40 kcal and each

red line provided 111 kcal and 9 g fat. In 1934, Lawrence, with the author H.G. Wells who also had type 1 diabetes, co-founded the Diabetic Association which became known as the British Diabetic Association and is now known as Diabetes UK.

The introduction of the 'free diets' during the 1930s caused acrimony and controversy for nearly 30 years. Some physicians believed that a rigid diet in children with diabetes was harmful to mental development and social adjustment, while others maintained a strict low carbohydrate diet [2–4].

2.1.4 Dietary management of type 2 diabetes

The link between obesity and type 2 diabetes was well observed in the twentieth century and outlined as early as 1919 in Frederick Allen's book 'The total regulation of diabetes' but not fully understood. The importance of weight management in type 2 diabetes was demonstrated by landmark studies, such as the UKPDS [5], which demonstrated the direct benefit of moderate weight reduction on improved metabolic control of blood sugar, blood pressure and cholesterol and led to published guidelines for weight management [6].

2.1.5 Carbohydrate counting and exchanges

In the 1960s carbohydrate counting and exchanges were developed by the American Diabetes Association (ADA) for people with diabetes, to help to control blood glucose levels. The carbohydrate exchange diet grouped all the carbohydrate-containing foods into one group. A serving of a carbohydrate-based food was called a carbohydrate exchange and contained 15 g carbohydrate. Standard advice recommended three to four carbohydrate exchanges (similar amounts) with each meal when starting the carbohydrate exchange diet. The number of carbohydrate exchanges could be increased or decreased depending on blood glucose levels, medication and activity.

In the early 1990s the Diabetes Control and Complications Trial (DCCT) used carbohydrate counting as one of its education tools in type 1 diabetes [7].

Carbohydrate counting became increasingly popular once the ADA revised dietary recommendations in 1994. Based on growing scientific evidence that sucrose affects blood glucose levels no differently than other carbohydrates, and that no single meal-planning method works for everyone, the new guidelines essentially lifted the ban on sugar-containing foods to focus attention on controlling total carbohydrate intake and individualising meal plans.

Carbohydrate counting was first embraced by individuals with type 1 diabetes on intensive insulin therapy who used an insulin pump or multiple daily insulin injections. Carbohydrate counting helped those who use insulin to tailor their mealtime dose or bolus of insulin to cover the amount of carbohydrate eaten at that meal. This allowed greater diet and lifestyle flexibility and freedom as the individual could vary the insulin doses depending on carbohydrate intake and activity levels.

Structured education programmes on insulin dose adjustment started in Germany in 1983 [8], and this idea was further developed in the UK as the DAFNE programme [9]. A number of similar education programmes have been developed around the world.

2.1.6 Glycaemic index

During the twentieth century it was observed that certain foods had less effect on blood glucose concentrations after eating, and these foods were identified as those high in protein and fat. Carbohydrate foods have the most significant effect on blood glucose concentrations, but even within this group there was great variation on the rate of the glycaemic effect. In 1981, David Jenkins and his team at the University of Toronto came up with an alternative system of classifying carbohydrate. He ranked the glycaemic effect of commonly eaten carbohydrates and compared them with pure glucose which had a score of 100. He called this the glycaemic index [10]. This system is now widely used and endorsed by all major diabetes authorities.

2.1.7 Development of nutritional guidelines for diabetes

The first position statement on diet and diabetes came from the British Diabetic Association (now known as Diabetes UK) in 1982 [1]. The emphasis of these recommendations was on healthy eating principles in line with those for the general population, which liberalised the diet for many individuals with diabetes. An update of these recommendations from the Nutrition Sub-Committee of the British Diabetic Association Professional Advisory Committee 10 years later in 1992 reinforced the high-carbohydrate low-fat diet [11]. These recommendations were followed by recommendations from the European Association for the Study of Diabetes (EASD) and the ADA in 2000 and 2002, respectively [12,13]. In 2003, Diabetes UK published a document entitled 'The implementation of nutritional advice for individuals with diabetes' [14] and this consensus-based paper built on the European and American reviews. The paper discussed the practical implementation of dietary advice for individuals with diabetes and described the provision of services needed to support this approach. The EASD guidelines were also updated and published in 2004 [15].

The move away from consensus-based guidelines towards those that were evidence-based began with dietary guidelines from the ADA in 2008 [16]. The Canadian dietary recommendations were updated in 2008 to reflect Health Canada's revised 'Eating well with Canada's food guide' and included more flexible recommendations on macronutrient distribution [17]. The most recent evidence-based guidelines from Diabetes UK were published in 2011 [18] and those from the ADA in 2013 [19].

2.1.8 Guidelines for low and middle income ountries

The International Diabetes Federation (IDF) developed a global guideline for the management of type 2 diabetes in 2005 [20]. Published national guidelines often come from relatively resource-rich countries, but the IDF guidelines focus on those that may also be relevant in less well resourced countries. The guidelines focus on physical activity in conjunction with nutrition education and are aimed at different groups in society including families, schools, groups and individuals.

2.1.9 Guidelines for children and adolescents

Children and adolescents have had specific guidelines developed for their use, and the third edition of the International Society for Pediatric and Adolescent Diabetes (ISPAD) Consensus Guidelines, now called "Clinical Practice Consensus Guidelines", was published in 2009 in conjunction with the IDF [21].

2.1.10 A change in emphasis

The ADA guidelines in 2008 [16] emphasised that nutrition counselling should be tailored to the individual, with encouragement of low GI carbohydrate foods and adequate vitamin and mineral intake. Low carbohydrate and restricted diets were recommended for weight loss in those with type 2 diabetes, but for 1 year only. Specific guidelines were included for physical activity.

The Diabetes UK 2011 guidelines [18] place an emphasis on carbohydrate management and a more flexible approach to weight loss, unlike previous guidelines which were expressed in terms of recommendations for individual nutrient intakes. These guidelines aim to support self-management, promote healthy lifestyles and reduce the risk of type 2 diabetes and the co-morbidities associated with diabetes. They encourage healthy eating and recommend effective strategies for weight management and glycaemic control.

2.1.11 Summary

Over the years, dietary management of diabetes has been subject to personal whim and anecdotal evidence. History has shown that complicated, restrictive diets are challenging, impractical and unsuccessful for the majority of people with diabetes. The development and improvement of evidence-based dietary recommendations have been important in understanding how to optimise metabolic control, but adherence to diet and lifestyle advice still proves challenging for many people with diabetes. It is essential to continue to develop skills and knowledge on how best to facilitate diet and lifestyle education, learning, motivation and support for individuals and groups with diabetes.

Key points

- Dietary treatment of diabetes dates from the Ancient Greeks.
- The first diets concentrated on severe carbohydrate restriction.
- Over the subsequent years, carbohydrate management was promoted, together with more emphasis on dietary management of cardiovascular risk and body weight.
- Today, an individualised, evidence-based approach is recommended by most authorities.

References

1. Nutrition sub-committee of the British Diabetic Association. Dietary recommendations for the 1980s. *Hum Nutr: Appl Nutr* 1987; **36**(5): 378–382.
2. Tattersall R. Diabetes, The Biography. Oxford University Press, Oxford, 2009.
3. Blades M, Morgan JB, Dickerson JW. Dietary advice in the management of diabetes mellitus – history and current practice. *JR Soc Health* 1997; **117**(3): 143–150.
4. Sanders LJ. *The Philatelic History of Diabetes.* Alexandria, VA: ADA, 2001.
5. King P, Peacock I, Donnelly R. The UK prospective diabetes study (UKPDS): clinical and therapeutic implications for type 2 diabetes. *Br J Clin Pharmacol* 1999; **48**(5): 643–688.

6. Campbell L, Rossner S. Management of obesity in patients with type 2 diabetes. *Diabet Med* 2001; **18**: 345–354.

7. The Diabetes Control and Complications Trial Research Group. The effect of intensive treatment of diabetes on the development and progression of long-term complications in insulin-dependent diabetes mellitus. *N Engl J Med* 1993; **329**(14): 977–986.

8. Muhlhauser I, Bruckner I, Berger M, Cheta D, Jorgens V, Ionescu-Tirqoviste C, et al. Evaluation of an intensified insulin treatment and teaching programme as routine management of type 1 (insulin-dependent) diabetes. The Bucharest-Düsseldorf Study. *Diabetologia* 1987; **30**(9): 681–690.

9. DAFNE study group. Training in flexible, intensive insulin management to enable dietary freedom in people with type 1 diabetes: dose adjustment for normal eating (DAFNE) randomised controlled trial. *BMJ* 2002; **325** (7367): 746.

10. Jenkins DJ, Wolever TM, Taylor RH, Barker H, Fielden H, Baldwin JM, et al. Glycemic index of foods: a physiological basis for carbohydrate exchange. *Am J Clin Nutr* 1981; **34**(3): 362–366.

11. Nutrition Sub Committee of the British Diabetic Association Professional Advisory Committee. Dietary recommendations for people with diabetes. An update for the 1990s. *Diabet Med* 1992; **9**: 189–202.

12. Diabetes and Nutrition Study Group of the European Association for the Study of Diabetes. Recommendations for the nutritional management of patients with diabetes mellitus. *Eur J Clin Nutr* 2000; **54**: 353–355.

13. Franz MJ, Bantle JP, Beebe CA, Brunzell JD, Chiasson JL, Garg A, et al. Evidence based nutrition principles and recommendations for the treatment and prevention of diabetes and related complications. *Diabetes Care* 2003; **26**(Suppl 1): S51–S61.

14. Nutrition sub-committee of the Diabetes Care Advisory Committee of Diabetes UK. The implementation of nutritional advice for people with diabetes. *Diabet Med* 2003; **20**(10): 786–807.

15. Mann JL, De Leeuw I, Hermansen K, Karamanos B, Karlstrom B, Katsilambros N, et al.; Diabetes and Nutrition Study Group (DNSG) of the European Association for the Study of Diabetes (ESAD). Evidence based nutrition approaches to the treatment and prevention of diabetes mellitus. *Nutr Metab Cardiovasc Dis* 2004; **14**: 373–394.

16. Bantle JP, Wylie-Rosett J, Albright AL, Apovian CM, Clarke NG, Franz MJ, et al. Nutrition recommendations and interventions for diabetes: A position statement from The American Diabetes Association. *Diabetes Care* 2008; **31**(Suppl 1): S61–S78.

17. Canadian Diabetes Association. 2008 Clinical practice guidelines for the prevention and management of diabetes in Canada. *Can J Diabetes* 2008; **32**(Suppl 1): 201.

18. Dyson PA, Kelly T, Deakin T, Duncan A, Frost G, Harrison Z, et al.; Diabetes UK Nutrition Working Group. Diabetes UK evidence-based nutrition guidelines for the prevention and management of diabetes. *Diabet Med* 2011; **28**(11): 1282–1288.

19. Evert AB, Boucher JL, Cypress M, Dunbar SA, Franz MJ, Mayer-Davis EJ, et al. Nutrition therapy recommendations for the management of adults with diabetes. *Diabetes Care* 2014; **37**(Suppl 1): S120–S143.

20. International Diabetes Federation Global Guideline for Type 2 Diabetes. Brussels: International Diabetes Federation, 2005.

21. Smart C, Aslander-van Vliet E, Waldron S. Ed Swift P. ISPAD Clinical Practice Consensus Guidelines 2009: Nutritional management. *Pediatric Diabetes* 2009; **10**(Suppl. 12): 100117.

Nutritional guidelines for diabetes

Marion J. Franz
Nutrition Concepts by Franz, Inc., Minneapolis, USA

Nutrition therapy can be defined as the implementation of evidence-based nutrition recommendations and guidelines. Evidence-based nutrition guidelines are defined as "a series of guiding statements and treatment algorithms that are developed using a systematic process for identifying, analyzing, and synthesizing scientific evidence. They are designed to assist practitioners and patients decisions about appropriate nutrition care for specific disease states or conditions in typical settings" [1].

To implement nutrition therapy for diabetes it is essential to have evidence for:

- The effectiveness of nutrition interventions
- The expected outcomes from implementation of nutrition interventions
- The types of nutrition interventions that are effective
- Timing of evaluation of outcomes.

These important questions and nutrition therapy guidelines for diabetes have been examined by a number of national expert committees including the UK Diabetes Nutrition Working Group [2], the Academy of Nutrition and Dietetics (formerly the American Dietetic Association) [3,4], the Canadian Diabetes Association Clinical Practice Expert Committee [5], the American Diabetes Association [6], the International Diabetes Federation Clinical Guidance Task Force [7], and the Diabetes and Nutrition Study Group of the European Association for the Study of Diabetes [8]. The primary goal for diabetes nutrition care is to integrate nutrition therapy into the management of diabetes in order to improve glycaemic control, lipid concentrations and blood pressure (BP) control and reduce the risk of potential diabetes-related complications. Weight management is another goal for the prevention of diabetes and the management of type 2 diabetes [9–11]. This chapter reviews evidence for the effectiveness of diabetes nutrition therapy and summarises evidence-based nutrition recommendations related to macronutrients in diabetes nutrition care.

2.2.1 Effectiveness of diabetes nutrition therapy

Diabetes nutrition therapy and glucose outcomes

Metabolic outcomes are improved in nutrition intervention studies, either when advice is provided by Registered Dietitians (RDs) as an independent therapy or when it is provided as part of overall diabetes self-management education [12]. Beneficial effects on haemoglobin A1c (HbA1c) are the most consistently reported outcome but other positive outcomes (lipids, BP, weight, quality of life) are also reported. Randomised controlled trials, cross-sectional studies, and non-randomised outcome studies report decreases in HbA1c of approximately 11–22 mmol/mol (1–2%,) with a range of 5–28 mmol/mol (0.5–2.6%), depending on the type and duration of diabetes, level of glycaemic control, and at what time point outcomes are reported [2–6]. These beneficial outcomes are similar to those from glucose-lowering medications.

The evidence suggests that nutrition therapy is most beneficial at initial diagnosis, but is effective at any time during the disease process, and that ongoing evaluation and intervention are essential. Outcomes from nutrition therapy interventions are generally known in six weeks to three months and evaluation should be done at this time. At three months, if no clinical improvement has occurred in metabolic outcomes (glucose, lipids, BP), usually a change in medication is required. Type 2 diabetes is a progressive disease and as β-cell function decreases, glucose-lowering medication, including insulin, must be combined with nutrition therapy to achieve target goals.

Of interest are several studies documenting the effectiveness of nutrition therapy conducted in the United Kingdom (UK). All treatment and control subjects in the UK Prospective Diabetes Study (UKPDS) received nutrition counselling at study entry and for the first three months, at which time they were randomised into the study arms and began taking medication. During this period, when nutrition therapy was the sole intervention, the mean HbA1c decreased by 22 mmol/mol (2%), from 75 to 53 mmol/mol (9 to 7%) [13,14]. At two years, the conventional therapy group, whose primary treatment was nutrition therapy, maintained an HbA1c of ~53 mmol/mol (~7%) and even after 15 years the HbA1c was still slightly less than at diagnosis.

In England and in newly diagnosed individuals with type 2 diabetes, the Early ACTID (Early Activity in Diabetes) trial compared usual care to intensive nutrition intervention with or without physical activity [15]. Baseline HbA1c levels of 49 mmol/mol (6.6%) in this study were considerably lower than in the UKPDS study. At six months, HbA1c had worsened in the usual care group but had improved in the two intensive nutrition interventions groups (–4 mmol/mol, –0.3%). These differences persisted to 12 months despite the use of fewer diabetes drugs. Improvements were also seen in body weight and insulin resistance between the intervention and control groups. Of interest, the addition of the physical activity program added no additional benefit.

In individuals with type 1 diabetes, the dose adjusted for normal eating (DAFNE) evaluated a five-day course teaching individuals how to adjust bolus or mealtime insulin based on carbohydrate intake on glucose control and quality of life compared to traditional treatment (insulin therapy determined first and carbohydrate intake matched to insulin therapy). In the group receiving DAFNE training, HbA1c levels were significantly reduced by 11 mmol/mol (1%) with no increase in severe hypoglycaemia. In addition, there were positive effects on quality of life, satisfaction with treatment and psychological well-being, despite an increase in the number of insulin injections (but not the total amount of insulin) and in blood glucose monitoring compared to controls [16]. A follow-up of the original participants at a mean of 44 months documented mean reduction in HbA1c from a baseline of approximately 4 mmol/mol (~0.4%) and with the improvements in quality of life seen at 12 months maintained [17].

Two other studies are of interest. In New Zealand, individuals with an average duration of type 2 diabetes of 9 years and who had HbA1c levels >53 mmol/mol (7%) despite optimised drug therapy were randomised to an intervention group who received intensive nutrition therapy or a control group. Nutrition therapy resulted in a highly significant difference in HbA1c (approximately 5 mmol/mol [0.5%], $p = 0.007$) compared to the control group at six months, documenting the effectiveness of nutrition therapy even in diabetes of long duration [18]. The reduction in HbA1c was comparable to adding a new drug, often a third agent, and at less cost.

A study documented the effectiveness of diabetes nutrition interventions in 'real world' clinical practice. Data were collected from 221 patients with type 2 diabetes who were referred for nutrition education and counselling to 59 RDs in 31 outpatient settings. To minimise selection bias, the RDs randomly recruited the first two patients meeting the inclusion criteria each day. 54% of the subjects were newly diagnosed and, in all subjects, HbA1c decreased by 15 mmol/mol (1.4%) over three months and by 20 mmol/mol (1.8%) at six months follow-up. Lipid concentrations, BP and weight also improved significantly [19].

Diabetes medical nutrition therapy and lipids and blood pressure outcomes

In studies done primarily in people without diabetes, cardioprotective nutrition therapy implemented by RDs resulted in a reduction of total cholesterol (TC) by 7% to 21%, LDL-cholesterol (LDL-C) by 17% to 22%, and triglycerides by 11% to 31% [20]. In patients with diabetes, reductions in TC have been shown to range from 0.2 to 0.71 mmol/l, in LDL-C by 0.2 to 0.42 mmol/l, and in triglycerides by 0.17 to 1.73 mmol/l [12]. Studies implementing nutrition therapy for hypertension by RDs report an average reduction in BP of ~5 mmHg in both systolic and diastolic BP [21].

Diabetes nutrition therapy and weight management outcomes

In weight loss trials conducted in subjects with diabetes of one-year duration or longer, approximately half of the studies reported improvements in HbA1c whereas half reported no improvement in HbA1c despite fairly similar weight losses [3,4]. However, the Look AHEAD (Action for Health in Diabetes) trial which is designed to assess if weight reduction combined with physical activity can reduce cardiovascular disease (CVD) morbidity and mortality in individuals with type 2 diabetes has reported very successful outcomes at one and four years follow-up (10,11). A very intensive lifestyle intervention compared to usual diabetes support and education reported reductions in HbA1c of 8 mmol/mol (0.7%) in the intensive group compared to 1 mmol/mol (0.1%) in the control group at one year. At four years follow-up, the intensive group showed a mean decrease of 4 mmol/mol (0.4%) versus 1 mmol/mol (0.1%) in the control group. It is well documented that in weight loss interventions, weight loss plateaus at approximately six months, and the goal then becomes to prevent weight regain. It is unclear if the benefits on glycaemia from weight management interventions are from the weight loss *per se* or from the reduced energy intake. In general, glucose concentrations improve

rapidly when energy intake is reduced and before much weight is lost.

The Diabetes UK nutrition guidelines recommend that to improve weight loss outcomes, individuals should be encouraged to adopt their diet of choice for weight loss [2]. They note that various nutrition strategies have been used to induce weight loss in people with type 2 diabetes and it is likely that a diet an individual enjoys and finds acceptable is more likely to succeed.

Summary

Although attempts are often made to identify one nutrition intervention for diabetes nutrition therapy, there is no evidence to support this. Many types of nutrition interventions have been shown to be effective. Interventions include reduced energy and/or fat intake, carbohydrate counting, simplified meal plans, healthy food choices, individualised meal planning strategies, exchange lists, insulin-to-carbohydrate ratios, physical activity and behavioral strategies [3,12]. Strategies used for successful nutrition interventions for individuals with type 2 diabetes consistently involve reducing the energy content of the usual food intake. For individuals with type 1 diabetes, adjusting insulin doses for planned carbohydrate intake is a consistent strategy. Also of importance are multiple encounters to provide nutrition education and counselling, initially and on a continuing basis. The Diabetes UK recommendations state that all people with diabetes and/or their carers should receive structured education at the time of diagnosis, with an annual follow-up [2]. The number and duration of nutrition care encounters may need to be greater if the patient has language, ethnic or cultural concerns, if there is a change in medications (such as addition of glucose-lowering medications or insulin therapy in type 2 diabetes or changes in insulin therapy in type 1 or type 2 diabetes), or for weight management [3,6]. It is essential that nutrition education and counselling be sensitive to the personal needs, learning styles and cultural preferences of individuals and their abilities to make lifestyle changes [2–8]. Even small changes in eating habits can result in beneficial outcomes.

2.2.2 Diabetes nutrition therapy and macronutrients

Historically, professional diabetes organisations such as Diabetes UK and the American Diabetes Association (ADA), attempted to identify ideal percentages of macronutrients for eating patterns of individuals with diabetes. However, just as there is no one type of nutrition therapy intervention appropriate for all people with diabetes, there is also no ideal percentage of macronutrients that applies to all people with diabetes. An extensive systematic review conducted by the ADA concluded: "Although in many instances there were not statistically differences between dietary approaches, improvements were often seen from baseline to follow-up in both intervention groups supporting the idea that several different macronutrient distributions may lead to improvements in glycaemic and/or cardiovascular disease risk factors" [22].

Carbohydrate

In people with diabetes on nutrition therapy alone, those taking oral glucose-lowering medications or those on fixed insulin doses, consistency in carbohydrate intake for meals (and snacks, if desired) is associated with improved blood glucose concentrations and this is recommended by most authorities. Concern is expressed that if the eating pattern is too low in carbohydrate, many foods that are important sources of vitamins, minerals, fibre and energy may be eliminated [2–7]. Generally, eating patterns that are low or very low in carbohydrate are high in fat, usually saturated fats, and over the long term this may reduce insulin sensitivity [8].

For people with type 1 diabetes on a basal prandial insulin regimen or who are on insulin pump therapy, insulin doses should be adjusted to match planned carbohydrate intake (insulin-to-carbohydrate ratios) [2–8]. To accomplish this requires comprehensive nutrition education on interpretation of blood glucose patterns, knowledge of medication adjustment and collaboration with the health care team. There is little evidence for this approach in people with type 2 diabetes who use a basal prandial insulin regimen, with only one study showing this strategy is as effective as an algorithm dosing approach [23].

Glycaemic index

Controversy exists regarding the usefulness of the glycaemic index (GI). There is conflicting evidence of effectiveness of this strategy as studies comparing high versus low GI diets report mixed effects on HbA1c concentrations [3,4,6,8]. An intervention review concluded that low GI diets compared to high GI diets can improve glycaemic control (decreasing HbA1c by up to 5 mmol/mol [0.5%]) [24]. However, the majority of studies included in this review were of short duration with a limited number of participants. The review did not include two one-year studies that reported no differences in HbA1c between low GI and control groups [25,26]. The ADA systematic review concluded: "In general, there is little difference in glycaemic control and CVD risk factors between low and high GI or other diets. A slight improvement in glycaemia may result from a lower GI diet, however, confounding by higher fiber must be accounted for in some of these studies" [22]. Although it appears that most individuals consume a moderate GI diet, individuals most likely to benefit from a low GI diet are those who consume a high GI diet [6].

Fibre and whole grains

In general, recommendations for fibre for people with diabetes are similar to the recommendations for the general public (UK Reference Intake: 18 g/day non-starch polysaccharide; United States Dietary Reference Intake: 14 g/1000 kcal). Although eating patterns containing 44–50 g fibre daily have been shown to improve glycaemic control in persons with diabetes, more usual fibre intakes (up to 24 g/day) have not shown beneficial effects on glycaemia [3,4,6]. It should be noted that the usual fibre intake is 12–17 g/day. Studies report that eating patterns high in total and soluble fibre, as part of a cardioprotective nutrition therapy, can reduce TC by 2% to 3% and LDL-C up to 7%, although the majority of the studies were not conducted specifically in persons with diabetes [20]. The ADA systematic review of fibre supplements concluded that the majority of the evidence supports that adding fibre supplements in moderate amounts (4–19 g) to a daily eating pattern leads to little improvement in glycaemia and CVD risk markers [22].

Consumption of whole grain foods may be of equal importance to fibre in reducing CVD risk. Whole grains contain fibre, vitamins, minerals, phenolic compounds, phytoestrogens and other unmeasured constituents, which have been shown to lower serum lipids and BP, improve glucose and insulin metabolism and endothelial function, and alleviate oxidative stress in the general population and in people with type 2 diabetes [27].

Protein

In persons with diabetes with normal renal function, there is not adequate evidence to support recommending a change in the usual protein intake of 15–20% of total energy intake [3,5,6,8]. In persons with type 2 diabetes, ingestion of protein results in acute insulin and glucagon responses with minimal, if any, postprandial glucose or lipid responses [3]. Studies lasting 5–12 weeks comparing high-protein diets to lower-protein diets showed no differences in long-term insulin response despite the acute insulin response. Studies done on protein intake and insulin needs are limited in persons with type 1 diabetes. Consuming large amounts of food protein appears to have the potential to modestly increase postprandial glucose concentrations and may require additional small amounts of bolus insulin [28]. It is clear that the usual bolus insulin doses cover the meal carbohydrate insulin needs and, therefore, it must be assumed that the protein (and fat) needs for insulin are covered by basal insulin doses. Generally an individual's protein intake is fairly consistent and extra insulin is only needed when excessive protein is consumed (or less insulin may be needed when protein consumed is less than usual). Because protein does not increase circulating blood glucose concentrations (and in persons with type 2 diabetes increases insulin levels), it

should not be used to treat acute hypoglycaemia or to prevent overnight hypoglycaemia (i.e. adding protein to bedtime snacks) [6].

Food fats

It is recommended that saturated fatty acid (SFA) intake should be less than 7% of total energy intake, intake of trans fats minimised, and dietary cholesterol intake be less than 200 mg/day [5,6,8]. Although reducing SFA may also reduce high density lipoprotein cholesterol (HDL-C), more importantly, the ratio of LDL-C to HDL-C does not change. SFA can be replaced with foods containing unsaturated fatty acids [2,5,6,8]. Saturated fats should be replaced by unsaturated fats [2,5,6,8].

A review by the Dietary Guidelines Advisory Committee 2010 of the evidence for the effect of SFA on type 2 diabetes and/or increased risk of CVD concluded that intake of SFA increases TC and LDL-C and the risk of CVD and increases markers of insulin resistance and type 2 diabetes risk [29]. A review of 12 studies published since 2000, and reviewed in the nutrition evidence library, provided evidence that a 5% energy decrease in SFA replaced by monounsaturated or polyunsaturated fatty acids decreases the risk of CVD and type 2 diabetes in healthy adults and improves insulin responsiveness in insulin resistant individuals and individuals with type 2 diabetes [30].

Summary

As no clear ideal percentages of carbohydrate, protein, and fat exist, the nutrition prescription for individuals with diabetes is best based on an appropriate energy intake and a healthy eating pattern. Individuals with both type 1 and type 2 diabetes report a moderate carbohydrate eating pattern (~45% of total energy intake) which appears to be of less importance than total energy intake. Therefore, for achieving glycaemic control, the focus is on total energy intake rather than the source of the energy in the eating pattern (macronutrient composition) [2]. However, the balance between carbohydrate consumed and available insulin does predict glycaemic response, so monitoring total carbohydrate intake, whether by use of exchanges, portions, carbohydrate counting or experience-based estimation, is also a key strategy in achieving glycaemic control [2,6].

2.2.3 Conclusion

Randomised controlled trials and outcome studies have demonstrated that nutrition therapy provided to people with diabetes by RDs improves glycaemic control as well as lipids, BP and quality of life, thus reducing the risk of potential diabetes related complications. A variety of nutrition therapy interventions have been shown to be effective. However, no ideal percentage of macronutrients exists for planning/implementing diabetes eating patterns. Evidence also demonstrates that the outcomes of nutrition therapy are evident by six weeks to three months, and at this time monitoring and evaluation of outcomes should be done. If goals for desired metabolic outcomes have not been met and individuals have made all the lifestyle changes they are willing or able to make, recommendations for the addition or changes in medication should be made, and these changes in medications should be combined with nutrition therapy.

Key points

- Nutrition therapy is effective for improving glycaemic control, promoting weight loss and reducing cardiovascular risk.
- There is no evidence for an ideal combination of macronutrients, and individualisation is recommended.
- Carbohydrate monitoring improves glycaemic control.

References

1. Academy of Nutrition and Dietetics. Evidence Analysis Library. Internet: https://www.andeal.org/ (accessed 9 June 2015).

2. Dyson PA, Kelly T, Deakin T, Duncan A, Frost G, Harrison Z, et al. on behalf of Diabetes UK Nutrition Working Group. Diabetes UK evidence-based nutrition guidelines for the prevention and management of diabetes. *Diabet Med* 2011; **28**: 1282–1288.

3. Academy of Nutrition and Dietetics Evidence Analysis Library. Diabetes type 1 and type 2 evidence-based nutrition practice guidelines for adults. Version current 2008. Internet: http://www.andeal.org/topic.cfm?cat=3252 (accessed 9 June 2015).

4. Franz MJ, Powers MA, Leontos C, Holzmeister LA, Kulkarni K, Monk A, et al. The evidence for medical nutrition therapy for type 1 and type 2 diabetes in adults. *J Am Diet Assoc* 2010; **110**: 1852–1859.

5. Gougeon R, Aylward N, Nichol H, Wuinn K, Whitham D. Nutrition therapy. In: Canadian Diabetes Association 2008 Clinical Practice Guidelines for the Prevention and Management of Diabetes in Canada. *Can J Diabetes* 2008; **32**: S40–S45.

6. Evert AB, Boucher JL, Cypress M, Dunbar SA, Franz MJ, Mayer-Davis EJ, et al. Nutrition therapy recommendations for the management of adults with diabetes. *Diabetes Care* 2014; **37**(Suppl 1): S120–S143.

7. Clinical Guidelines Task Force. Lifestyle management. In: Global Guidelines for Type 2 Diabetes, International Diabetes Federation 2005: 22–5.

8. Mann JI, De Leeuw I, Hermansen K, Karamanos B, Karlström B, Katsilambros N, et al.; Diabetes and Nutrition Study Group of the European Association for the Study of Diabetes. Evidence-based nutritional approaches to the treatment and prevention of diabetes mellitus. *Nutr Metab Cardiovasc Dis* 2004; **14**: 373–394.

9. Franz MJ. The evidence is in: lifestyle interventions can prevent diabetes. *AJLM* 2007; **1**: 113–121.

10. Look AHEAD Research Group. Reduction in weight and cardiovascular disease risk factors in individuals with type 2 diabetes: one year results of the Look AHEAD trial. *Diabetes Care* 2007; **30**: 1374–1382.

11. Look AHEAD Research Group. Long-term effects of a lifestyle intervention on weight and cardiovascular risk factors in individuals with type 2 diabetes mellitus: four-year results of the Look AHEAD trial. *Arch Intern Med* 2010; **170**: 1566–1575.

12. Pastors JG, Franz MJ. Effectiveness of medical nutrition therapy in diabetes. In: Franz MJ, Evert AB, eds. American Diabetes Association Guide to Nutrition Therapy, 2nd edn. Alexandria, VA: American Diabetes Association, 2012, pp. 1–18.

13. UK Prospective Diabetes Study 7. Response of fasting glucose to diet therapy in newly presenting type II diabetic patients. *Metabolism* 1990; **39**: 905–912.

14. UK Prospective Diabetes Study Group prepared by Manley SE, Stratton IM, Cull CA, Frighi V, Eeley A,

Matthews DR, et al. Effects of three months' diet after diagnosis of type 2 diabetes on plasma lipids and lipoproteins (UKPDS 45). *Diabet Med* 2000; **17**: 518–523.

15. Andrews RC, Cooper AR, Montgomery AA, Norcross AJ, Peters TJ, Sharp DJ, et al. Diet or diet plus physical activity versus usual care in patients with newly diagnosed type 2 diabetes: the Early ACTID randomized controlled trial. *Lancet* 2011; **378**: 129–139.

16. DAFNE Study Group. Training in flexible, intensive insulin management to enable dietary freedom in people with type 1 diabetes. Dose Adjusted for Normal Eating (DAFNE) randomized controlled trial. *BMJ* 2002; **325**: 746–752.

17. Speight J, Amiel SA, Bradley C, Heller S, Oliver L, Roberts S, et al. Long-term biomedical and psychosocial outcomes following DAFNE (Dose Adjustment for Normal Eating) structured education to promote intensive insulin therapy in adults with sub-optimally controlled type 1 diabetes. *Diabetes Res Clin Pract* 2010; **89**: 22–29.

18. Coppell KJ, Kataolka M, Williams SM, Chisholm AW, Vorgers SM, Mann JI. Nutritional interventions in patients with type 2 diabetes who are hyperglycaemic despite optimized drug treatment – Lifestyle Over and Above Drugs in Diabetes (LOADD) study: randomized controlled trial. *BMJ* 2010; **341**: 746–752.

19. Lemon CC, Lacey K, Lohse B, Hubacher DO, Klawitter B, Palta M. Outcomes monitoring health, behavior, and quality of life after nutrition interventions in adults with type 2 diabetes. *J Am Diet Assoc* 2004; **104**: 1805–1815.

20. Academy of Nutrition and Dietetics Evidence Analysis Library. Disorders of lipid metabolism. Version current 2011. Internet: http://www.andeal.org/topic.cfm?=2875 (accessed 9 June 2015).

21. Academy of Nutrition and Dietetics Evidence Analysis Library. Effectiveness of MNT for hypertension. Version current 2008. Internet: http://www.andeal.org/topic.cfm?conclusion_statement_id=251204 (accessed 9 June 2015).

22. Wheeler ML, Dunbar SA, Jaacks LM, Karmally W, Mayer-Davis EJ, Wylie-Rosett J, et al. Macronutrients, food groups and eating patterns in the management of diabetes mellitus: a systematic review of the literature, 2010. *Diabetes Care* 2012; **35**: 434–445.

23. Bergenstal R, Johnson M, Powers M, Wynne A, Vlajnic A, Hollander P, et al. Adjust to target in Type 2 diabetes. Comparison of a simple algorithm with carbohydrate counting for adjustment of mealtime insulin glulisine. *Diabetes Care* 2008; **31**(7); 1305–1310.

24. Thomas D, Elliott EJ. Low glycaemic index, or low glycemic load, diets for diabetes mellitus. *Cochrane Database Syst Rev* 2009, Issue 1. Art. No: CD006296.

25. Wolever TMS, Gibbs AL, Mehling C, Chiasson J-L, Connelly PW, Josse RG, et al. The Canadian Trial of Carbohydrates in Diabetes (CCD), a 1-y controlled trial of low-glycemic-index dietary carbohydrate in type 2 diabetes. No effect on glycated hemoglobin but reduction in C-reactive protein. *Am J Clin Nutr* 2008; **87**: 114–125.

26. Ma Y, Olendzki BC, Merriam PA, Chiriboga DE, Culver AL, Li W, et al. A randomized clinical trial comparing low-glycemic index versus ADA dietary education among individuals with type 2 diabetes. *Nutrition* 2008; **24**: 45–56.

27. He M, van Dam RM, Rimm E, Hu FB, Qi L. Whole-grain, cereal fiber, bran, and germ intake and the risks of all-cause and cardiovascular disease-specific mortality among women with type 2 diabetes mellitus. *Circulation* 2010; **121**: 2162–2168.

28. Pańkowska E, Blazik M, Groele L. Does the fat-protein meal increase postprandial glucose levels in type 1 diabetes patients on insulin pump: the conclusion of a randomized study. *Diabetes Technol Ther* 2012; **14**: 16–22.

29. Dietary Guidelines Advisory Committee Report on the Dietary Guidelines for Americans, 2010. Version current 2010. Internet: http://www.health.gov/dietaryguidelines/dga2010/dietaryguidelines2010.pdf (accessed 9 June 2015).

30. USDA's Nutrition Evidence Library (NEL). Version current 2010. Internet: http://nel.gov/topic.cfm?cat2862 (accessed 26 January 2012).

Chapter 2.3

Carbohydrates

Kimber L. Stanhope
University of California, Davis, USA

2.3.1 Introduction

Types of dietary carbohydrates

Dietary carbohydrate is a broad category that includes 'simple' carbohydrates, 'complex' carbohydrates and dietary fibre. The simple carbohydrates, which are also called sugars, include the monosaccharides glucose, fructose and galactose, and the disaccharides maltose (glucose–glucose), sucrose (glucose–fructose), and lactose (glucose–galactose). The complex carbohydrates include the oligosaccharides, that consist of three to ten attached monosaccharide units, and polysaccharides that contain more than ten monosaccharide units. Starch, the predominant dietary polysaccharide, consists only of glucose units as opposed to inulin, a polysaccharide that consists of fructose units. Dietary fibre is commonly defined as "all plant polysaccharides and lignins which are resistant to hydrolysis by the digestive enzymes of man" [1]. Humans in the Western countries typically obtain approximately half their daily energy requirements from dietary carbohydrate.

Naturally-occurring sources of simple carbohydrate

Honey is nature's most concentrated source of simple carbohydrate (or sugar), containing about 40% fructose, 30% glucose, 7% maltose and 1% sucrose (by weight). Sugar beets and sugar cane contain about 20% and 10% sucrose, respectively. The sugar content in fruit ranges from 4 to 12%, consisting of mainly fructose, glucose and sucrose, with only trace amounts of galactose and maltose. Milk, the only significant dietary source of naturally-occurring lactose, contains about 5% lactose by weight.

Consumption of naturally-occurring sources of simple carbohydrate

Typically, Americans consume about 45 kcal/day as naturally-occurring sugar from fruit [2]. While this results from a level of fruit consumption that is only 38% of the recommended amount (2 cups/day, USDA MyPlate) [2], the global per capita fruit consumption is even lower by approximately 35% [3]. However, there are several countries, including Canada, Italy, Greece, Norway, Ghana and Iran, in which fruit consumption exceeds the global average by more than 100%. Fruit consumption in South Africa, Ukraine and India is approximately half the global average [3].

Americans consume 63% of the recommended amount of vegetables (2.5 cups/day, USDA MyPlate includes potato and corn) [2], thus only about 30 kcal/day as naturally-occurring sugar from vegetables. This level of vegetable consumption is very similar to the global average [3]. Countries that consume at least 80% more vegetables than the global average include China, Greece, Iran and Turkey. Countries in which vegetable consumption is less than half the global average include Colombia, Brazil, South Africa, Indonesia and Pakistan [3].

Advanced Nutrition and Dietetics in Diabetes, First Edition. Edited by Louise Goff and Pamela Dyson.
© 2016 John Wiley & Sons, Ltd. Published 2016 by John Wiley & Sons, Ltd.

The main source of dietary lactose is milk, the majority or all of the lactose is removed when milk is processed into cheese, butter and yogurt. Milk consumption varies greatly by country, with some of the variability being accounted for by lactose non-persistence [4]. Intestinal absorption of lactose requires that the disaccharide be hydrolysed by the enzyme lactase to its component monosaccharides. Infants have high concentrations of lactase, however, after weaning lactase synthesis decreases in about 30% of the white population and up to 70% of the nonwhite and Hispanic white populations. This lactase non-persistence causes incomplete digestion of lactose within the intestine, resulting in lactose intolerance. Lactose intolerance is characterised by abdominal pain, bloating, excess flatulence, and diarrhoea [4]. Americans consume about 75 litres of milk/year (5), which provides 40 kcal/day of lactose. China, Japan, Mexico and India, which have greater prevalence of lactase non-persistence, consume less than or about half this amount. Ireland, Finland, United Kingdom and Australia consume approximately 50% more [5].

The total amount of energy consumed from the naturally-occurring sugars in fruit, vegetable and milk in the American diet is 115 kcal, which is less than 5% of total daily energy. Generally, unless one eats a great deal of honey, it is difficult to consume excessive amount of simple carbohydrate from unprocessed foods. An average size man would have to eat an apple, peach, orange, 2 plums, 3 apricots, 16 strawberries, ½ cantaloupe, 1/8 watermelon and 4 slices of pineapple to consume 25% of his energy as naturally-occurring sugar.

Sources of processed simple carbohydrate

The predominant source of added sugar throughout the world is sucrose, which is extracted and purified from sugar cane and sugar beets. However, in the United States (US), an equal amount of the added sugar energy is provided by high fructose corn syrup (HFCS). HFCS is derived from the hydrolysis of cornstarch that produces glucose syrup, and then isomerisation of glucose syrup to produce syrup containing 42% fructose. The fructose in this syrup can be extracted to produce syrup that is 90% fructose. Analyses of popular sugar-sweetened beverages have shown the mean fructose content of HFCS used in production was 59% (range 47–65%) and several major brands appear to be produced with HFCS that is 65% fructose [6].

Consumption of processed sugar

Americans consume more than three times more energy as processed sugar, 368 kcal/day, than naturally-occurring sugar [2]. Sugar-sweetened beverages contribute 33% of this energy, sugar and candy contribute 16%, cakes and other baked goods contribute 13% and ice cream and dairy desserts contribute 9% [7]. Self-reported food intake data suggest that 13% of the US population consume 25% or more of their daily energy as added, processed sugar [8]. This may be an underestimate, as self-reported food intake is often under-reported [9], and sugar is one of the foods most likely to be under-reported [10]. The US leads the world in sugar consumption with levels more than double the world average. Sugar consumption in Brazil, Australia, Argentina and Mexico is close to the US level, while it is 75% lower in China and Africa [11].

Whole-grain and refined starch

More than half of the total carbohydrate consumed is in the form of starch. The most concentrated sources of starch are grains, such as wheat, oats, barley, rye and rice. Whole-grain wheat, oats, barley and rye are 69–73% starch, 12–16% protein and 10–16% dietary fibre by weight. Refined starch is made from grains that have been significantly altered from their natural composition, generally by removal of the bran and germ. In the case of wheat, refining increases the proportion of starch to 76% and decreases the proportions of protein from 14 to 10% and fibre from 12 to 2%. The loss of fibre is especially important because only 12% of the total grain consumed in the US is from whole grain and 88% is consumed as refined grain. Americans consume approximately 140 g/day as wheat flour [2]. If 100% of that wheat flour were consumed as a whole grain, the daily fibre intake from the flour would be 17 g. Instead, due to the substitution of refined for whole wheat flour, the daily fibre intake from wheat flour is 5 g. The average American adult consumes only 15 g of dietary fibre per day, well short of the Institute of Medicine recommendation that they consume 14 g of fibre for every 1000 kcal [12].

Potatoes, corn and legumes, such as pinto bean, black bean, navy bean, peas and chickpeas, are concentrated sources of starch that are often grouped as vegetables. Whole grain corn flour and potato flour contain 7% protein and 7% fibre. The legumes (mature, dry) are especially significant sources of protein (19–24%), fibre (15–25%) and micronutrients.

Carbohydrates and health

Adherence to diets that include high amounts of vegetables, fruit, legumes and whole grains, as well as fish and poultry, is associated with decreased mortality compared with diets that include high amounts of refined grains, french fries, sweets/desserts, red meat and processed meat in non-diabetic subjects [13,14]. There is much evidence that consumption of unrefined carbohydrates, such as whole grains, legumes, vegetables and fruit, and dietary fibre; promotes more healthful outcomes in diabetic patients than consumption of refined starches and sugar [15,16]. It was recently reported that the inverse association between dietary intake of fruit, legumes, nuts, seeds and pasta and mortality risk tended to be even stronger in people with diabetes than in those without [17]. It was also reported that the positive association between intake of butter and margarine and mortality risk tended to be stronger in people with diabetes than in those without. The authors conclude that people with diabetes may benefit more from a healthy diet than people without, and that dietary advice with respect to mortality for patients with diabetes should not differ from recommendations for the general population [17]. There is evidence to suggest that consumption of dietary fibre [18], whole grains [19], and vegetables and fruit [20] is associated

with preventing diabetes onset, while consumption of refined starch [21] and sugar [22,23] is associated with increased incidence of diabetes. Furthermore, many of the adverse metabolic outcomes that are associated with the diabetic state have also been shown to be related to excessive sugar consumption, including dyslipidemia [24], fatty liver [25], cardiovascular disease (CVD) [26], hyperuricemia [27] and chronic kidney disease [28].

Fructose – potential mediator

It has been suggested that the adverse metabolic outcomes associated with consumption of refined starch and sugar are mediated by their effects to increase glucose responses [29]. However, our group has reported that overweight to obese adult men and women (40–72 years of age) consuming fructose-sweetened beverages at 25% of energy requirements for 10 weeks exhibited increased visceral adipose deposition and *de novo* lipogenesis (DNL), decreased fatty acid oxidation, dyslipidemia and decreased glucose tolerance/insulin sensitivity; whereas subjects consuming glucose-sweetened beverages did not, even though both groups of subjects gained comparable amounts of body weight (~1.4 kg) [30,31]. These adverse effects of fructose consumption were not mediated by glycaemic response. Consumption of the fructose-sweetened beverages lowered postprandial glucose exposure (24-h area under the curve) and post-meal glucose peaks compared to consumption of the baseline diet, which contained refined starch in place of fructose [32]. In contrast, consumption of the glucose-sweetened beverages increased postprandial glucose exposure and post-meal glucose peaks compared to the baseline diet [32]. This suggests that fructose may be an important mediator and/or contributor to the association between the consumption of the rapidly absorbed carbohydrates, specifically sugar, and adverse metabolic outcomes. In support of this, we have shown in the University of California that for Davis-type 2 diabetes rats, a model of polygenic obese type 2 diabetes, sustained fructose consumption at 20% of energy sped the onset of diabetes

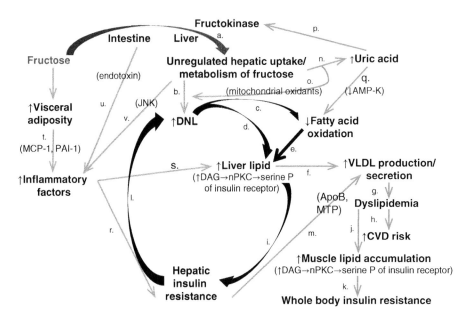

Figure 2.3.1 Potential mechanism by which consumption of fructose affects lipid metabolism and insulin sensitivity: Unregulated fructose uptake by the liver, mediated primarily by phosphorylation via fructokinase (**a**), leads to increased DNL (**b**). DNL increases the intra-hepatic lipid supply directly, via synthesis of fatty acids (**d**), and indirectly, by inhibiting fatty acid oxidation (**c**)(**e**). Increased levels of intra-hepatic lipid content promote VLDL production and secretion (**f**), which leads to dyslipidemia (**g**) and increased CVD risk (**h**). Increased levels of hepatic lipids may also promote hepatic insulin resistance by increasing levels of DAG, which activates nPKC and leads to serine phosphorylation of the insulin receptor and IRS-1 and impaired insulin action (**i**). Increased exposure to circulating triglyceride may lead to the accumulation of intramyocellular lipid in skeletal muscle (**j**), impaired DAG-mediated insulin signalling, and whole body insulin resistance (**k**). This sequence of events is likely to be exacerbated by hepatic insulin resistance, uric acid production, and inflammatory factors. Due to selective insulin resistance, DNL is even more strongly activated in the insulin resistant liver DNL (**l.**), which has the potential to generate a vicious cycle (black arrows). This cycle would be expected to further exacerbate VLDL production and secretion by increasing the intra-hepatic lipid supply. Hepatic insulin resistance also exacerbates VLDL production/secretion by increasing apoB availability and MTP expression (**m**).The unregulated fructose uptake by the liver, mediated by fructokinase, also leads to increased production of uric acid via the purine degradation pathway (**n**). This pathway may indirectly contribute to the liver lipid supply by concurrently generating mitochondrial oxidants that up-regulate DNL (**o**). Uric acid may also promote fructose uptake into the liver by up-regulating expression of fructokinase (**p**) and may contribute to the accumulation of lipid in the liver by inhibiting AMP-activated kinase, an activator of fatty acid oxidation (**q**). Inflammatory responses to fructose may impair hepatic insulin signalling (**r**) or increase hepatic lipid levels (**s**).These may be mediated by fructose-induced increases of visceral adipose which increase MCP-1 and PAI-1 (**t**), or fructose exposure to intestine which increases translocation of bacterial endotoxin (**u**), or exposure to hepatocytes which increases JNK activation (**v**)

by 2.6 months and markedly increased fasting and postprandial triglyceride levels compared with control diet [33]. In this chapter we will review the potential metabolic pathways by which fructose may specifically promote metabolic disease (Figure 2.3.1), and the direct experimental evidence that suggests these pathways are relevant to the fructose-containing sugars, sucrose and HFCS.

2.3.2 Adverse effects of fructose: potential metabolic pathways

Regulation by hepatic energy status

Hepatic glucose metabolism is regulated by phosphofructokinase, which is inhibited by adenosine triphosphate (ATP) and citrate when hepatic energy status is elevated, thereby limiting hepatic uptake of dietary glucose. This allows much of the ingested glucose arriving via the portal vein to bypass the liver and reach the systemic circulation and raise blood concentrations of glucose and insulin.

The initial phosphorylation of dietary fructose is largely catalysed by fructokinase, which is not regulated by hepatic energy status. The result is unregulated fructose uptake by the liver, resulting in most of the ingested fructose being metabolised in the liver (see path [a] in Figure 2.3.1) and very little reaching the systemic circulation. This is illustrated in the 24-h fructose and glucose profiles in subjects who consumed fructose- or glucose-sweetened beverages with 3 meals in a 24-h crossover trial [34]. When the subjects consumed the glucose-sweetened beverages, post-meal glucose peaks increased over fasting levels by 4 to 5 mmol; when they consumed the fructose-sweetened beverages, post-meal fructose peaks increased by less than 0.4 mmol [34]. Accordingly, postprandial increases of plasma glucose and insulin concentrations were substantially lower when subjects consumed fructose along with mixed meals compared with a baseline diet containing refined starch, and compared with the increases observed in subjects consuming isocaloric amounts of glucose [32,35].

The ability of fructose to lower post-meal glucose responses compared to an isocaloric amount of complex carbohydrate would be of potential benefit for maintaining glucose control in patients with diabetes. Indeed, aggregate analyses of short-term controlled feeding trials showed that isocaloric fructose replacement of other carbohydrates resulted in clinically significant improvements in glycaemic control, equivalent to a ~0.53% reduction in haemoglobin A_{1c}, without significantly affecting insulin in diabetic individuals. This benefit was seen across a full dose range of 20–160 g fructose/day [36]. However, given one of the goals of maintaining tight glycaemic control is to lower the risk of cardiovascular disease, the major cause of death in patients with type 2 diabetes, it is extremely important to investigate the potential effects of the unregulated hepatic uptake of high doses of fructose beyond its benefits on glycaemic control.

The unregulated hepatic metabolism of fructose

The unlimited hepatic uptake of fructose results in increased production of lipogenic precursors, thereby leading to increased DNL (path b in Figure 2.3.1). We have shown that the rate of fractional DNL was increased in subjects consuming meals containing 25% of energy as fructose-sweetened beverages under steady state conditions compared with when they consumed meals high in complex carbohydrate, and also compared with subjects consuming 25% of energy as glucose-sweetened beverages [31]. Additionally, as upregulation of hepatic DNL limits fatty acid oxidation in the liver (path c in Figure 2.3.1), the same subjects who exhibited fructose-induced increases of fractional DNL also exhibited markedly inhibited post-meal fatty acid oxidation compared with the subjects consuming glucose [30]. Thus by two mechanisms, increased production of fatty acids via DNL [31] (path d in Figure 2.3.1) and DNL-induced inhibition of oxidation of endogenous and exogenous fatty acids [30] (path e in Figure 2.3.1), consumption of fructose may increase levels of liver lipid. This is supported by the results from a diet intervention study in which overweight and obese men and women (age 20–50 years) consumed 1 l/d of sucrose-sweetened soda (~20% energy requirements), isocaloric amounts of low-fat milk, 1 l/d aspartame-sweetened beverages or 1 l/d water for 6 months. Liver lipid was significantly increased in the group consuming sucrose compared with the 3 other groups [37]).

Hepatic lipid and VLDL production

Liver lipid content is involved in the regulation of very low density lipoprotein (VLDL) production and secretion, which is expected given it is the role of VLDL to transport excess triglyceride out of the liver [38] (path f in Figure 2.3.1). Increased levels of hepatic triglyceride provide the lipid substrate that is packaged into VLDL, and also lead to increased availability of apolipoprotein B100 (apoB) by preventing its post-translational degradation [39]. ApoB is essential for the intracellular assembly of triglyceride into VLDL. Increased availability of hepatic lipid has also been described as a driver of the overproduction of large VLDL1 particles [40], which contain more triglyceride than the smaller VLDL2 particles.

Dyslipidaemia

Increased production and secretion of VLDL1 into the circulation, reduced lipoprotein lipase (LPL) activation by insulin, and competition for LPL-mediated triglyceride hydrolysis by chylomicrons can all contribute to a longer VLDL residence time, resulting in increased postprandial triglyceride concentrations following consumption of fructose. Dietary interventions studies, ranging from 24 hours to 10 weeks, demonstrate that postprandial hypertriglyceridaemia is the earliest lipid perturbation associated with fructose consumption [31,34,35,41–43]. Studies have also shown that consumption of sucrose [44–46] or HFCS [35,41] increase postprandial triglyceride concentrations compared with consumption of starch, glucose or non-nutritive sweeteners. An analysis of trials in which isocaloric fructose was exchanged for complex carbohydrate showed a triglyceride-raising effect in patients with type 2 diabetes when the daily dose exceeded 60 g [47].

While overproduction/secretion of VLDL1 has been described as the underlying defect that leads to the dyslipidemia that is characteristic of patients with type 2 diabetes and metabolic syndrome [48] (path g in Figure 2.3.1), it is controversial as to whether high triglyceride levels are a mediator or a marker [49]. Nevertheless, a number of studies have documented increases of established and potential risk factors for CVD in subjects consuming fructose or fructose-containing sugars compared with glucose or complex carbohydrate [31,35,50–53], including fasting and postprandial levels of apoB, low density lipoprotein-cholesterol (LDL-C), and small

dense LDL-C . Elevated plasma levels of LDL-apoB100 are strongly associated with increased risk of coronary artery disease [39] (path h in Figure 2.3.1). This risk involves the retention of LDL within the arterial wall due to an ionic interaction between basic amino acids in apoB and negatively charged sulfate groups on the artery wall proteoglycans [54]. Nevertheless, authors of a systematic review and meta-analysis reported that fructose has a cholesterol-lowering effect in diabetic patients compared to starch or sucrose [47]. However, only one of the included studies investigated the effects of isocaloric exchange of 20% of energy fructose for starch for a period longer than 8 days. This 4-week, diet-controlled, crossover study showed that in both subjects with type 1 and type 2 diabetes, the fructose diet improved glycaemic control, but circulating levels of total and LDL-cholesterol were increased [55].

Hepatic lipid and insulin sensitivity

The fructose-induced increase of hepatic lipid may also lead to hepatic insulin resistance [56] (path i in Figure 2.3.1). A potential mechanism involves increased intra-hepatic levels of diacylglycerol (DAG), which activates novel-protein kinase C (nPKC), a serine phosphorylator of the insulin receptor and insulin receptor substrate-1 (IRS-1) [57]. Aeiberli et al. have reported that hepatic insulin sensitivity, indexed by endogenous glucose production during euglycemic-hyperinsulinaemic clamps, was decreased in healthy young men who consumed 80 g of fructose/day as sweetened beverages for 3 weeks, compared with when they consumed 80 g of glucose/day [51]. These young men did not exhibit decreases in whole body insulin sensitivity, which suggests that the development of hepatic insulin resistance on high sugar diets occurs prior to the development of whole body insulin resistance.

Whole body insulin sensitivity

Our group has reported that older, overweight and obese men and women who consumed an average of 167 g of fructose/day for 9 weeks exhibited decreased whole body insulin sensitivity [31]. This suggests that when the period of exposure exceeds 3 weeks and/or the dose exceeds 80 g, consumption of fructose can lead to whole body insulin resistance downstream of hepatic insulin resistance. It may be caused by sustained exposure to postprandial triglycerides leading to increased intramyocellular lipid concentrations (path j in Figure 2.3.1), which have been shown to be correlated with reduced whole body insulin sensitivity in humans [58]. In the study described above, in which subjects consumed 1 l/d of sucrose-sweetened cola, low-fat milk, aspartame-sweetened cola, or water for 6 months, muscle lipid content was increased compared with baseline only in subjects consuming sucrose [37]. As suggested for hepatic insulin resistance, the relationship between intramyocellular lipid concentrations and whole body insulin sensitivity may be mediated by activation of nPKC by DAG, resulting in serine phosphorylation of the insulin receptor or IRS-1 [59] (path k in Figure 2.3.1). It is also possible that other factors, such as inflammation and oxidative stress [60], are involved [61].

2.3.3 Contributors to the adverse effects of fructose

It is likely the sequence of events described above is an oversimplified explanation of the potential mechanisms by which fructose may promote the development of metabolic disease. It is more likely there are other contributors to and/or mediators of this process.

Hepatic insulin resistance and DNL

The factor that has the greatest potential to contribute to the adverse effects of fructose is hepatic insulin resistance via its effects on DNL and VLDL production. DNL is an insulin-activated process in the normal liver that is, paradoxically, even more strongly activated in the insulin-resistant liver [62] (path l in

Figure 2.3.1). This has the potential to set up a vicious cycle (black arrows in Figure 2.3.1) in which the resulting increase of hepatic lipid content exacerbates the insulin resistance, which further activates DNL and further increases hepatic lipid accumulation. This vicious cycle may also exacerbate VLDL production/secretion due to the increasing liver lipid accumulation. However, VLDL production/secretion is also increased in the insulin resistant liver because insulin negatively regulates VLDL production by targeting apoB for post-translational degradation and inhibiting microsomal triglyceride-transfer protein (MTP) expression [62]. Impairment of these actions in the insulin-resistant liver leads to increased availability of apoB and chronic up-regulation of MTP expression and protein levels, which may further promote increased production of VLDL [62] (path m in Figure 2.3.1). Thus, there is the potential that the insulin resistance that is already present in diabetic patients would make them more vulnerable to the adverse effects of excessive fructose consumption than healthy, insulin-sensitive subjects. This suggestion is supported by a recent study in which the 24-h triglyceride profile was measured in children, with or without non-alcoholic fatty liver disease (NAFLD), during consumption of fructose and glucose in crossover feeding trials [63]. Postprandial TG levels were higher during fructose compared with glucose consumption in all children, but the fructose-induced increases in TG were higher in children with NAFLD than in those without NAFLD. Baseline insulin resistance was a highly significant contributor to the increases in 24-h triglyceride [63].

Uric acid

Uric acid is also a potential contributor to the adverse effects of fructose. Both published [64] and unpublished data from our clinical studies show that increases in both fasting uric acid and 24-h uric acid exposure (the mean plasma concentration of samples collected every 30–60 minutes over a 24-h period) are among the most consistent and significant effects of fructose, HFCS or sucrose consumption. They are consequential to the fructokinase-catalysed phosphorylation of fructose to fructose-1-phosphate, which results in conversion of ATP to adenosine monophosphate (AMP) and a depletion of inorganic phosphate. The degradation of AMP leads to increased uric acid production [65] (path n in Figure 2.3.1).The research group of Richard Johnson has shown that the purine degradation pathway that generates uric acid also upregulates DNL in hepatocytes, via the generation of mitochondrial oxidants [66] (path o in Figure 2.3.1). Furthermore, uric acid may amplify the lipogenic effects of fructose by activating fructokinase (path p in Figure 2.3.1) and inhibiting AMP-activated kinase (AMPK), an activator of fatty acid oxidation [66] (path q in Figure 2.3.1). It has also been suggested that uric acid is a mediator of diabetic nephropathy [67] and that high levels of uric acid are an independent risk factor for developing type 2 diabetes [68].

Inflammatory factors

Inflammation may contribute to the processes by which fructose may promote the development of metabolic disease. Data from studies in rodents suggest that fructose increases levels or expression of inflammatory factors in the liver, which may adversely affect hepatic insulin signalling (path r in Figure 2.3.1) or increase hepatic lipid levels (path s in Figure 2.3.1) [69]. In humans, direct experimental data that dietary fructose induces inflammation and oxidative stress are limited due to constraints regarding clinical liver sampling and the fact that plasma levels of inflammatory markers may not adequately reflect tissue-specific inflammation. However, we have reported that fasting concentrations of markers of inflammation; monocyte chemoattractant protein-1 (MCP-1), and plasminogen activator inhibitor-1 (PAI-1), and E-selectin were increased in older, overweight/obese subjects consuming fructose for 10 weeks [70]. These increases could be related to the fructose-induced increase in visceral adipose deposition observed in these same subjects [31], as MCP-1 and PAI-1 are both preferentially secreted by visceral fat compared with subcutaneous fat [70] (path t in Figure 2.3.1).

It is also possible that inflammatory responses to fructose are mediated through its direct exposure to the intestine or liver. In animals, fructose consumption has been shown to increase intestinal translocation of bacterial endotoxin, hepatic tumour necrosis factor-α, and liver lipid accumulation [69,71] (path u in Figure 2.3.1). In isolated hepatocytes, fructose exposure, compared with glucose exposure, leads to activation of c-jun NH_2-terminal kinase (JNK) (path v in Figure 2.3.1), increased serine phosphorylation of IRS-1 and reduced insulin-stimulated tyrosine phosphorylation of IRS-1 and IRS-2 [72].

2.3.4 Conclusion

The direct experimental data and potential mechanisms discussed above suggest that the relationship between sugar consumption and diabetes incidence could be causal. Furthermore, they suggest that adding up to 160 g fructose/day to the diet of diabetic patients in order to achieve a glucose lowering effect [36] would not prove beneficial to the health of diabetic patients. Many of the dysregulated processes that are potentially induced by excess fructose consumption are associated with the diabetic state due to the insulin resistance that underlies the disease [73]. It is reasonable to assume that excessive fructose consumption would exacerbate the dysregulation, and/or the already present insulin resistance would exacerbate the adverse effects of fructose. More long-term studies are needed to determine the level of dietary fructose that lowers glycaemic exposure without promoting lipid dysregulation in diabetic patients. In the meantime, it would appear prudent that both diabetic and nondiabetic patients consume diets that are low in fructose, sucrose and HFCS.

Key points

- Dietary carbohydrates include monosaccharides (simple sugars), disaccharides, oligosaccharides (starch and complex carbohydrates) and dietary fibre.
- Epidemiological evidence suggests that diets high in unrefined carbohydrate are associated with better health.
- There is growing evidence that there is a causal relationship between sugar intake and metabolic disorders.
- High intakes of fructose (usually derived from sugar-sweetened beverages) appear to be associated with adverse metabolic outcomes.
- For people with diabetes, recent evidence suggests that diets that are low in fructose, sucrose and HFCS are of benefit.

References

1. Trowell H, Southgate DA, Wolever TM, Leeds AR, Gassull MA, Jenkins DJ. Letter: Dietary fibre redefined. *Lancet* 1976; **1**(7966): 967. Epub 1976/05/01.
2. United States Department of Agriculture Economic Research Service. Food Availability (Per Capita) Data System. Version 13 September 2013. Internet: http://www.ers.usda.gov/data-products/food-availability-(per-capita)-data-system.aspx (accessed 4 December 2013).
3. Helgi Library. Fruit Consumption Per Capita. Version 2007 [database on the Internet]. Internet: http://www.helgilibrary.com/indicators/index/fruit-consumption-per-capita (accessed 7 December 2013).
4. Wilt TJ, Shaukat A, Shamliyan T, Taylor BC, MacDonald R, Tacklind J, et al. Lactose intolerance and health. *Evid Rep Technol Assess* 2010; **192**: 1–410. Epub 2010/07/16.
5. Canadian Dairy Information Centre. Global Consumption of Dairy Products by Country (Annual). Version 12 November 2013. Internet: http://www.dairyinfo.gc.ca/index_e.php?s1=dff-fcil&s2=cons&s3=consglo (accessed 7 December 2013).
6. Ventura EE, Davis JN, Goran MI. Sugar content of popular sweetened beverages based on objective laboratory analysis: focus on fructose content. *Obesity (Silver Spring)* 2011; **19**(4): 868–874. Epub 2010/10/16.
7. Johnson RK, Appel LJ, Brands M, Howard BV, Lefevre M, Lustig RH, et al. Dietary sugars intake and cardiovascular health: a scientific statement from the American Heart Association. *Circulation* 2009; **120**(11): 1011–1020. Epub 2009/08/26.
8. Marriott BP, Olsho L, Hadden L, Connor P. Intake of added sugars and selected nutrients in the United States, National Health and Nutrition Examination Survey (NHANES) 2003-2006. *Crit Rev Food Sci Nutr* 2010; **50**(3): 228–258. Epub 2010/03/20.
9. Livingstone MB, Black AE. Markers of the validity of reported energy intake. *J Nutr* 2003; **133**(Suppl. 3): 895S–920S.
10. Rangan A, Allman-Farinelli M, Donohoe E, Gill T. Misreporting of energy intake in the 2007 Australian Children's Survey: differences in the reporting of food types between plausible, under- and over-reporters of energy intake. *J Hum Nutr Diet* 2013. Epub 2013/11/12.
11. Sugar consumption at a crossroads. Version September 2013. Accessed 9 December 2013. Available from: https://publications.credit-suisse.com/tasks/render/file/index.cfm?fileid=780BF4A8-B3D1-13A0-13A0-D2514E21EFFB0479.
12. Satija A, Hu FB. Cardiovascular benefits of dietary fiber. *Curr Atheroscler Rep* 2012; **14**(6): 505–514. Epub 2012/08/09.
13. Heidemann C, Schulze MB, Franco OH, van Dam RM, Mantzoros CS, Hu FB. Dietary patterns and risk of mortality from cardiovascular disease, cancer, and all causes in a prospective cohort of women. *Circulation* 2008; **118**(3): 230–237. Epub 2008/06/25.
14. Ford DW, Jensen GL, Hartman TJ, Wray L, Smiciklas-Wright H. Association between dietary quality and mortality in older adults: a review of the epidemiological evidence. *J Nutr Gerontol Geriatr* 2013; **32**(2): 85–105. Epub 2013/05/15.
15. Lazarou C, Panagiotakos D, Matalas AL. The role of diet in prevention and management of type 2 diabetes: implications for public health. *Crit Rev Food Sci Nutr* 2012; **52**(5): 382–389. Epub 2012/03/01.
16. Wolfram T, Ismail-Beigi F. Efficacy of high-fiber diets in the management of type 2 diabetes mellitus. *Endocr Pract* 2011; **17**(1): 132–142. Epub 2010/08/18.
17. Sluik D, Boeing H, Li K, Kaaks R, Johnsen NF, Tjonneland A, et al. Lifestyle factors and mortality risk in individuals with diabetes mellitus: are the associations different from those in individuals without diabetes? *Diabetologia* 2013. Epub 2013/10/18.
18. Hopping BN, Erber E, Grandinetti A, Verheus M, Kolonel LN, Maskarinec G. Dietary fiber, magnesium, and glycemic load alter risk of type 2 diabetes in a multiethnic cohort in Hawaii. *J Nutr* 2010; **140**(1): 68–74. Epub 2009/11/06.

19. Aune D, Norat T, Romundstad P, Vatten LJ. Whole grain and refined grain consumption and the risk of type 2 diabetes: a systematic review and dose-response meta-analysis of cohort studies. *Eur Epidemiol* 2013. Epub 2013/10/26.

20. Cooper AJ, Forouhi NG, Ye Z, Buijsse B, Arriola L, Balkau B, et al. Fruit and vegetable intake and type 2 diabetes: EPIC-InterAct prospective study and meta-analysis. *Eur J Clin Nutr* 2012; **66**(10): 1082–1092. Epub 2012/08/03.

21. Mohan V, Radhika G, Sathya RM, Tamil SR, Ganesan A, Sudha V. Dietary carbohydrates, glycaemic load, food groups and newly detected type 2 diabetes among urban Asian Indian population in Chennai, India (Chennai Urban Rural Epidemiology Study 59). *Br J Nutr* 2009; **102**(10): 1498–1506. Epub 2009/07/10.

22. Bhupathiraju SN, Pan A, Malik VS, Manson JE, Willett WC, van Dam RM, et al. Caffeinated and caffeine-free beverages and risk of type 2 diabetes. *Am J Clin Nutr* 2013; **97**(1): 155–166. Epub 2012/11/16.

23. de Koning L, Malik VS, Rimm EB, Willett WC, Hu FB. Sugar-sweetened and artificially sweetened beverage consumption and risk of type 2 diabetes in men. *Am J Clin Nutr* 2011; **93**(6): 1321–1327. Epub 2011/03/25.

24. Welsh JA, Sharma A, Abramson JL, Vaccarino V, Gillespie C, Vos MB. Caloric sweetener consumption and dyslipidemia among US adults. *JAMA* 2010; **303**(15): 1490–1497. Epub 2010/04/22.

25. Assy N, Nasser G, Kamayse I, Nseir W, Beniashvili Z, Djibre A, et al. Soft drink consumption linked with fatty liver in the absence of traditional risk factors. *Can J Gastroenterol* 2008; **22**(10): 811–816. Epub 2008/10/18.

26. de Koning L, Malik VS, Kellogg MD, Rimm EB, Willett WC, Hu FB. Sweetened beverage consumption, incident coronary heart disease, and biomarkers of risk in men. *Circulation* 2012; **125**(14): 1735–1741, S1. Epub 2012/03/14.

27. Choi JW, Ford ES, Gao X, Choi HK. Sugar-sweetened soft drinks, diet soft drinks, and serum uric acid level: the Third National Health and Nutrition Examination Survey. *Arthritis Rheum* 2008; **59**(1): 109–116. Epub 2008/01/01.

28. Bomback AS, Derebail VK, Shoham DA, Anderson CA, Steffen LM, Rosamond WD, et al. Sugar-sweetened soda consumption, hyperuricemia, and kidney disease. *Kidney Int* 2010; **77**(7): 609–616. Epub 2009/12/25.

29. Ludwig DS. The glycemic index: physiological mechanisms relating to obesity, diabetes, and cardiovascular disease. *JAMA* 2002; **287**(18): 2414–2423. Epub 2002/05/04.

30. Cox CL, Stanhope KL, Schwarz JM, Graham JL, Hatcher B, Griffen SC, et al. Consumption of fructose-sweetened beverages for 10 weeks reduces net fat oxidation and energy expenditure in overweight/obese men and women. *Eur J Clin Nutr* 2012; **m66**(2): 201–208. Epub 2011/09/29.

31. Stanhope KL, Schwarz JM, Keim NL, Griffen SC, Bremer AA, Graham JL, et al. Consuming fructose-sweetened, not glucose-sweetened, beverages increases visceral adiposity and lipids and decreases insulin sensitivity in overweight/obese humans. *J Clin Invest* 2009; **119**(5): 1322–1334. Epub 2009/04/22.

32. Stanhope KL, Griffen SC, Bremer AA, Vink RG, Schaefer EJ, Nakajima K, et al. Metabolic responses to prolonged consumption of glucose- and fructose-sweetened beverages are not associated with postprandial or 24-h glucose and insulin excursions. *Am J Clin Nutr* 2011; **94**(1): 112–119. Epub 2011/05/27.

33. Cummings BP, Stanhope KL, Graham JL, Evans JL, Baskin DG, Griffen SC, et al. Dietary fructose accelerates the development of diabetes in UCD-T2DM rats: amelioration by the antioxidant, alpha-lipoic acid. *Am J Physiol Regul Integr Comp Physiol* 2010; **298**(5): R1343–1350. Epub 2010/02/12.

34. Teff KL, Grudziak J, Townsend RR, Dunn TN, Grant RW, Adams SH, et al. Endocrine and metabolic effects of consuming fructose- and glucose-sweetened beverages with meals in obese men and women: influence of insulin resistance on plasma triglyceride responses. *J Clin Endocrinol Metab* 2009; **94**(5): 1562–1569. Epub 2009/02/12.

35. Stanhope KL, Bremer AA, Medici V, Nakajima K, Ito Y, Nakano T, et al. Consumption of fructose and high fructose corn syrup increase postprandial triglycerides, LDL-cholesterol, and apolipoprotein-B in young men and women. *J Clin Endocrinol Metab* 2011; **96**(10): E1596–1605. Epub 2011/08/19.

36. Cozma AI, Sievenpiper JL, de Souza RJ, Chiavaroli L, Ha V, Wang DD, et al. Effect of fructose on glycemic control in diabetes: a systematic review and meta-analysis of controlled feeding trials. *Diabetes Care* 2012; **35**(7): 1611–1620. Epub 2012/06/23.

37. Maersk M, Belza A, Stodkilde-Jorgensen H, Ringgaard S, Chabanova E, Thomsen H, et al. Sucrose-sweetened beverages increase fat storage in the liver, muscle, and visceral fat depot: a 6-mo randomized intervention study. *Am J Clin Nutr* 2012; **95**(2): 283–289. Epub 2011/12/30.

38. Choi SH, Ginsberg HN. Increased very low density lipoprotein (VLDL) secretion, hepatic steatosis, and insulin resistance. *Trends Endocrinol Metab* 2011; **22**(9): 353–363. Epub 2011/05/28.

39. Olofsson SO, Boren J. Apolipoprotein B secretory regulation by degradation. *Arterioscler Thromb Vasc Biol* 2012; **32**(6): 1334–1338. Epub 2012/05/18.

40. Adiels M, Taskinen MR, Packard C, Caslake MJ, Soro-Paavonen A, Westerbacka J, et al. Overproduction

of large VLDL particles is driven by increased liver fat content in man. *Diabetologia* 2006; **49**(4): 755–765. Epub 2006/02/08.

41. Stanhope KL, Griffen SC, Bair BR, Swarbrick MM, Keim NL, Havel PJ. Twenty-four-hour endocrine and metabolic profiles following consumption of high-fructose corn syrup-, sucrose-, fructose-, and glucose-sweetened beverages with meals. *Am J Clin Nutr* 2008; **87**(5): 1194–1203.

42. Swarbrick MM, Stanhope KL, Elliott SS, Graham JL, Krauss RM, Christiansen MP, et al. Consumption of fructose-sweetened beverages for 10 weeks increases postprandial triacylglycerol and apolipoprotein-B concentrations in overweight and obese women. *Br J Nutr* 2008; **100**(5): 947–952.

43. Teff KL, Elliott SS, Tschop M, Kieffer TJ, Rader D, Heiman M, et al. Dietary fructose reduces circulating insulin and leptin, attenuates postprandial suppression of ghrelin, and increases triglycerides in women. *J Clin Endocrinol Metab* 2004; **89**(6): 2963–2972.

44. Mann JI, Truswell AS. Effects of isocaloric exchange of dietary sucrose and starch on fasting serum lipids, postprandial insulin secretion and alimentary lipaemia in human subjects. *Br J Nutr* 1972; **27**(2): 395–405. Epub 1972/03/01.

45. Raben A, Moller BK, Flint A, Vasilaris TH, Christina Moller A, Juul Holst J, et al. Increased postprandial glycaemia, insulinemia, and lipidemia after 10 weeks' sucrose-rich diet compared to an artificially sweetened diet: a randomised controlled trial. *Food Nutr Res* 2011; **55**. Epub 2011/07/30.

46. Raben A, Vasilaras TH, Moller AC, Astrup A. Sucrose compared with artificial sweeteners: different effects on ad libitum food intake and body weight after 10 wk of supplementation in overweight subjects. *Am J Clin Nutr* 2002; **76**(4): 721–729. Epub 2002/09/27.

47. Sievenpiper JL, Carleton AJ, Chatha S, Jiang HY, de Souza RJ, Beyene J, et al. Heterogeneous effects of fructose on blood lipids in individuals with type 2 diabetes: systematic review and meta-analysis of experimental trials in humans. *Diabetes Care* 2009; **32**(10): 1930–1937. Epub 2009/07/14.

48. Adiels M, Olofsson SO, Taskinen MR, Boren J. Overproduction of very low-density lipoproteins is the hallmark of the dyslipidemia in the metabolic syndrome. *Arterioscler Thromb Vasc Biol* 2008; **28**(7): 1225–1236. Epub 2008/06/21.

49. Goldberg IJ, Eckel RH, McPherson R. Triglycerides and heart disease: still a hypothesis? *Arterioscler Thromb Vasc Biol* 2011; **31**(8): 1716–1725. Epub 2011/04/30.

50. Aeberli I, Gerber PA, Hochuli M, Kohler S, Haile SR, Gouni-Berthold I, et al. Low to moderate sugar-sweetened beverage consumption impairs glucose and lipid metabolism and promotes inflammation in healthy young men: a randomized controlled trial. *Am J Clin Nutr* 2011. Epub 2011/06/17.

51. Aeberli I, Hochuli M, Gerber PA, Sze L, Murer SB, Tappy L, et al. Moderate Amounts of Fructose Consumption Impair Insulin Sensitivity in Healthy Young Men: A randomized controlled trial. *Diabetes Care* 2012. Epub 2012/08/31.

52. Hallfrisch J, Reiser S, Prather ES. Blood lipid distribution of hyperinsulinemic men consuming three levels of fructose. *Am J Clin Nutr* 1983; **37**(5): 740–748. Epub 1983/05/01.

53. Reiser S, Powell AS, Scholfield DJ, Panda P, Fields M, Canary JJ. Day-long glucose, insulin, and fructose responses of hyperinsulinemic and nonhyperinsulinemic men adapted to diets containing either fructose or high-amylose cornstarch. *Am J Clin Nutr* 1989; **50**(5): 1008–1014.

54. Boren J, Olin K, Lee I, Chait A, Wight TN, Innerarity TL. Identification of the principal proteoglycan-binding site in LDL. A single-point mutation in apo-B100 severely affects proteoglycan interaction without affecting LDL receptor binding. *J Clin Invest* 1998; **101**(12): 2658–2664. Epub 1998/06/24.

55. Bantle JP, Swanson JE, Thomas W, Laine DC. Metabolic effects of dietary fructose in diabetic subjects. *Diabetes Care* 1992; **15**(11): 1468–1476.

56. Morino K, Petersen KF, Shulman GI. Molecular mechanisms of insulin resistance in humans and their potential links with mitochondrial dysfunction. *Diabetes* 2006; **55**(Suppl. 2): S9–S15.

57. Jornayvaz FR, Shulman GI. Diacylglycerol activation of protein kinase Cepsilon and hepatic insulin resistance. *Cell Metab* 2012; **15**(5): 574–584. Epub 2012/05/09.

58. Krssak M, Falk Petersen K, Dresner A, DiPietro L, Vogel SM, Rothman DL, et al. Intramyocellular lipid concentrations are correlated with insulin sensitivity in humans: a 1H NMR spectroscopy study. *Diabetologia* 1999; **42**(1): 113–116.

59. Samuel VT, Shulman GI. Mechanisms for insulin resistance: common threads and missing links. *Cell* 2012; **148**(5): 852–871. Epub 2012/03/06.

60. Anderson EJ, Lustig ME, Boyle KE, Woodlief TL, Kane DA, Lin CT, et al. Mitochondrial H2O2 emission and cellular redox state link excess fat intake to insulin resistance in both rodents and humans. *J Clin Invest* 2009; **119**(3): 573–581. Epub 2009/02/04.

61. Coen PM, Goodpaster BH. Role of intramyocelluar lipids in human health. *Trends Endocrinol Metab* 2012; **23**(8): 391–398. Epub 2012/06/23.

62. Lewis GF, Carpentier A, Adeli K, Giacca A. Disordered fat storage and mobilization in the pathogenesis of insulin resistance and type 2 diabetes. *Endocr Rev* 2002; **23**(2): 201–229.

63. Jin R, Le NA, Liu S, Farkas Epperson M, Ziegler TR, Welsh JA, et al. Children with NAFLD are more sensitive to the adverse metabolic effects of fructose beverages than children without NAFLD. *J Clin Endocrinol Metab* 2012; **97**(7): E1088–1098. Epub 2012/05/01.

64. Cox CL, Stanhope KL, Schwarz JM, Graham JL, Hatcher B, Griffen SC, et al. Consumption of fructose- but not glucose-sweetened beverages for 10 weeks increases circulating concentrations of uric acid, retinol binding protein- 4, and gamma-glutamyl transferase activity in overweight/obese humans. *Nutr Metab (Lond.)* 2012; **9**(1): 68. Epub 2012/07/26.

65. Mayes PA. Intermediary metabolism of fructose. *Am J Clin Nutr* 1993; **58**(5 Suppl): 754S–765S.

66. Johnson RJ, Nakagawa T, Sanchez-Lozada LG, Shafiu M, Sundaram S, Le M, et al. Sugar, uric acid, and the etiology of diabetes and obesity. *Diabetes* 2013; **62**(10): 3307–3315. Epub 2013/09/26.

67. Jalal DI, Maahs DM, Hovind P, Nakagawa T. Uric acid as a mediator of diabetic nephropathy. *Semin Nephrol* 2011; **31**(5): 459–465. Epub 2011/10/18.

68. Lv Q, Meng XF, He FF, Chen S, Su H, Xiong J, et al. High serum uric acid and increased risk of type 2 diabetes: a systemic review and meta-analysis of prospective cohort studies. *PLoS ONE* 2013; **8**(2): e56864. Epub 2013/02/26.

69. Dekker MJ, Su Q, Baker C, Rutledge AC, Adeli K. Fructose: a highly lipogenic nutrient implicated in insulin resistance, hepatic steatosis, and the metabolic syndrome. *Am J Physiol Endocrinol Metab* 2010; **299**(5): E685–694. Epub 2010/09/09.

70. Cox CL, Stanhope KL, Schwarz JM, Graham JL, Hatcher B, Griffen SC, et al. Circulating concentrations of monocyte chemoattractant protein-1, plasminogen activator inhibitor-1, and soluble leukocyte adhesion molecule-1 in overweight/obese men and women consuming fructose- or glucose-sweetened beverages for 10 weeks. *J Clin Endocrinol Metab* 2011; **96**(12): E2034–2038. Epub 2011/10/01.

71. Kavanagh K, Wylie AT, Tucker KL, Hamp TJ, Gharaibeh RZ, Fodor AA, et al. Dietary fructose induces endotoxemia and hepatic injury in calorically controlled primates. *Am J Clin Nutr* 2013; **98**(2): 349–357. Epub 2013/06/21.

72. Wei Y, Wang D, Topczewski F, Pagliassotti MJ. Fructose-mediated stress signaling in the liver: implications for hepatic insulin resistance. *J Nutr Biochem* 2007; **18**(1): 1–9.

73. Verges B. Abnormal hepatic apolipoprotein B metabolism in type 2 diabetes. *Atherosclerosis* 2010; **211**(2): 353–360. Epub 2010/03/02.

Chapter 2.4

Glycaemic index and glycaemic load in diabetes

C. Jeya Henry[1] and P. Sangeetha Thondre[2]

[1] National University of Singapore, Singapore
[2] Oxford Brookes University, Oxford, UK

2.4.1 Introduction

Glycaemic index (GI) is the concept developed in the 1980s as a physiological basis for carbohydrate classification, recognising that carbohydrate-containing foods with the same amount of available carbohydrate produce different glycaemic responses [1]. The concept of glycaemic load (GL) was first introduced by researchers at Harvard University to quantify the glycaemic impact of a portion of food. The GL of a typical serving of food is essentially the product of the glycaemic index of the food and the quantity of available carbohydrate in that serving, and can be considered a more practical method of assessing the impact of carbohydrate on glycaemia [2].

2.4.2 Measurement of glycaemic index and glycaemic load

Glycaemic index

The GI of a food is determined by comparing its blood glucose response with the blood glucose response after a standard amount of a reference food (either white bread or glucose) [1]. It is expressed as a percentage of the incremental area under the glycaemic response curve elicited by a portion of food containing 50 g available carbohydrate in comparison with the area under the curve elicited by 50 g carbohydrate in the reference food in the same subject. The GI of a food is calculated as follows:

$$\text{Glycaemic index} = \frac{\text{Incremental blood glucose area of 50g carbohydrate test food}}{\text{Incremental blood glucose area of 50g carbohydrate reference food}} \times 100$$

A recent review that discusses the GI methodology recommends that a minimum of 10 healthy human volunteers need to be tested after 10–14 hour overnight fasting to determine the GI of a food [3]. Blood sampling (venous or capillary) should be done before and at 15, 30, 45, 60, 90 and 120 min after consuming the test meal. In the event of testing multiple foods, the testing period should not exceed four months and the test foods should be randomised in blocks of six with a reference food tested before and after each block [3]. Although most of the earlier reports on GI were based on testing carried out on Europeans, North Americans or Australians, more recent studies have been focusing on Asian and African populations. Most of the studies using subjects of various ethnic origins have found no difference in GI values for the same foods [4,5], allowing the use of the GI concept worldwide.

Advanced Nutrition and Dietetics in Diabetes, First Edition. Edited by Louise Goff and Pamela Dyson.
© 2016 John Wiley & Sons, Ltd. Published 2016 by John Wiley & Sons, Ltd.

Table 2.4.1 Glycaemic index and glycaemic load classification

	Glycaemic index	Glycaemic load
High	>70	≥20
Medium	55–70	11–19
Low	<55	≤10

Source: Atkinson et al. 2008 [9] and Henry and Thondre 2011 [10]

International tables of GI and GL values published to date list 2487 different items across a range of globally produced food groups and brands [6]. The vast majority of published GI values are Australasian, British or Canadian in origin, with some Danish, French and Swedish values. There are a few published GI values for Chinese foods [7], mixed meals and speciality products such as weight management meals added to the database [8].

Table 2.4.1 shows the values for categories of high, medium and low GI foods.

Glycaemic load

GL is calculated as the quantity of carbohydrate in a food (g/serving) multiplied by the quantity of food eaten (weight [g] or volume [ml]) and by its GI value and is represented by the following equation:

$$\text{Glycaemic load} = \sum(\text{quantity of food consumed (g or mL)} \times \text{carbohydrate content of food (g / serving)} \times \text{GI})$$

Table 2.4.1 shows the values for categories of high, medium and low GL foods.

The GL of a diet can be lowered by choosing foods with low GI or by reducing the quantities of carbohydrates consumed or by a combination of both. GL is more relevant to clinical practice as it provides the glycaemic effect of realistic portion sizes of different foods, for example water melon has a high GI but a low GL, whereas cornflakes have high values for both GI and GL (Table 2.4.2).

Table 2.4.2 Comparison of the glycaemic index and glycaemic load of some common foods

Food	GI	Serving size (g)	GL
White baguette	57	30	10
Corn flakes	93	30	23
Baked potato	69	150	19
Water melon	72	120	4
White bread	75	30	9
Crisps, salted	51	50	12
Rice, white, boiled	69	150	36
Porridge made from rolled oats	63	250	19
Pizza, cheese	36	100	9
Rice, brown, boiled	66	150	21
Pineapple pieces, canned in natural fruit juice	55	120	10
Bran flakes	50	30	10
Ice cream	32	50	1
Spaghetti, white, boiled	51	180	24
Apple	39	120	6
Lentils	29	150	5
Barley, pearled	35	150	15

Source: Atkinson et al. 2008 [6].

2.4.3 Factors affecting glycaemic index and glycaemic load

Many factors influence the GI value of foods, including the nature of the starch, the ratio of amylose to amylopectin, the degree of retrogradation, the degree of hydration (method of cooking), particle size, food form, protein–starch interaction, fibre, antinutrients and acidity of foods [9]. In addition, other dietary factors that affect nutrient digestibility or insulin secretion, such as the fat or protein content, also influence the GI of a food [10]. Food processing methods at high temperatures and high pressure extrusion technology, which are commonly used in breakfast cereal and snack production, can increase the degree of starch gelatinisation, resulting in quick digestion and a high GI [11]. High amylose starches tend to have lower GI as they are digested more slowly than amylopectin-rich starches [12]. There are a number of ingredients that can lower the GI of foods. Some, for example soluble fibre, delay carbohydrate digestion and absorption from the gut by increasing the viscosity of the stomach and intestinal contents and forming a protective layer incorporating readily digestible carbohydrates [13]. Other food components, such as fats, delay the rate of gastric emptying or result in the secretion of gut hormones which result in a faster clearance of glucose through an increase in insulin response [14]. The addition of protein to a carbohydrate food results in the formation of a protective network around the carbohydrate molecule thereby preventing the action of glycolytic enzymes [15].

Compounds such as polyphenols attenuate postprandial glycaemic response by inhibiting carbohydrate digestion and glucose absorption in the intestine, stimulating insulin secretion from the pancreatic β-cells, modulating glucose release from the liver, activating insulin receptors and glucose uptake in the insulin sensitive tissues and modulating intracellular signalling pathways and gene expression [10,16].

2.4.4 GI, GL and diabetes

The relevance of GI and GL to both the prevention and management of diabetes has received much attention; high GI foods may increase the risk of type 2 diabetes by over stimulating insulin secretion or contributing to pancreatic β-cell dysfunction, which can result in impaired glucose tolerance [17]. Low GI diets have additionally been shown to limit reductions in insulin sensitivity [17,18]. GI is not only relevant to type 2 diabetes due to its direct effects on blood glucose and insulin sensitivity but also has therapeutic potential in hyperlipidaemia and weight management [18,19].

Epidemiological evidence supports a positive relationship between GI and risk of type 2 diabetes. In a Dutch population, the risk of developing type 2 diabetes was increased by 37% in men and women in the highest GI quintile [20]. However, in the Iowa Women's Health Study no relationship was found between GI and the risk of type 2 diabetes in a 6-year follow-up of 35 988 post-menopausal women [2]; these inconsistent results may be explained by methodological differences between the studies.

The EURODIAB study showed that in the lowest GI quartile, HbA1c concentrations were 11% lower in individuals with type 1 diabetes from Southern Europe and 6% lower in individuals from the rest of Europe [21].

International diabetes organisations including the Canadian Diabetes Association [18], Diabetes Australia [22], Diabetes UK [23] and the European Association for the Study of Diabetes [24] currently recommend GI as a strategy for diabetes management in type 2 diabetes.

Intervention studies

Type 2 diabetes

The results of two systematic reviews have demonstrated the clinical utility of low GI diets in the management of type 2 diabetes, with studies showing a reduction in HbA1c of 5 mmol/mol (0.4%) [25,26]. The American Diabetes Association (ADA) has recommended that low GI diets can produce a modest benefit in controlling postprandial hyperglycaemia in individuals who normally consume a high GI diet [27].

Randomised controlled trials of very short duration of up to four weeks have demonstrated the beneficial effects of low GI diets in type 2 diabetic men [28,29]. The main improvements observed were in fasting plasma glucose, HbA1c, whole body glucose utilisation (measured by the euglycaemic-hyperinsulinaemic clamp), lipid profiles and the capacity for fibrinolysis. Consumption of a low GI Mexican-style diet consisting of corn tortillas and legumes for six weeks resulted in improved metabolic parameters such as fasting serum glucose, HbA1c and Body Mass Index (BMI) in overweight and obese subjects with type 2 diabetes. This study showed the possibility of adapting the concept of low GI into different cultures [30]. Longer term studies have also demonstrated a protective effect of a low GI diet in older women followed up for six years [31].

There is still some debate about the relative effects of altering the type or the amount of carbohydrate in the diet. In one study comparing a low carbohydrate and a low GI diet, both diets improved HbA1c, fasting glucose, fasting insulin and body weight in obese type 2 diabetes subjects, but diabetes medications were reduced or eliminated in 33% more participants in the low carbohydrate group compared to the low GI group [32].

Gestational diabetes

Low GI diets during pregnancy in normoglycaemic women have been shown to reduce HbA1c and glucose concentrations [33] and increase birth weight and ponderal index in their offspring [34]. There is some evidence for the role of low GI diets in preventing gestational diabetes (GDM), with an 8-year follow-up of subjects in the Nurses Health Study showing a 26% reduction in the risk of developing GDM with each 10 g/day increment in total fibre intake, predominantly from dark breads. High GL and low fibre intakes were risk factors associated with the risk of developing GDM [35].

A further study of women with GDM showed that a low GI diet during a 12-month period did not make any significant differences in obstetric and foetal outcomes when compared to a high GI diet. However, the low GI diet was effective in reducing the number of women needing to use insulin by 50%, with no compromise of obstetric or foetal outcomes [36].

Type 1 diabetes

The majority of studies investigating the effect of low GI diets on diabetes outcomes have taken place in those with type 2 diabetes, with a Cochrane review of 12 studies including only one in adults with type 1 diabetes [26]. This study in type 1 diabetes showed that a fibre-rich low GI diet improved blood glucose concentrations and reduced hypoglycaemia [37]. In adults treated with continuous subcutaneous insulin infusion, low GI meals were associated with significantly lower postprandial blood glucose concentrations than high GI meals [38]. In addition, knowledge about the GI of foods aids determination of pre-meal bolus type and optimises post-prandial glycaemia in patients using subcutaneous infusion.

In children with type 1 diabetes who were given a low GI diet and a standard diet on two separate days, the low GI diet improved daytime blood glucose control and glucose metabolism, reduced fat intake and increased fibre intake [39]. Advice on low GI food choices was also reported to help children with type 1 diabetes with improvements in quality of life and HbA1c concentration [40]. The beneficial effects of diets with low GI and medium GL were also observed in the glycaemic control of children and teenagers with type 1 diabetes. Almost 74% of subjects in this study who showed good glycaemic control consumed a diet of mean GI 54.8 [41].

2.4.5 GI, GL and obesity

Epidemiological studies have shown an inverse relation between carbohydrate consumption and BMI [42,43]. Low GI foods may benefit weight regulation by promoting prolonged feeling of fullness and satiety and promoting fat oxidation at the expense of carbohydrate oxidation. Increased food residence time of low GI foods in the gut lumen can also trigger the stimulation of satiety hormones such as cholecystokinin [44].

In a systematic review, 12 out of 18 studies using subjective methods of appetite assessment reported an increase in satiety with low glycaemic meals. In addition, 4 out of 7 studies using objective methods of appetite assessment also showed that low GI meals delayed the first food request and decreased the subsequent and cumulative energy intake [45]. Many low-GI foods are high in fibre, which prolongs distension of the gastrointestinal tract, causing increased and prolonged secretion of the gut peptides cholecystokinin, ghrelin, glucagon, glucagon-like-peptide-1 and glucose-dependent insulinotropic polypeptide, all of which have been suggested as satiety factors [46].

In children, the ARCA project reported that the risk of overweight/obesity or of central fat distribution was almost two-fold higher in the upper quartile in comparison to the lowest quartile of dietary GI. In children, the prevalence of obesity showed an increasing trend in German children associated with an increase in dietary GI from 1990 to 2002 [47]. An increase of six units in dietary GI was associated with a two-fold increased risk of the occurrence of overweight/obesity and of abdominal adiposity. Intervention studies in obese children have reported that low GI diets are associated with lower energy intake, and low GI foods eaten at breakfast were found to have a significant impact on reducing food intake at lunch in preadolescent children [48].

Although short-term studies have shown that low GI foods have greater satiogenic effect than high GI foods, there is no evidence showing an effect of low GI foods on long-term energy intake and body weight regulation [45,46], and no evidence that low GI diets have any effect on body weight in people with type 2 diabetes [49].

2.4.6 Metabolic effects of low glycaemic index and glycaemic load diets

Low GI diets improve insulin sensitivity in patients with advanced coronary heart disease (CHD) and those at increased risk of CHD, suggesting that those subjects who already have some extent of insulin resistance might get the most benefit from a low GI diet [50]. In some studies, a low GI diet, in subjects with impaired glucose tolerance, improved insulin secretion from pancreatic β-cells [42]. An attenuated glucose response regulates the responses of other hormones, such as insulin and glucagon, whereas high GI foods that result in large insulin responses increase the glucose uptake and glycogen synthesis in skeletal muscle and liver, and lipogenesis in adipose tissue but suppress gluconeogenesis, glucose output by liver and lipolysis. The rapid absorption of nutrients following a high GI meal slows down the rate of entry of exogenous glucose into the circulation. Glucose mobilisation from tissues remains suppressed due to the effects of high insulin and glucagon concentrations, resulting in rapid decline in blood glucose below fasting concentration. This triggers release of counter-regulatory hormones,

including glucagon, adrenaline and growth hormone, that act to restore circulating glucose concentration by increasing hepatic glucose output and decreasing glucose uptake by skeletal muscle. They also trigger lipolysis and fatty acids release by adipose tissue, causing a rebound in circulating fatty acid concentration. Following a low GI meal, the prolonged and continued absorption of nutrients from the gastrointestinal tract does not result in hypoglycaemia. This allows adjustment of hepatic glucose output to maintain circulating glucose concentration without dramatic rises and falls, or a large rebound in fatty acid concentrations. Thus a more stable diurnal profile is maintained following low GI diets [42].

2.4.7 GI and GL in real life situations

Controversy in nutrition research surrounds the use of GI due to the variability and inconsistency of results from studies and the perceived difficulty of application to real life situations. A recent report argued that GI is more of a personal attribute rather than a universal measurement, with the authors finding up to five-fold differences in area under the curve between individuals testing the same food [51]. The shape of the postprandial glycaemic curve has been reported as similar for foods categorised as having low, medium or high GI, contradicting the general belief that low GI foods produce sustained rise in blood glucose [52]. The validity of the GI concept is often challenged on the grounds of individual variability, changes due to cooking, processing or ripeness of food and other factors such as the rate of gastrointestinal motility, digestion and absorption. The application of GI to people with diabetes has been questioned due to the effect of the fat, protein and total energy content of a meal [53], although there is evidence that the carbohydrate content and GI were the only determinants of glycaemic response of mixed meals [54]. The practical application of GI has also been questioned, although advice for using GI in practice is widely available [55], and an example of low,

Table 2.4.3 Practical application of the glycaemic index – low, medium and high GI foods

Food	Low glycaemic index (<55)	Medium glycaemic index (56–69)	High glycaemic index (>70)
Bread	Multigrain, seeded, granary and rye		All wholemeal, brown and white bread including French bread and naan bread
Breakfast cereals	All-Bran, Special K, muesli and porridge	Other bran cereals	All other cereals including cornflakes, puffed rice, Shredded Wheat, Weetabix and sugared cereals
Potatoes	Sweet potato, yams	New potatoes, crisps	Old potatoes including baked, boiled, mashed, roast and chips
Pasta and rice	All types of pasta and egg noodles	Basmati rice, egg noodles	Brown and white rice, rice pasta
Vegetables	Pulses including lentils, beans, peas and sweetcorn		
Fruit	Apples, pears, citrus fruit, berries and stone fruit including peaches, cherries, apricots	Tropical fruit including melon, pineapple, mango, banana and grapes	
Dairy products	All milk and yogurt, whether full fat, semi-skimmed or skimmed	Ice cream	
Cakes and biscuits	Plain sponge cake, fruit and malt bread	Plain, semi-sweet biscuits, crackers	Doughnuts, scones
Savoury snacks	Maize or corn chips, cashews, peanuts	Potato crisps	Extruded potato snacks including hoops and puffs and pretzels

medium and high GI foods is shown in Table 2.4.3. There may be errors in calculating the GI of composite meals, with one study showing that the method of calculating the GI of meals using published individual GI values of foods will overestimate the GI of the meal by 22–50% [56]. Nevertheless, there are arguments in favour of GI in terms of its robustness in predicting response to mixed meals, ease of implementation and benefits to type 2 diabetes management, as evidenced from epidemiological studies, clinical trials and basic research.

2.4.8 Conclusion

In conclusion, GI and GL play a role in determining food choices to manage the postprandial hyperglycaemia which is a characteristic feature of diabetes, and GI and GL are important concepts to guide consumers towards choosing the right type of carbohydrates. Many low GI foods are high in fibre, antioxidants and phytochemicals that are beneficial to health. In general, most of the foods already labelled as healthy (whole grains, milk, fruits, vegetables, legumes) are low GI foods. Although there are some exceptions to this general consensus, for example food formulated with added fat to develop energy dense foods with low GI and GL, adverse health effects could be alleviated by using healthier monounsaturated and polyunsaturated fats instead of undesirable saturated fats. No negative effects have been demonstrated so far by following a low GI or low GL diet with healthy ingredients. Consumption of low GI foods may be effective in the prevention and management of type 2 diabetes, and may have a role in reducing the co-morbidities associated with diabetes, such as cardiovascular diseases and obesity.

Key points

- GI of carbohydrate foods can only be measured practically in the laboratory.
- GL of foods can be calculated from the GI.
- Randomised, controlled trials and intervention studies in children and adults with diabetes have reported benefits in terms of glycaemic control and cardiovascular risk.
- There is little evidence of the effect of low GI diets on body weight in people with diabetes.
- Controversy still remains, with some authorities recommending low GI diets as a primary strategy and others suggesting that the amount rather than the type of carbohydrate is of most importance.

References

1. Jenkins DJA, Wolever TMS, Taylor RH, Barker H, Fielden H, Baldwin JM, et al. Glycemic index of foods: a physiological basis for carbohydrate exchange. *Am J Clin Nutr* 1981; **34**: 362–366.
2. Willett W, Manson J, Liu S. Glycemic index, glycemic load and risk of type 2 diabetes. *Am J Clin Nutr* 2002; **76**: 274S–280S.
3. Brouns F, Bjorck I, Frayn KN, Gibbs AL, Lang V, Slama G, et al. Glycaemic index methodology. *Nutr Res Rev* 2005; **18**: 145–171.
4. Chan HMS, Brand-Miller J, Holt SHA, Wilson D, Rozman M, Petocz P. The glycemic index values of Vietnamese foods. *Eur J Clin Nutr* 2001; **55**: 1076–1083.
5. Henry CJK, Lightowler HJ, Newens K, Sudha V, Radhika G, Sathya RM, et al. Glycemic index of common foods tested in the UK and India. *Br J Nutr* 2008; **99**: 840–845.
6. Atkinson FS, Foster-Powell K, Brand-Miller JC. International Table of glycemic index and glycemic load values: 2008. *Diabetes Care* 2008; **31**: 2281–2283.
7. Lok KY, Chan R, Chan D, Li L, Leung G, Woo J, et al. Glycemic index and glycemic load values of a selection of popular foods consumed in Hong Kong. *Br J Nutr* 2010; **103**: 556–560.
8. Henry CJK, Lightowler HJ, Dodwell LM, Wynne JM. Glycaemic index and glycaemic load values of cereal products and weight-management meals available in the UK. *Br J Nutr* 2007; **98**:147–153.
9. Arvidsson-Lenner R, Asp NG, Axelsen M, Bryngelsson S, Haapa E, Jarvi A, et al. Glycemic index. *Scand J Nutr* 2004; **48**: 84–89.
10. Henry CJK, Thondre PS. The glycaemic index: concept, recent developments and its impact on diabetes and obesity. in: Pasternak CA, ed. *Access not Excess*. St Ives, Cambridgeshire: Smith-Gordon, 2011: 154–175.
11. Brand JC, Nicholson PL, Thorburn AW, Truswell AS. Food processing and the glycemic index. *Am J Clin Nutr* 1985; **42**: 1192–1196.
12. Åkerberg A, Liljeberg H, Björck I. Effects of amylose/amylopectin ratio and baking conditions on resistant starch formation and glycaemic indices. *J Cereal Sci* 1998; **28**: 71–80.
13. Holt S, Heading RC, Cater DC, Prescott LF, Tothill P. Effect of gel-forming fibre on gastric emptying and absorption of glucose and paracetamol. *Lancet* 1979; **1**: 636–639.
14. Frost GS, Brynes AE, Dhillo WS, Bloom SR, McBurney MI. The effects of fiber enrichment of pasta and fat content on gastric emptying, GLP-1, glucose, and insulin responses to a meal. *Eur J Clin Nutr* 2003; **57**: 293–298.
15. Linn T, Santosa B, Gronemeyer D, Aygen S, Scholz N, Busch M, et al. Effect of long-term dietary protein intake on glucose metabolism in humans. *Diabetologia* 2000; **43**: 1257–1265.
16. Hanhineva K, Torronen R, Bondia-Pons I, Pekkinen J, Kolehmainen M, Mykkanen H, et al. Impact of dietary polyphenols on carbohydrate metabolism. *Int J Mol Sci* 2010; **11**: 1365–1402.
17. Barclay AW, Petocz P, Mc-Millan Price J, Flood VM, Prvan T, Mitchell P, et al. Glycemic index, glycemic load and chronic disease risk – a meta-analysis of observational studies. *Am J Clin Nutr* 2008; **87**: 627–637.
18. Wolever TMS, Barbeau MC, Charron S, Harrington K, Leung S, Madrick B, et al. Guidelines for the nutritional management of diabetes mellitus in the new millennium: a position by the Canadian Diabetes Association. *Can J Diabetes Care* 2000; **23**: 56–69.
19. Goff LM, Cowland DE, Hooper L, Frost GS. Low glycemic index diets and blood lipids: a systematic review and meta-analysis of randomized controlled trials. *Nutr Metab Cardiovasc Dis* 2013; **23**(1): 1–10.
20. Du H, van der ADL, van Bakel MME, van der Kallen CJH, Blaak EE, van Greevenbroek MMJ, et al. Glycemic index and glycemic load in relation to food and nutrient intake and metabolic risk factors in a Dutch population. *Am J Clin Nutr* 2008; **87**: 655–661.
21. Buyken AE, Toeller M, Heitkamp G, Karamanos B, Rottiers R, Muggeo M, et al. Glycemic index in the diet of European outpatients with type 1 diabetes: relations to glycated hemoglobin and serum lipids. *Am J Clin Nutr* 2001; **73**: 574–581.

22. Diabetes Australia. National Evidence based guidelines for the management of type 2 diabetes mellitus. Part 2: Evidence based guidelines for the primary prevention of type 2 diabetes. Dec 2001, http://www.diabetesaustralia.com.au/education_info/nebg.html.

23. Dyson PA, Kelly T, Deakin T, Duncan A, Frost G, Harrison Z, et al.; Diabetes UK Nutrition Working Group. Diabetes UK evidence-based nutrition guidelines for the prevention and management of diabetes. *Diabet Med* 2011; **28**: 1282–1288.

24. The Diabetes and Nutrition Study Group (DNSG) of the European Association for the Study of Diabetes (EASD). Recommendations for the nutritional management of patients with diabetes mellitus. *Eur J Clin Nutr* 2000; **54**: 353–355.

25. Brand-Miller J, Hayne S, Petocz P, Colagiuri S. Low glycemic diets in the management of diabetes: a meta-analysis of randomized controlled trials. *Diabetes Care* 2003; **26**(8): 2466–2468.

26. Thomas D., Elliott EJ. Low glycaemic index, or low glycaemic load, diets for diabetes mellitus. *Cochrane Database Syst Rev* 2009; **1**: CD006296.

27. Evert AB, Boucher JL, Cypress M, Dunbar SA, Franz MJ, Mayer-Davis EJ, et al. Nutrition therapy recommendations for the management of adults with diabetes. *Diabetes Care* 2014; **37**(Suppl. 1): S120–143.

28. Jenkins DJA, Kendall CWC, McKeown-Eyssen G, Josse RG, Silverberg J, Booth GL, et al. Effect of a low-glycemic index or a high-cereal fiber diet on type 2 diabetes A randomized trial. *J Am Med Assoc* 2008; **300**: 2742–2753.

29. Rizkalla SW, Boillot J, Taghrid L, Rigoir A, Laromiguiere M, Elgrably F, et al. Improved plasma glucose control whole-body glucose utilization, and lipid profile on a low glycemic index diet in type 2 diabetic men. *Diabetes Care* 2004; **27**: 1866–1872.

30. Jimenez-Cruz A, Rosales-Garay P, Bacardi-Gascon M, Severino-Lugo I, and Turnbull WH. A flexible, low glycemic index Mexican-style diet in overweight and obese subjects with type 2 diabetes improves metabolic parameters during a 6-week treatment period. *Diabetes Care* 2003; **26**: 1967–1970

31. Meyer KA, Kushi LH, Jacobs DR, Slavin J, Sellers TA, Folsom AR. Carbohydrates, dietary fibre and incident type 2 diabetes in older women. *Am J Clin Nutr* 2000; **71**: 921–930.

32. Westman EC, Yancy WS, Mavropoulos JC, Marquart M, McDuffle JR. The effect of a low-carbohydrate, ketogenic diet versus a low-glycemic index diet on glycemic control in type 2 diabetes mellitus. *Nutr Metab* 2008; **5**: 36.

33. Scholl TO, Chen X, Khoo CS, Lenders C. The dietary glycemic index during pregnancy: Influence on infant birth weight, fetal growth, and biomarkers of carbohydrate metabolism. *Am J Epidemiol* 2004; **159**: 467–474.

34. Moses RG, Luebcke M, Davis WS, Coleman KJ, Tapsell LC, Petocz P, et al. Effect of a low glycemic index diet during pregnancy on obstetric outcomes. *Am J Clin Nutr* 2006; **84**: 807–812.

35. Zhang C, Liu S, Solomon CG, Hu FB. Dietary fiber intake, dietary glycemic load and the risk of gestational diabetes mellitus. *Diabetes Care* 2006; **29**: 2223–2230.

36. Moses RG, Barker M, Winter M, Petocz P, Brand-Miller JC. Can a low glycemic index diet reduce the need for insulin in gestational diabetes mellitus? A randomized trial. *Diabetes Care* 2009; **32**: 996–1000.

37. Giacco R, Parillo M, Rivellese AA, Lasorella G, Giacco A, D'Episcopo L, et al. Long-term dietary treatment with increased amounts of fiber-rich low-glycemic index natural foods improves blood glucose control and reduces the number of hypoglycemic events in type 1 diabetic patients. *Diabetes Care* 2000; **23**: 1461–1466.

38. Parillo M, Annuzzi G, Rivellese AA, Bozzetto L, Alessandrini R, Riccardi G, et al. Effects of meals with different glycaemic index on postprandial blood glucose response in patients with type 1 diabetes treated with continuous subcutaneous insulin infusion. *Diabetic Med* 2011; **28**: 227–229.

39. O'Connell MA, Gilbertson HR, Donath SM, Cameron FJ. Optimizing postprandial glycemia in pediatric patients with type 1 diabetes using insulin pump therapy. impact of glycemic index and prandial bolus type. *Diabetes Care* 2008; **31**: 1491–1495.

40. Gilbertson HR, Brand-Miller JC, Thorburn AW, Evens S, Chondros P, Werther G. The effect of flexible low glycemic index dietary advice versus measured carbohydrate exchange diets on glycemic control in children with type 1 diabetes. *Diabetes Care* 2001; **24**: 1137–1143.

41. Queiroz KC, Novato Silva I, Goncalves Alfenas RD. Influence of the glycemic index and glycemic load of the diet in the glycemic control of diabetic children and teenagers. *Nutr Hosp* 2012; **27**:510–515

42. Aston LM. Glycemic index and metabolic disease risk. *Proc Nutr Soc* 2006; **65**: 125–134.

43. Gaesser GA. Carbohydrate quantity and quality in relation to body mass index. *J Am Diet Assoc* 2007; **107**: 1768–1780.

44. Brand-Miller JC, Holt SH, Pawlak DB, MacMillan J. Glycemic index and obesity. *Am J Clin Nutr* 2002; **76**: 281S–285S.

45. McMillan-Price J, Brand-Miller J. Low-glycaemic index diets and body weight regulation. *Int J Obes* 2006; **30**: S40–46.

46. Bornet FRJ, Jardy-Gennetier A, Jacquet N, Stowell J. Glycaemic response to foods: impact on satiety and long-term weight regulation. *Appetite* 2007; **49**: 535–553.

47. Barba G, Sieri S, Dello Russo M, Donatiello E, Formisano A, Lauria F, et al. Glycaemic index and body fat distribution in children: The results of the ARCA project, *Nutr Metab Cardiovasc Dis* 2012; **22**: 28–34.

48. Warren JM, Henry CJK, Simonite V. Low glycemic index breakfasts and reduced food intake in preadolescent children. *Paediatrics* 2003; **112**: e414–419.

49. Ajala O, English P, Pinkney J. Systematic review and meta-analysis of different dietary approaches to the management of type 2 diabetes. *Am J Clin Nutr* 2013; **97**: 505–516.

50. Marsh K, Barclay A, Colagiuri S, Brand-Miller J. Glycemic index and glycemic load of carbohydrates in the diabetes diet. *Curr Diab Rep* 2011; **11**(2): 120–127.

51. Whelan WJ, Hollar D, Agatston A, Dodson HJ, Tahal DS. The glycmeic response is a personal attribute. *IUBMB Life* 2010; **62**: 637–641.

52. Brand-Miller JC, Stockmann K, Atkinson F, Petocz P, Denyer G. Glycemic index, postprandial glycemia, and the shape of the curve in healthy subjects: analysis of a database of more than 1000 foods. *Am J Clin Nutr* 2009; **89**: 97–105.

53. Kalergis M, De Grandpre E, Andersons C. The role of glycemic index in the prevention and management of diabetes: A review and discussion. *Can J Diabetes* 2005; **29**: 27–38.

54. Wolever TMS, Yang M, Zeng XY, Atkinson F, Brand-Miller JC. Food glycemic index, as given in glycemic index tables, is a significant determinant of glycemic responses elicited by composite breakfast meals. *Am J Clin Nutr* 2006; **83**: 1306–1312.

55. The University of Sydney, 2011, updated 8 August, 2014, http://www.glycemicindex.com/.

56. Dodd H, Williams S, Brown R, Venn B. Calculating meal glycemic index by using measured and published food values compared with directly measured meal glycemic index. *Am J Clin Nutr* 2011; **94**: 992–996.

SECTION 3

Type 1 diabetes

Chapter 3.1

Epidemiology and pathogenesis of type 1 diabetes

Sathish Parthasarathy[1] and Pratik Choudhary[1,2]
[1]King's College Hospital NHS Foundation Trust, London, UK
[2]King's College London, London, UK

3.1.1 Epidemiology

Type 1 diabetes is caused by autoimmune destruction of islet β-cells leading to a complete deficiency of insulin. This affects about 0.3% of the worldwide population, making up about 10% of those with diabetes [1].

Incidence of type 1 diabetes

Approximately 479 600 children aged 0–14 years have type 1 diabetes amongst 1.7 billion children worldwide with annual incidence of 3% [2]. The incidence of type 1 diabetes increases with age, the highest incidence being observed in 10–14 year olds (Figure 3.1.1). Indeed, diagnosis is made in 50–60% of cases before the age of 15 years [2]. Type 1 diabetes affects male and females roughly equally [2].

Geographical variation in incidence

There is marked geographical variation in the incidence of type 1 diabetes (Figure 3.1.2). China and South America have a low incidence (<1/100 000) with the highest incidence (>20/100 000) in Western European nations, such as Finland, Sweden, Norway, Portugal, United Kingdom (UK) and Canada and New Zealand [3]. The sentinel data comes from a World Health Organisation (WHO) project, DiaMond, which evaluated the worldwide patterns of incidence of type 1 diabetes in children (aged <15 years) from 1990 for a period of 5 years with a sample population of 75.1 million. The incidence varies from <1/100 000 (China, Venezuela) to 36/100 000 (Sardinia, Finland) with European countries having higher incidence in general [3] (Figure 3.1.3). Although essential, neither the presence of an insulin autoantibody nor the presentation and phenotype alone confers the diagnosis of type 1 diabetes in an adult population, given the presence of other forms of diabetes such as latent autoimmune diabetes of adults (LADA) [4], ketosis prone diabetes [5] and monogenic diabetes [6], respectively, making true incidence difficult to predict.

The incidence of type 1 diabetes in the adult population aged between 20 and 100 is noted to be around 25.1/100 000 with 83% of cases diagnosed above the age of 40 years [7].

Incidence rates in South Asia and Africa are much lower, with estimates of just 18 000 new cases/year in South East Asia, and incidence rates of 3.5–12/100–000 population in sub-Saharan Africa. This may reflect true differences in incidence in different populations, but may also be due to high mortality of young children with type 1 diabetes in countries with poor health facilities as well as diagnostic discrepancies, as there is a higher proportion of patients with ketosis prone type 2 diabetes and young onset type 2 diabetes in these regions [5].

Advanced Nutrition and Dietetics in Diabetes, First Edition. Edited by Louise Goff and Pamela Dyson.
© 2016 John Wiley & Sons, Ltd. Published 2016 by John Wiley & Sons, Ltd.

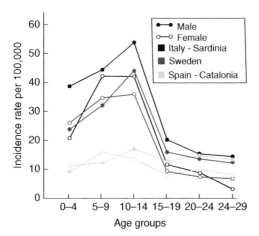

Figure 3.1.1　Incidence rates of type 1 diabetes with onset in the age range 0–29 years in 1996–1997 for three European countries. Source: Diabetes Atlas 3rd edn, © International Diabetes Federation, 2006.

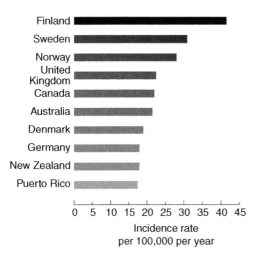

Figure 3.1.2　Top 10 countries incidence rate for type 1 diabetes in children (0–14 years). Only countries where studies have been carried out in that country are included. Source: Diabetes Atlas 3rd edn, © International Diabetes Federation, 2006.

The rising tide of type 1 diabetes

Just as there has been an exponential increase in the incidence of type 2 diabetes, there has been a marked increase in the incidence of type 1 diabetes across the world. In most populations the incidence increases with age and is highest in the 10–14 years age group [3]. However, given the magnitude of increase in type 2 diabetes, the overall proportion of those with type 1 is likely to fall.

Between 1991 and 2008, data collected from a UK primary care database suggested that incidence of type 1 diabetes in the UK increased from 11 to 24/100 000 person years in boys and from 15 to 20/100 000 person years in girls. In adults aged 15–34, the incidence increased from 13 to 20/100 000 person years in men and from 7 to 10/100000 person years in women. The prevalence of type 1 diabetes in the UK is estimated at 1 per 700–1000 with 25 000 people under the age of 25 years living with the disease [8].

The rise in rate was greatest in those with the lowest incidence and also in younger patients. Trends for increased incidence of type 1 diabetes have been seen across the world in the populations studied (4.0% in Asia, 3.2% in Europe and 5.3% in North America) with the exception of Central America and the West Indies, where type 1 is less prevalent, and where the trend was a decrease of 3.6% [9]. Projections from these data suggest an increase in new cases across Europe from 15 000 in 2005 to 24 000 in 2020. The prevalence of type 1 diabetes in those <15 years is predicted to rise from 94 000 in 2005 to 160 000 in 2020. Based on the SEARCH study from North America, a 23% rise in incidence over the next 40 years is projected, mainly related to an increase in incidence in Hispanic people that will grow to make up 50% of those with type 1 diabetes by 2050 [10].

Reports from China project a potential doubling in incidence over the next 10 years [11]. The exact projections of incidence of type 1 diabetes in adults are not clear but a peak has been demonstrated at ages between 50 and 80 years with no difference between the three decades in the Swedish population [7].

Although some studies have identified a slight male preponderance, which is more marked after puberty, the reasons for this are unclear [12], other studies have found an equal male: female split [13].

3.1.2 Pathogenesis of type 1 diabetes

Type 1 diabetes is an autoimmune condition, characterised by immune-mediated destruction of β-cells in pancreatic islets (Figure 3.1.4). Most of the pancreas is made of exocrine tissue, which secretes various digestive enzymes, but

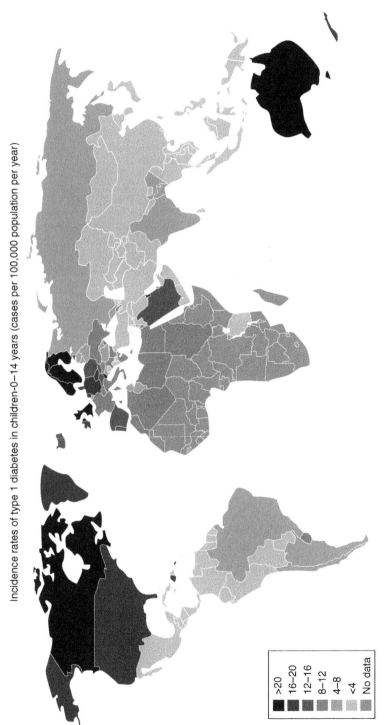

Incidence rates of type 1 diabetes in children-0–14 years (cases per 100,000 population per year)

■	>20
■	16–20
■	12–16
■	8–12
■	4–8
■	<4
■	No data

Figure 3.1.3 Incidence of type 1 diabetes in children 0–14 years worldwide (cases per 100 000 population per year. Source: Diabetes Atlas 3rd edn. © International Diabetes Federation, 2006.

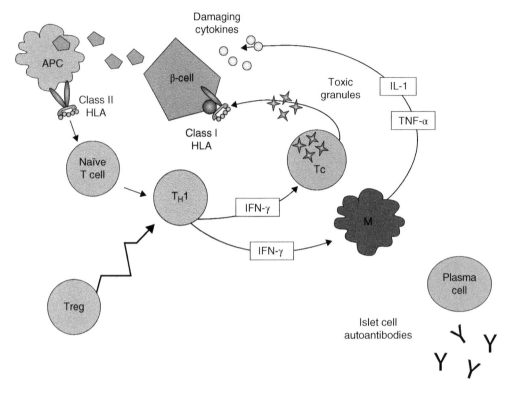

Figure 3.1.4 Immunological basis for type 1 diabetes. Source: Ref. [18].

2% of the cells are arranged in small islands called Islets of Langerhans. Each islet has a combination of insulin-producing β-cells, glucagon-producing alpha cells and somatostatin-producing delta cells [14]. The islets are richly vascularised and innervated with sympathetic and parasympathetic neurons [15]. Pathological evaluation of specimens from patients who died soon after developing type 1 diabetes reveal a characteristic picture of infiltration of the islets with macrophages and CD4 and CD8+ve T cells [16], that show auto-reactivity against islet antigens such as glutamic acid decarboxylase (GAD), islet antigen-2, insulin and Zn Transporter 8 [17].

Immunological basis for type 1 diabetes

The trigger for the inflammatory reaction against the β-cells, leading to their destruction, is unknown. One hypothesis is that antigen presenting cells such as macrophages present specific islet autoantigens to T cells in the pancreatic lymph nodes and activate them. These activated T cells then invade the islets and secrete cytokines that may play a role in destroying the β-cells directly, but also serve to attract cytotoxic T cells that can destroy β-cells as well. Interestingly, other cells within the islets are not affected [18].

The four main auto-antibodies namely insulin antibody (IAA), glutamic acid decarboxylase 65 (GAD), a tyrosine phosphatase-like molecule called IA-2 (IA-2A) and Zn transporter 8 are not pathogenic, and indeed are not all present in every patient. Most patients (>70%) are GAD +ve, but there are subgroups of patients who only have antibodies against one of the other antigens. Greater titres and number of antibodies are associated with earlier onset of disease. The insidious type 1 diabetes process usually starts a number of years before clinical presentation, with studies showing most patients have evidence of abnormal glucose tolerance a few years before [19].

This autoimmune process usually happens in the setting of a predisposing HLA (human leucocyte antigen) type, and more than 60 genes have been identified that affect the risk of developing type 1 diabetes, with HLA DR3 and DR4 having the greatest impact on susceptibility [20]. Twin studies suggest that about 80% of the susceptibility can be explained by these susceptibility genes [21]. However, fewer than 5% of those with HLA conferred genetic susceptibility actually develop clinical disease and the vast majority of patients with type 1 diabetes do not have a family history.

Individuals with a first degree relative with type 1 diabetes have a 1 in 20 lifetime risk compared to a 1 in 300 risk for the general population. Concordance between monozygotic twins is >60% if followed long enough, but <10% with dizygotic twins. Siblings of children with onset of type 1 diabetes before the age of 5 years have a three- to five-fold greater cumulative risk by age 20 compared to siblings of children diagnosed between 5 and 15 years of age. Diabetes with onset before age 5 years is a marker of high familial risk and suggests a major role for genetic factors. The offspring of affected mothers have a 2 to 3% risk, whereas offspring of affected fathers have a 7% risk [22].

An association between type 1 diabetes and other autoimmune diseases, such as autoimmune thyroid disease, Addison's disease, coeliac disease and autoimmune gastritis, is well established, as they share the same susceptibility genes within the HLA complex [23].

Antibodies against specific antigens are seen in over 95% of those with type 1 diabetes, with a greater number of antibodies generally conferring an earlier age of onset [24].

3.1.3 Environmental Triggers

A number of potential triggers have been suggested, that may induce the disease in genetically susceptible patients. Patterns in the seasonality of detection for type 1 diabetes, with increases particularly in April to July births are more clearly seen in northern latitudes, suggesting possible associations with maternal vitamin D levels [25], or with seasonal viral infections [26]. Increased maternal vitamin D intake has also been associated with decreased risk of type 1 diabetes [27].

Viral infections such as enteroviruses and cytomegalovirus (CMV) have long been proposed as potential triggers of the autoimmune process, with the body producing antibodies against the viruses that cross-react with proteins on β-cells and destroy them [28].

Insufficient exposure to early infections may increase the risk of type 1 diabetes by reducing maturation of immune regulation [29].

Cows milk is one of the mostly widely studied triggers and is implicated in the increasing incidence of type 1 diabetes. However, evidence that early introduction of cows milk may predispose to type 1 diabetes is equivocal [30]. Timing of introduction of gluten may also affect autoimmunity and there is a clear association with increased risk for coeliac disease and type 1 diabetes [31].

The accelerator hypothesis postulates insulin resistance as a trigger for β-cell loss in an individual already susceptible to autoimmune insult [32]. Obesity, which is commonly associated with insulin resistance, serves as a trigger in the genetically susceptible individuals (HLA DR3/DR4) and there is increasing evidence to suggest the causal association between the two [33].

3.1.4 Summary

Type 1 diabetes represents around 10% of all diabetes, but the incidence is increasing rapidly, especially in areas such as South East Asia and Africa. It is caused by autoimmune destruction of insulin-producing β-cells in a genetically susceptible individual. Making correct diagnoses becomes important, as classical differences of age, weight and ethnicity become less relevant, and auto-antibody tests can help clarify diagnosis. Similarly, the known auto-immune targets can offer potential therapeutic strategies, in identifying and possibly eventually treating those with type 1 diabetes.

Key points

- Type 1 diabetes is an autoimmune condition requiring insulin replacement.
- It is most commonly diagnosed in children and young people, but can occur at any age.
- Globally, the prevalence of type 1 diabetes differs between different ethnic groups and rates are increasing.
- The cause of type 1 diabetes is unknown, but genetic and environmental factors, including exposure to viral infections, may all play a part.

References

1. Diabetes UK. Diabetes in the UK 2012. Key statistics on diabetes. Diabetes UK 2012; London.
2. Gyula Soltesz CP, Dahlquist G. Diabetes in the Young: a Global Perspective. Global trends in childhood type 1 diabetes. *IDF Diabetes Atlas*, 4th edn. Brussels, Belgium: International Diabetic Federation, 2009.
3. Karvonen MM, Viik-Kajander, Moltchanova E, Libman I, LaPorte R, Tuomilehto J. Incidence of childhood type 1 diabetes worldwide. Diabetes Mondiale (DiaMond) Project Group. *Diabetes Care* 2000; **23**(10): 1516–1526.
4. Fourlanos S. A clinical screening tool identifies autoimmune diabetes in adults. *Diabetes Care* 2006; **29**(5): 970–975.
5. Mauvais-Jarvis F, Sobngwi E, Porcher R, Riveline JP, Kevorkian JP, Vaisse C, et al. Ketosis-prone type 2 diabetes in patients of Sub-Saharan African origin: Clinical pathophysiology and natural history of β-cell dysfunction and insulin resistance. *Diabetes* 2004; **53**(3): 645–653.
6. Murphy R, Ellard S, Hattersley AT. Clinical implications of a molecular genetic classification of monogenic beta-cell diabetes. *Nat Clin Pract Endocrinol Metab* 2008; **4**(4): 200–213.
7. Thunander M, Petersson C, Jonzon K, Fornander J, Ossiansson B, Torn C, et al. Incidence of type 1 and type 2 diabetes in adults and children in Kronoberg, Sweden. *Diabetes Res Clin Pract* 2008; **82**(2): 247–255.
8. Imkampe AK, Gulliford MC. Trends in Type 1 diabetes incidence in the UK in 0- to 14-year-olds and in 15- to 34-year-olds, 1991–2008. *Diabet Med* 2011; **28**(7): 811–814.
9. DIAMOND Project Group Incidence and trends of childhood Type 1 diabetes worldwide 1990–1999. *Diabet Med* 2006; **23**(8): 857–866.
10. Imperatore G, Boyle JP, Thompson TJ, Case D, Dabelea D, Hamman RF, et al. Projections of type 1 and type 2 diabetes burden in the U.S. population aged <20 years through 2050: dynamic modeling of incidence, mortality, and population growth. *Diabetes Care* 2012; **35**(12): 2515–2520.
11. Gong C, Meng X, Saenger P, Wu D, Cao B, Wu D, et al. Trends in the incidence of childhood type 1 diabetes mellitus in Beijing based on hospitalization data from 1995 to 2010. *Horm Res Paediatr* 2013; **80**(5): 328–334.
12. Kyvik KO, Nystrom L, Gorus F, Songini M, Oestman J, Castell C, et al. The epidemiology of Type 1 diabetes mellitus is not the same in young adults as in children. *Diabetologia* 2004; **47**(3): 377–384.
13. Rojnic Putarek N, Ille J, Spehar Uroic A, Skrabic V, Stipancic G, Krnic N, et al. Incidence of type 1 diabetes mellitus in 0 to 14-yr-old children in Croatia – 2004 to 2012 study. *Pediatr Diabetes* 2014, DOI: 10.1111/pedi.12197.
14. Atkinson MA, Maclaren NK. Islet cell autoantigens in insulin dependent diabetes. *J Clin Invest* 1993; **92**: 1608–1616.
15. Ahren B, Wierup N, Sundler F. Neuropeptides and the regulation of islet function *Diabetes* 2006; **55**(Supplement_2): S98-S107.
16. Willcox A, Richardson SJ, Bone AJ, Foulis AK, Morgan NG. Analysis of islet inflammation in human type 1 diabetes. *Clin Exp Immunol* (2009); **155**(2): 173–181.
17. Roep BO, Peakman M. Antigen targets of type 1 diabetes autoimmunity. (2012) *Cold Spring Harb Perspect Med* **2**(4): a007781.
18. Marcovecchio L, Dunger DB, Peakman M, Taylor KW. Aetiology of type 1 diabetes mellitus – genetics, autoimmunity and trigger factors. In Allgrove J, Swift PGF, Greene S (eds). Evidence-based Paediatric and Adolescent Diabetes, Blackwell Publishing Ltd, 2007, pp. 26–41.
19. Colman PG, McNair P, Margetts H, Schmidli RS, Werther GA, Alford FP, et al. The Melbourne Pre-Diabetes Study: prediction of type 1 diabetes mellitus using antibody and metabolic testing. *Med J Aust* 1998; **169**(2): 81–84.
20. Bradfield JP, Qu HQ, Wang K, Zhang H, Sleiman PM, Kim CE, et al. A genome-wide meta-analysis of six type 1 diabetes cohorts identifies multiple associated loci. *PLoS Genet* 2011; **7**(9): e1002293.
21. Morahan, G, Mehta M, James I, Chen WM, Akolkar B, Erlich HA, et al. Tests for genetic interactions in type 1 diabetes: Linkage and stratification analyses of 4,422 affected sib-pairs. *Diabetes* 2011; **60**(3): 1030–1040.
22. Hamalainen AM, Knip M. Autoimmunity and familial risk of type 1 diabetes. *Curr Diab Rep* 2002; **2**(4): 347–353.

23. Gough SCLS, Simmonds MJ. The HLA region and autoimmune disease: Associations andmechanisms of action. *Curr Genomics* 2007; **8**(7): 453–465.

24. Siljander H T, Simell S, Hekkala A, Lähde J, Simell T, Vähäsalo P, et al. Predictive characteristics of diabetes-associated autoantibodies among children with HLA-conferred disease susceptibility in the general population. *Diabetes* 2009; **58**(12): 2835–2842.

25. The EURODIAB Substudy 2 Study Group EURODIAB Substudy2. Vitamin D supplement in early childhood and risk for Type I (insulin-dependent) diabetes mellitus. *Diabetologia* 1999; **42**(1): 51–54.

26. van der Werf N, Kroese FGM, Rozing J, Hillebrands JL. Viral infections as potential triggers of type 1 diabetes. *Diabetes Metab Res Rev* 2007; **23**(3): 169–183.

27. Hypponen E, Laara E, Reunanen A, Järvelin MR, Virtanen SM. Intake of vitamin D and risk of type 1 diabetes: a birth-cohort study. *Lancet* 2001; **358**(9292): 1500–1503.

28. van der Werf N, Kroese FGM, Rozing J, Hillebrands JL. Viral infections as potential triggers of type 1 diabetes. *Diabetes Metab Res Rev* 2007;23(3): 169–183.

29. Egro FM. Why is type 1 diabetes increasing? *J Mol Endocrinol* 2013; **51**(1): R1–R13.

30. Harrison LC, Honeyman MC. Cow's milk and type 1 diabetes: the real debate is about mucosal immune function. *Diabetes* 1999; **48**(8): 1501–1507.

31. Levy-Shraga Y, Lerner-Geva L, Boyko V, Graph-Barel C, Mazor-Aronovitch K, Modan-Moses D, et al. Type 1 diabetes in pre-school children—long-term metabolic control, associated autoimmunity and complications. *Diabet Med* 2012; **29**(10): 1291–1296.

32. Wilkin TJ. The convergence of type 1 and type 2 diabetes in childhood. *Pediatr Diabetes* 2012; **13**(4): 334–339.

33. Verbeeten KC, Elks CE, Daneman D, Ong KK. Association between childhood obesity and subsequent Type 1 diabetes: a systematic review and meta-analysis. *Diabet Med* 2011; **28**(1): 10–18.

Chapter 3.2

Clinical management of type 1 diabetes

Ahmed Iqbal and Simon Heller
University of Sheffield, Sheffield, UK

3.2.1 Introduction

Type 1 diabetes is a multi-system disorder with immune-mediated destruction of beta cells in the pancreatic islets [1]. The resultant hyperglycaemia is responsible for clinical symptoms of the disease and causes a plethora of complications affecting both large and small blood vessels, known as macro and microvascular complications, respectively [2].

3.2.2 Clinical presentation

The peak age of onset for type 1 diabetes in children is puberty [3] and presentation often follows a fulminant course presenting with weight loss, marked polyuria and thirst. Presentation in adults can also be acute, but is often more insidious with weight loss and lethargy the key initial indicators of the underlying metabolic imbalance.

Type 1 diabetes may also present as an acute medical emergency, diabetic ketoacidosis (DKA), although the incidence of this is unknown [4]. DKA can be precipitated by an intercurrent infection. Patients typically present with anorexia, nausea, vomiting and abdominal pain with the clinical features of the underlying infection often masked. In severe cases, the fluid and electrolyte imbalances resulting from DKA can result in coma and death.

3.2.3 Medical management of hyperglycaemia

The immediate aim of medical management in the short term is to prevent DKA, and the long-term aim is to maintain near normal glucose values to prevent tissue complications. The key to successful treatment is to engage the person themselves in the management of their condition, as it is they who have to apply treatment 24 hours a day for the rest of their lives. The responsibility of the professional is first to equip the patient with the skills to achieve this, and second to provide on-going support and encouragement.

Diabetic ketoacidosis, whether occurring at diagnosis or as a result of illness or lack of insulin, is a life-threatening condition. Treatment is focused on addressing the three main biochemical disorders of hyperglycaemia, acidaemia and ketonaemia by administering fluids and insulin to correct these abnormalities. A number of national and international guidelines have been published for the intensive management of DKA [4–7].

As the key metabolic derangement in type 1 diabetes is hyperglycaemia, the core aim of medical management is to maintain glucose concentrations as near to the normal range as possible [8–10]. In order to achieve this, a multidisciplinary team (MDT) approach is needed, with key roles played by dietitians, diabetes nurses and physicians, with patient education and empowerment as a cornerstone of disease

Advanced Nutrition and Dietetics in Diabetes, First Edition. Edited by Louise Goff and Pamela Dyson.
© 2016 John Wiley & Sons, Ltd. Published 2016 by John Wiley & Sons, Ltd.

management. There is now strong evidence emphasising the importance of structured training courses to support effective self-management (see Chapter 3.3).

Historically, animal data [11,12] have suggested that tight control of glucose concentrations may be mechanistically associated with reduced long-term complications and better outcomes for those with type 1 diabetes. Further evidence from epidemiological studies [13,14] supported the role of tight glycaemic control in reducing long term complications. The Diabetes Control and Complications Trial (DCCT) [15] was a landmark study completed in 1993 that studied 1441 patients with type 1 diabetes and randomly assigned subjects to intensive glucose control or conventional therapy. Over a mean follow up of six and a half years, with 99% subjects completing the study, the trial group was able to demonstrate a statistically significant reduction in retinopathy, neuropathy and nephropathy in those subjects randomised to intensive control. There was also a reported 41% reduction in macrovascular events in the DCCT cohort randomised to intensive control [16], however, this was not statistically significant. Longer-term follow-up of the subjects taking part in DCCT has shown that the benefit of intensive control remained after 18 years, despite convergence in glycosylated haemoglobin (HbA1c) following the end of the study [17]. A recent Cochrane review has confirmed the role of intensive glycaemic control in risk reduction for microvascular disease in those with type 1 diabetes [18].

Treatment targets

The key recommendation for individuals with type 1 diabetes is to treat blood glucose concentrations intensively, aiming for the normal (non-diabetic) range, in order to reduce the risk of microvascular complications.

Guidelines from the American Diabetes Association (ADA) [8] and the American Association of Clinical Endocrinologists (AACE) [19], which are widely acknowledged internationally with respect to HbA1c targets, are summarised in Table 3.2.1.

The ADA guidelines are clear in recommending less stringent glycaemic targets in those that

Table 3.2.1 ADA and AACE guidelines for target HbA1c.

Parameter	ADA	ACE
HbA1c mmol/l (%)	53 (<7)	48 (≤6.5)

have a propensity to severe hypoglycaemia, limited life expectancy, advanced microvascular and macrovascular complications and difficulty in close monitoring of blood glucose. Conversely, targets <53mmol/mol (7%) are recommended for those that are recently diagnosed with diabetes, have a long life expectancy and no previous history of hypoglycaemia and cardiovascular events.

Insulin treatment

Exogenous insulin replacement to substitute loss of endogenous insulin production from pancreatic islets is the mainstay of the treatment of type 1 diabetes. Recent advances in biotechnology have meant a complete transition from animal (bovine or porcine) insulin treatment to insulin derived from recombinant DNA technology that closely mimics human insulin in its chemical structure [20].

Insulin treatments are broadly divided into: rapid-acting, short-acting, intermediate-acting and long-acting depending on their pharmacokinetic properties. In addition, mixed insulin is available, but this is now rarely prescribed for those with type 1 diabetes. Table 3.2.2 summarises the key characteristics of available insulin for the treatment of type 1 diabetes.

Rapid- and short-acting insulin

Rapid-acting insulin can be further divided into regular insulin (short-acting) and insulin analogues (rapid-acting). Regular insulin is characterised by zinc-insulin crystals [21] that result in delayed absorption and hence a delayed onset of action. This renders regular insulin somewhat limited in its ability to counteract postprandial hyperglycaemia and the prolonged duration of action (up to eight hours) can result in an increased risk of hypoglycaemia.

Table 3.2.2   Characteristics of insulin for treating type 1 diabetes.

Insulin Type	Administration	Onset (h)	Peak (h)	Duration (h)
Rapid acting analogues	Before, with or after food	0.25–0.5	1–1.5	4
Short acting	30 minutes before food	0.5–1	2–4	6 - 8
Intermediate acting	Various – either before food or before bed	1–4	6–8	8–12
Long acting	Once or twice daily	Varies	Analogues have no peak	20–24

Insulin analogues differ from regular insulin in that their relatively less complex chemical structure allows rapid absorption (within 15 minutes compared to 30–60 minutes with regular insulin) and a peak of action at 1 hour compared to 2–4 hours with regular insulin. This rapidity of onset, coupled with a quick peak and shorter overall duration of action, renders insulin analogues less likely to cause hypoglycaemia and more efficacious in controlling postprandial hyperglycaemia. Insulin analogues have thus been shown to reduce hypoglycaemia and result in significant reductions in HbA1c in comparison to regular insulin [22].

Intermediate-acting and long-acting insulins

Intermediate- and long-acting insulin have a significantly longer duration of action, typically 8–12 hours, when compared to rapid-acting insulin.

NPH insulin

Neutral Protamine Hagedorn (NPH) insulin is an intermediate-acting insulin which contains insulin in a crystalline association with zinc and protamine. Owing to its chemical structure, NPH insulin has an onset of peak at 1–3 hours, peak at 6–8 hours and duration of effect lasting 24 hours.

Long-acting analogue insulin

Long-acting analogue insulin is recombinant insulin that provides up to 24 hour cover, mimicking the basal insulin produced by the healthy pancreas in between meals or during periods of fasting, such as overnight. It has been suggested

that insulin detemir has a more predictable glucose lowering effect in patients with type 1 diabetes compared to NPH insulin and insulin glargine[23], and that there is reduction in weight gain and fewer episodes of hypoglycaemia when comparing insulin determir to NPH insulin.

Clinical approaches to insulin dosing

Basal/prandial-bolus treatment

A combination of rapid-acting insulin with meals (breakfast, lunch and dinner) and long-acting insulin once daily (in total four injections daily), the so-called 'basal/prandial-bolus' regimen aims to emulate the naturally occurring peaks and troughs of endogenous insulin production in response to feeding and fasting. In clinical practice, the basal/prandial-bolus regimen has largely superseded the previously used combination of mixed rapid and intermediate-acting insulin taken twice daily before breakfast and the evening meal.

Insulin dosing

The majority of people with type 1 diabetes require 0.5–1 unit insulin per kilogramme of body weight, but insulin sensitivity can differ significantly both between and within individuals [24]. Most people with type 1 diabetes begin with small doses of insulin and titrate up until target blood glucose levels are achieved. Recently, it was suggested that the balance between the amount of basal or background (long-acting) insulin and the amount of rapid-acting insulin taken with meals is predictive of glycaemic control, and that the ideal balance is 47% of total insulin dose as background or basal [25]. Once individuals are familiar with diabetes management, carbohydrate counting and insulin adjustment are the preferred option for increasing flexibility and quality of life and for improving glycaemic control [26].

Insulin Pumps

An alternative to basal-bolus treatment is the use of rapid-acting insulin analogues that are administered by means of a continuous subcutaneous infusion of insulin (CSII) using an insulin pump. Figure 3.2.1 illustrates an insulin pump device.

The pump can be pre-programmed to deliver insulin at a fixed basal rate or to vary with levels of activity and energy intake and thus anticipate glycaemic excursion. New generation insulin pump devices allow multiple pre-determined profiles of basal insulin infusion to anticipate known trends in glucose variation from past experience, for example for intense sporting or social activity.

Key advantages of an insulin pump in comparison to multiple daily injections (MDI) of insulin are improvement in glycaemic control, reductions in hypoglycaemia and, arguably, increased patient flexibility [27]. As only rapid-acting insulin analogues are used in insulin pumps, changes to basal rates of insulin are more readily and dynamically reflected with changes in blood glucose levels whilst, in comparison, changes to long-acting preparations of insulin are reflected many hours later in blood glucose levels. Individuals with type 1 diabetes who have a propensity to hypoglycaemia and have developed unawareness of the symptoms of hypoglycaemia due to recurrent severe episodes may derive significant benefit from CSII. Moreover, there is a suggestion that long term CSII may be superior to MDI in reducing the risk of severe hypoglycaemia without compromising glycaemic control [28]. There are, nevertheless, disadvantages to CSII including: risk of infection at the catheter site, the need to re-prime the pump every 24–48 hours and significant costs to less developed health care systems. In addition, because only rapid-acting insulin is used as part of CSII in pump devices, an inadvertent failure of the device or dislodged tubing can quickly result in hyperglycaemia and potentially DKA in the absence of intermediate or long-acting insulin cover. It is, therefore, important that patients receiving CSII are also proficient in self-monitoring of blood glucose to detect and act on glycaemic variations.

Other treatment modalities

Closed-loop systems

Closed-loop insulin delivery, that is 'the artificial pancreas', is a unique way of approaching the management of glycaemic control in type 1 diabetes. In a closed-loop system, a continuous glucose monitor measures interstitial glucose readings every one to five minutes whilst a portable computer controlled algorithm increases or decreases the rate of subcutaneous insulin delivery from a pump device depending on real-time glucose values [29]. It has been demonstrated that unsupervised closed-loop insulin delivery is feasible at home and may improve glycaemic targets in adult patients with type 1 diabetes [30]. However, data from additional studies are needed to replicate these results and demonstrate the efficacy and reliability of this emerging technology-based treatment modality for type 1 diabetes.

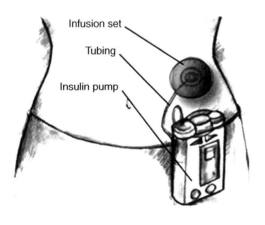

Figure 3.2.1 This cartoon illustrates the key components of an insulin pump device as would be worn by a patient. A reservoir pumps insulin through tubing into a subcutaneous catheter at a predetermined rate.

Immunotherapy and vaccine

Given the auto-immune basis for the pathogenesis of type 1 diabetes, much work has focussed on immunomodulatory therapies to halt the progressive destruction of beta cells and to potentially prevent the disease altogether by means of a vaccination [31]. A number of trials are underway examining the role of immunosuppression and of a potential vaccine, the results of which are eagerly awaited.

Islet cell and pancreatic transplantation

Transplantation of the whole pancreas or islet cells in isolation has generated interest in the treatment of type 1 diabetes as a means of curative treatment. However, the auto-immune nature of the disease and graft rejection means that diabetes can recur even after successful transplantation [32]. There is, however, at least one report of insulin independence at one year post-operatively with surgery done in expert hands, utilising a modified immunosuppressive regimen [33].

3.2.4 Cardiovascular risk and type 1 diabetes

The Joint British Societies' guidelines recognise that type 1 diabetes confers significant cardiovascular risk [34]. Consequently, specific measures are advised to address the risk, including lifestyle modifications and pharmacological therapy.

Lifestyle modifications

All patients with type 1 diabetes are encouraged to give up smoking, engage in regular aerobic exercise and adopt a healthy diet. In addition, optimal weight targets are recommended for all patients.

Pharmacological therapy

Blood pressure

The optimal blood pressure targets for those with diabetes, including type 1 diabetes, are ≤130 mmHg systolic, 80 mmHg diastolic, which are lower than for the general population

[34]. If lifestyle measures fail then treatment with appropriate antihypertensive medications, including beta-blockers, calcium channel blockers and angiotensin converting enzyme inhibitors (ACE-I) or angiotensin receptor blockers is recommended. Blockade of the renin–angiotensin–aldosterone axis by the latter two classes of drugs in particular appears to confer additional renal protective benefits to patients with type 1 diabetes [35]. For this reason, ACE-I are designated first choice agents.

Lipid-lowering therapy

The optimal cholesterol targets for those with diabetes are:

- Total cholesterol < 4.0 mmol/l
- Low density lipoprotein (LDL) cholesterol < 2.0 mmol/l

Statin therapy is recommended for all patients with T1DM aged ≥50 years. In addition, treatment is recommended for most of those aged 40–50 years. Those aged 30–40 years are recommended statin treatment in the presence of a long duration of diabetes in addition to poor glycaemic control and established microvascular complications, with risk factors for macrovascular disease, including a family history. Lastly, treatment is recommended for those aged 18–30 years of age in the presence of significant microalbuminuria [34].

3.2.5 Hypoglycaemia

Hypoglycaemia is a common side-effect of intensive glycaemic control in the context of type 1 diabetes. In the DCCT [15] cohort, patients in the intensive treatment group had a three-fold higher incidence of hypoglycaemia compared to conventional treatment, with certain severe episodes of hypoglycaemia requiring hospitalisation.

In addition, hypoglycaemia has been associated with increased mortality in those with type 1 diabetes and is thought to cause abnormal cardiac electrophysiology [36] with resultant sudden cardiac death, often described as the 'dead in bed' syndrome [37–39].

All people with type 1 diabetes, and their carers, require education about the symptoms and treatment of hypoglycaemia. Fast-acting carbohydrate (preferably glucose) should be kept readily available to reverse the effects of hypoglycaemia as needed. Home glucagon emergency kits also provide effective treatment of hypoglycaemia for those unable to take oral treatment.

3.2.6 Conclusion

Type 1 diabetes is a multifaceted disease that requires a holistic approach to management, addressing both the biology and the associated psychosocial morbidity. An MDT approach to the care of the patient is needed to ensure good glycaemic control and appropriate management of cardiovascular risk factors and to prevent and retard the development of both micro- and macrovascular complications.

Key points

- Clinical management of type 1 diabetes should address glycaemic control and cardiovascular risk using a patient-centred approach.
- The aim of glycaemic control is to lower HbA1c levels in order to reduce the risk of long-term complications.
- Insulin replacement is necessary and can be administered by injection or pump therapy.
- Hypoglycaemia is a common side-effect of insulin therapy requiring management and education.

References

1. Todd JA. Etiology of type 1 diabetes. *Immunity* 2010; **32**: 457–467.
2. Bluestone JA, Herold K, Eisenbarth G. Genetics, pathogenesis and clinical interventions in type 1 diabetes. *Nature* 2010; **464**: 1293–1300.
3. Tuomilehto J. The emerging global epidemic of type 1 diabetes. *Curr Diab Rep* 2013; **13**(6): 795–804.

4. Savage MW, Dhatariya KK, Kilvert A, Rayman G, Rees JA, Courtney CH, et al.; Joint British Diabetes Societies. Joint British Diabetes Societies guideline for the management of diabetic ketoacidosis. *Diabet Med* 2011; **28**(5): 508–515.
5. McGeoch SC, Hutcheon SD, Vaughan SM, John K, O'Neill NP, Pearson DWM. Development of a national Scottish diabetic ketoacidosis protocol. *Pract Diabetes Int* 2007; **24**: 257–261.
6. Savage M, Kilvert A; ABCD. ABCD guidelines for the management of hyperglycaemic emergencies in adults. *Pract Diabetes Int* 2006; **23**: 227–231.
7. Kitabchi AE, Umpierrez GE, Miles JM, Fisher JN. Hyperglycemic crises in adult patients with diabetes: a consensus statement from the American Diabetes Association. *Diabetes Care* 2009; **32**: 1335–1343.
8. American Diabetes Association. Standards of medical care in diabetes – 2014. *Diabetes Care* 2014; **37**(Suppl. 1): S14–S80.
9. European Society of Cardiology/European Association for the Study of Diabetes. ESC guidelines on diabetes, pre-diabetes, and cardiovascular disease developed in conjunction with the EASD - summary. *Eur Heart J* 2013; **34**(39): 3035–3087.
10. National Institute for Health and Care Excellence. Type 1 diabetes (GC15). NICE 2004, London.
11. Engerman R, Bloodworth JM, Nelson S. Relationship of microvascular disease in diabetes to metabolic control. *Diabetes* 1977; **26**(8): 760–769.
12. Engerman RL, Kern TS. Progression of incipient diabetic retinopathy during good glycemic control. *Diabetes* 1987; **36**(7): 808–812.
13. Klein R, Klein BE, Moss SE, Davis MD, DeMets DL. Glycosylated hemoglobin predicts the incidence and progression of diabetic retinopathy. *JAMA* 1988; **260**(19): 2864–2871.
14. Chase HP, Jackson WE, Hoops SL, Cockerham RS, Archer PG, O'Brien D. Glucose control and the renal and retinal complications of insulin-dependent diabetes. *JAMA* 1989; **261**(8): 1155–1160.
15. The Diabetes Control and Complications Trial Research Group. The effect of intensive treatment of diabetes on the development and progression of long-term complications in insulin-dependent diabetes mellitus. *N Engl J Med* 1993; **329**(14): 977–986.
16. The Diabetes Control and Complications Trial Research Group. Effect of intensive diabetes management on macrovascular events and risk factors in the Diabetes Control and Complications Trial. *Am J Cardiol* 1995; **75**(14): 894–903.
17. Nathan DM; DCCT/EDIC Research Group. The diabetes control and complications trial/epidemiology of diabetes interventions and complications study at 30 years: overview. *Diabetes Care* 2014; **37**(1): 9–16.

18. Fullerton B, Jeitler K, Seitz M, Horvath K, Berghold A, Siebenhofer A. Intensive glucose control versus conventional glucose control for type 1 diabetes mellitus. *Cochrane Database Syst Rev* 2014 Feb 14; **2**: CD009122.

19. American Association of Clinical Endocrinologists. Medical guidelines for clinical practice for developing a diabetes mellitus comprehensive care plan. *Endocr Pract* 2011; **17**(Suppl. 2).

20. Owns DR. The quest for physiologic insulin replacement. *Postgrad Med* 2004; **116**(Suppl. 5): 4–12.

21. Hirsch IB. Intensive treatment of type 1 diabetes. *Med Clin North Am* 1998; **82**(4): 689–719.

22. Jacobsen IB, Henriksen JE, Hother-Nielsen O, Vach W, Beck-Nielsen H. Evidence-based insulin treatment in type 1 diabetes mellitus. *Diabetes Res Clin Pract* 2009; **86**(1): 1–10.

23. Heise T, Nosek L, Rønn BB, Endahl L, Heinemann L, Kapitza C, et al. Lower within-subject variability of insulin detemir in comparison to NPH insulin and insulin glargine in people with type 1 diabetes. *Diabetes* 2004; **53**(6): 1614–1620.

24. Hirsch I. Type 1 diabetes mellitus and the use of felxible insulin regimens. *Am Fam Physician* 1999; **60**(8): 2343–2352.

25. Davidson PC, Hebblewhite HR, Steed RD, Bode BW. Analysis of guidelines for basal-bolus insulin dosing: basal insulin, correction factor, and carbohydrate-to-insulin ratio. *Endocr Pract* 2008; **14**(9): 1095–1101.

26. Cooke D, Bond R, Lawton J, Rankin D, Heller S, Clark M, et al.; U.K. NIHR DAFNE Study Group. Structured type 1 diabetes education delivered within routine care: impact on glycemic control and diabetes-specific quality of life. *Diabetes Care* 2013; **36**(2): 270–272.

27. Pickup JC. Insulin-pump therapy for type 1 diabetes mellitus. *N Engl J Med* 2012; **366**: 1616–1624.

28. Yeh HC, Brown TT, Maruthur N, Ranasinghe P, Berger Z, Suh YD, et al. Comparative effectiveness and safety of methods of insulin delivery and glucose monitoring for diabetes mellitus: a systematic review and meta-analysis. *Ann Intern Med* 2012; **157**: 336–347.

29. Hovorka R. Closed-loop insulin delivery: from bench to clinical practice. *Nat Rev Endocrinol* 2011; **7**(7): 385–395.

30. Thabit H, Elleri D, Leelarathna L, Allen JM, Lubina-Solomon A, Stadler M, et al. Unsupervised home use of overnight closed-loop system over 3 to 4 weeks - Pooled analysis of randomized controlled studies in adults and adolescents with type 1 diabetes. *Diabetes Obes Metab* 2015; **17**(5): 452–458.

31. Bach JF, Chatenoud L. A historical view from thirty eventful years of immunotherapy in autoimmune diabetes. *Semin Immunol* 2011; **23**: 174–181.

32. Nakhleh RE, Gruessner RW, Swanson PE, Tzardis PJ, Brayman K, Dunn DL, et al. Pancreas transplant pathology. A morphologic, immunohistochemical, and electron microscopic comparison of allogeneic grafts with rejection, syngeneic grafts, and chronic pancreatitis. *Am J Surg Pathol* 1991; **15**(3): 246–256.

33. Shapiro AM, Lakey JR, Ryan EA, Korbutt GS, Toth E, Warnock GL, et al. Islet transplantation in seven patients with type 1 diabetes mellitus using a glucocorticoid-free immunosuppressive regimen. *N Engl J Med* 2000; **343**(4): 230–238.

34. JBS3 Board. Joint British Societies' consensus recommendations for the prevention of cardiovascular disease (JBS3). *Heart* 2014; **100**(Suppl. 2): ii1–ii67.

35. Cherney DZI, Zinman B, Kennedy CRJ, Moineddin R, Lai V, Yang S, et al. Long-term hemodynamic and molecular effects persist after discontinued renin-angiotensin system blockade in patients with type 1 diabetes mellitus. *Kidney Int* 2013; **84**(6): 1246–1253.

36. Marques JL, George E, Peacey SR, Harris ND, Macdonald IA, Cochrane T, et al. Altered ventricular repolarization during hypoglycaemia in patients with diabetes. *Diabet Med* 1997; **14**(8): 648–654.

37. Little SA, Leelarathna L, Barendse SM, Walkinshaw E, Tan HK, Lubina Solomon A, et al. Severe hypoglycaemia in type 1 diabetes mellitus: underlying drivers and potential strategies for successful prevention. *Diabetes Metab Res Rev* 2014; **30**(3): 175–190.

38. Heller SR. Abnormalities of the electrocardiogram during hypoglycaemia: the cause of the dead in bed syndrome? *Int J Clin Pract Suppl* 2002; **129**: 27–32.

39. Robinson RTCE, Harris ND, Ireland RH, Lee S, Newman C, Heller SR. Mechanisms of abnormal cardiac repolarization during insulin-induced hypoglycemia. *Diabetes* 2003; **52**(6): 1469–1474.

Chapter 3.3

Nutritional management of glycaemia in type 1 diabetes

Lindsay Oliver
North Tyneside General Hospital, North Shields, UK

3.3.1 Introduction

This chapter aims to explore the evidence and practical application of nutritional strategies employed in the management of glycaemia in type 1 diabetes. In the last decade, the clinical practice of dietitians working with people with type 1 diabetes has moved from a qualitative approach incorporating nutritional advice which focused on healthy eating and glycaemic index, to an approach which now almost exclusively focuses on quantitative practical methods of carbohydrate estimation.

There is good clinical evidence demonstrating both the value of implementing this approach and the benefit of dietetic interventions in type 1 diabetes management. Structured education programs, such as dose adjustment for normal eating (DAFNE), which focuses on the development of self-management skills [1], can improve intermediate risk factors and quality of life for people with type 1 diabetes, and has been shown to be cost-effective [2]. In one study comparing people with newly diagnosed type 1 diabetes who received nutritional advice with a control group, an additional 8 mmol/mol (0.7%) HbA1c improvement was gained in the intervention group [3].

3.3.2 Nutrition and glucose management – the evidence

Carbohydrate

Carbohydrate counting

Recently published guidelines and recommendations from the American Diabetes Association (ADA) and from Diabetes UK [4,5] focus on carbohydrate as the main determinant of postprandial glucose in people with diabetes. Most authorities now agree that monitoring and regulating carbohydrate intake is a key strategy for glycaemic control in people with type 1 diabetes. Table 3.3.1 summarises the main recommendations for carbohydrate management.

Carbohydrate counting has been shown to be an effective strategy in managing glucose control in type 1 diabetes, when combined with flexible insulin therapy. The Diabetes Control and Complication Trial (DCCT) demonstrated that carbohydrate counting was an effective approach in achieving glycaemic control [8]. HbA1c was reduced when carbohydrate counting was implemented with intensive insulin treatment and these benefits were maintained over the long term [9]. In addition, randomised controlled trials from Europe have shown that carbohydrate

Advanced Nutrition and Dietetics in Diabetes, First Edition. Edited by Louise Goff and Pamela Dyson.
© 2016 John Wiley & Sons, Ltd. Published 2016 by John Wiley & Sons, Ltd.

Table 3.3.1 Summary of key recommendations for carbohydrate management in type 1 diabetes

Recommendation	American Diabetes Association [4]	Diabetes UK [5]	Canadian Diabetes Association [6]	European Association [7]
Total daily intake of carbohydrate	Minimum of 130 g/day	No specific recommendation	≥45% of total energy intake	45–60% of total energy intake
Insulin regimen: MDI or CSII	Individuals should adjust prandial doses based on carbohydrate content of meals and snacks	Individuals benefit from adjusting insulin to carbohydrate intake and should be offered education to support this	Insulin should be adjusted based on the carbohydrate content of meals	In those treated with insulin, timing and dosage of medication should match amount and nature of carbohydrate
Fixed regimens	Carbohydrate intake on a day-to-day basis should be kept consistent with respect to time and amount	Consistent quantities of carbohydrate on a day-to-day basis	Consistency in carbohydrate intake with spacing and regularity in meal consumption	
Sucrose	Can be included, but care taken to avoid excessive intake	No specific recommendation	≤10% of total energy intake	Total free sugars should not exceed ≤10% of total energy intake
Glycaemic index/load (GI/GL)	Use of the glycaemic load may provide additional benefit	No specific recommendation	Replace high GI foods with low GI foods	Carbohydrate-rich low GI foods are suitable as carbohydrate-rich choices

counting can improve glycaemic control and [10–13] quality of life and general wellbeing, without increasing severe hypoglycaemia, body weight or blood lipid concentrations.

Further evidence in people with type 1 diabetes illustrates that the quantity of carbohydrate consumed does not affect glycaemic control if carbohydrate counting is implemented in conjunction with an algorithm of units of insulin per 10 g of carbohydrate. A study has shown that wide variations in carbohydrate intake (20–180 g) did not change basal insulin requirements [14].

For those treated with fixed biphasic insulin regimes, studies demonstrate that day-to-day consistency in carbohydrate is positively associated with improvements in HbA1c [15].

Type of carbohydrate

The amount of carbohydrate ingested is usually the primary determinant of postprandial glucose response in type 1 diabetes, but the type of carbohydrate also affects this response.

Glycaemic index

Most trials of low glycaemic index (GI) diets have focused on type 2 diabetes, and it is difficult to extrapolate these findings of modest improvement in HbA1c (3–5 mmol/mol or 0.3–0.5% reduction) into constructive guidance for type 1 diabetes [16–18]. Observational studies have shown that dietary GI is independently associated with HbA1c, with intakes of high GI foods showing a positive association with higher HbA1c levels [19]. However, there is little evidence to support the use of low glycaemic index diets as a primary nutritional strategy in type 1 diabetes.

GI may be useful in the fine-tuning of glucose control, particularly in pregnancy, where postprandial blood glucose concentrations are targeted, and also with pump therapy, where the infusion of mealtime insulin can be altered according to the glycaemic profile of the meal.

Sugars and artificial sweeteners

Sucrose, Glucose, Fructose and Lactose

A technical review by the ADA concluded that sucrose does not affect glycaemic control in diabetes differently from other types of carbohydrates [20]. The same review demonstrated that ingestion of a variety of sugars and starches produced no differences in glycaemic control when the total amount of carbohydrate was similar. Fructose may reduce postprandial glycaemia when it is used as a replacement for sucrose or starch, although large amounts of fructose may be associated with increased CVD risk and nonalcoholic fatty liver disease (NAFLD) [21].

Polyols

The glycaemic index of polyols (maltitol, isomalt, lactitol) is significantly lower than other forms of carbohydrate, with only maltitol having any significant impact on glycaemia [22].

Non-nutritive sweeteners

There are five non-nutritive sweeteners permitted for use in the United Kingdom (UK): aspartame, saccharin, acesulfame potassium (acesulfame K), cyclamate and sucralose. Only very small amounts are needed because they are so intensely sweet. They are virtually free of energy and do not affect blood glucose concentrations.

In conclusion, in type 1 diabetes sucrose, glucose and lactose should be treated as any other type of carbohydrate, with associated adjustments in insulin therapy to compensate for their carbohydrate value. Polyols and other sugar substitutes have little to no impact on glycaemia and do not require additional insulin adjustment.

Carbohydrate and principles of insulin dose adjustment

There are two core insulin regimens and they are either fixed regimens (commonly twice daily premixed insulin) or multiple injection regimens (also known as basal bolus or basal prandial regimens), and both of these require regular monitoring and adjustments to maintain glycaemic targets. For both approaches it is invaluable to know the carbohydrate value of different types and amounts of food. This is normally calculated using a system of carbohydrate portions or exchanges. In the UK a system of carbohydrate portions has been adopted, where one carbohydrate portion (CP) is an amount of food containing 10 g of carbohydrate. In the United States (US), a carbohydrate portion or exchange typically contains 15 g carbohydrate.

The fixed insulin regimen is best suited to an individual who tends to eat at similar times and with very little difference in the quantity of carbohydrate at each meal or snack from day-to-day. For individuals adopting a fixed regimen, it is important that they eat meals with consistent amounts of carbohydrate and may need to include snacks to prevent hypoglycaemia.

A multiple injection system or basal bolus regimen is more flexible and can allow a much more varied approach to eating, including ease in terms of eating out or working shifts. On this system, short-acting insulin is taken to match the quantity of carbohydrate in the meal or snack (the bolus) and a long-acting insulin is used to provide the background insulin requirements (the basal). If more carbohydrate is eaten, then more short-acting insulin is needed to counteract it. Most regimes work on ratios of insulin to carbohydrate portions, with the needs of individuals being worked out through dose adjustment algorithms.

Other nutritional factors and glycaemia

In the past, it was not uncommon for people with type 1 and type 2 diabetes to receive similar nutritional education, which would have focused on healthy eating and weight management. There is little, if any evidence to support this approach when focusing on glycaemic management in type 1 diabetes. There are other factors which may have an impact on insulin requirements and glycaemic control, and they include body weight, macronutrient intake and dietary fibre intake.

Body weight

The relationship between type 1 diabetes and body weight is not straightforward. A high HbA1c is often associated with weight loss [23] and so improvement in glucose control without some reduction in energy intake is usually associated with weight gain. Although there is no published evidence of a direct relationship between absolute body weight and glycaemic control in people with type 1 diabetes, it may be true that planned weight loss in the overweight or obese individual may improve glycaemic control by reducing insulin resistance. Body weight does have an impact on the insulin requirements of an individual with most adults (non-pregnant) requiring 0.6–0.8 units of insulin per kg body weight.

Proportion of macronutrients in the diet

There is little evidence to suggest that the proportion of total macronutrients consumed on a daily basis has any impact on long-term glucose control in the management of type 1 diabetes. A small 6 month trial evaluated a 43–46% carbohydrate, 20% monounsaturated fat diet compared with a 54–57% carbohydrate, 10% monounsaturated fat diet in well-controlled patients and found no difference in HbA1c [24]. Five year cohort evidence from people previously intensively treated in the DCCT show that lower carbohydrate and higher saturated, monounsaturated and total fat intakes were associated with higher HbA1c levels, but failed to reach significance after adjustment was made for baseline HbA1c and insulin dose [8]. Smaller, short-term studies from the 1970s and 1980s found no adverse effects on glycaemic control and promoted the idea that carbohydrate intake in people with type 1 diabetes could be liberalised [25–27]. In conclusion, there is no recommended proportion or amount of daily carbohydrate that should be recommended for good glycaemic outcomes in type 1 diabetes and there is no evidence to support the routine use of low or restricted carbohydrate diets.

Dietary fibre

The effect of dietary fibre on glycaemic control in type 1 diabetes is controversial. Evidence from EURODIAB [28], a large epidemiological study of type 1 diabetes and its complications, highlights the observation that a higher intake of fibre was independently related to lower HbA1c, with an additional benefit of reduced risk of severe ketoacidosis. There was no difference in the type of dietary fibre on the relationship to HbA1c. However a 24-week parallel randomised control trial in people with type 1 diabetes showed that a high fibre diet providing 50 g fibre, emphasising water-soluble fibre, was effective in reducing blood glucose concentration and hypoglycaemic events but did not affect HbA1c independently of weight and insulin dose in the intention-to-treat analysis [29]. Long-term evidence (>6 months) of the benefits of fibre is lacking and high fibre diets are unlikely to confer benefit in terms of the glycaemic management of type 1 diabetes.

Hypoglycaemia

Hypoglycaemia is a common and wide-spread side-effect of insulin therapy in people with type 1 diabetes and is widely reported, with a recent study showing that 87% of those with type 1 diabetes reported mild hypoglycaemia and 46% reported severe hypoglycaemia [30].

Oral treatments for hypoglycaemia

The goal of hypoglycaemia treatment is to restore glucose concentrations to normal as rapidly as possible, relieve symptoms and limit the risk of injury, whilst avoiding over-treatment. Glucose is the preferred treatment for hypoglycaemia with a 10 g and 20 g dose of oral glucose increasing blood glucose concentrations by approximately 2 mmol/l and 5 mmol/l, respectively [31]. Depending on the insulin regime, glucose concentrations may continue to fall approximately 60 minutes after glucose ingestion [31] and often a longer-acting carbohydrate snack may be advised, despite the lack of evidence to support this practice. More flexible insulin regimens, such as MDI and CSII, may not require additional longer-acting carbohydrate compared with fixed insulin regimens. Clearly, if the hypoglycaemic episode occurs during physical activity or following alcohol consumption, where the glucose levels will continue to fall, additional carbohydrate may well be needed to prevent further hypoglycaemia.

Hypoglycaemia should be treated immediately by administration of oral glucose, and although there is little evidence for the most effective treatment Diabetes UK, the Canadian Diabetes Association and the International Diabetes Federation all propose the 15 rule [5,6,32], which states that 15 g glucose should be taken immediately, and if glucose concentrations do not rise above 4 mmol/l after 15 minutes, the treatment should be repeated. A follow-up snack containing 15–20 g carbohydrate may be necessary to reduce the risk of further hypoglycaemia.

Key points

- Carbohydrate counting and insulin adjustment improves glycaemic control in type 1 diabetes.
- The ideal amount of macronutrients is unknown.
- There is a lack of evidence for the role of low GI or high fibre diets.
- Hypoglycaemia is common in type 1 diabetes and it is recommended that oral glucose is used to treat mild hypoglycaemia.

References

1. DAFNE Study Group. Training in flexible, intensive insulin management to enable dietary freedom in people with type 1 diabetes: dose adjustment for normal eating (DAFNE) randomised controlled trial. *BMJ* 2002; **325**: 746–752.
2. Shearer A, Bagust A, Sanderson D, Heller S, Roberts S. Cost effectiveness of flexible intensive insulin management to enable dietary freedom in people with Type 1 diabetes in the UK. *Diabetic Med* 2004; **21**(5): 460–467.
3. Kulkarni K, Castle G, Gregory R, Holmes A, Leontos C, Powers M, et al. Nutrition practice guidelines for type 1 diabetes mellitus positively affect dietitian practices and patient outcomes. *J Am Diet Assoc* 1998; **98**: 62–70.
4. Bantle JP, Wylie-Rosett J, Albright AL, Apovian CM, Clark NG, Franz MJ, et al. Nutrition recommendations and interventions for diabetes: a position statement of the American Diabetes Association. *Diabetes Care* 2008; **31**(Suppl. 1): S61–S78.
5. Dyson PA, Kelly T, Deakin T, Duncan A, Frost G, Harrison Z, et al. Evidence-based nutrition guidelines

for the prevention and management of diabetes. *Diabet Med* 2011; **28**(11): 1282–1288.

6. Canadian Diabetes Association. 2008 Clinical practice guidelines for the prevention and management of diabetes in Canada. *Can J Diabetes* 2008; **32**(Suppl. 1): S40–S45.

7. Mann JI, de Leeuw I, Hernansen K, Karamanos B, Karlsrom B, Katsilambros N, et al.; Diabetes and Nutrition Study Group (DNSG) of the European Association for the Study of Diabetes (EASD). Evidence-based nutritional approaches to the treatment and prevention of diabetes mellitus. *Nutr Metab Cardiovasc Dis* 2004; **14**(6): 373–394.

8. The DCCT Research Group. Nutrition interventions for intensive therapy in the Diabetes Control and Complications Trial. *J Am Diet Assoc* 1993; **93**: 768–772.

9. Delahanty L, Nathan D, Lachin J, Hu FB, Cleary PA, Ziegler GK, et al. Association of diet with glycated haemoglobin during intensive treatment of type 1 diabetes in the Diabetes Control and Complications Trial. *Am J Clin Nutr* 2009; **89**: 518–524.

10. Muhlhauser I, Jorgens V, Berger M, Graninger W, Gurtler W, Hornke L, et al. Bicentric evaluation of a teaching and treatment programme for type 1 (insulin-dependent) diabetic patients: improvement of metabolic control and other measures of diabetes care for up to 22 months. *Diabetologia* 1983; **25**: 470–476.

11. Muhlhauser I, Bruckner I, Berger M, Cheta D, Jorgens V, Ionescu-Tirgoviste C, et al. Evaluation of an intensified insulin treatment and teaching programme as routine management of Type 1 (insulin-dependent) diabetes. The Bucharest-Düsseldorf Study. *Diabetologia* 1987; **30**: 681–690.

12. Bott S, Bott U, Berger M, Muhlhauser I. Intensified insulin therapy and the risk of severe hypoglycaemia. *Diabetologia* 1997; **40**: 926–932.

13. Trento M, Borgo E, Kucich C, Passera P, Trinette A, Charrier L, et al. Quality of life, coping ability, and metabolic control in patients with type 1 diabetes managed by group care and a carbohydrate counting program. *Diabetes Care* 2009; **32**(11): e134.

14. Rabasa-Lhoret R, Garon J, Langelier H, Poisson D, Chiasson JL. Effects of meal carbohydrate content on insulin requirements in type 1 diabetic patients treated intensively with the basal-bolus (Ultralente-Regular) insulin regimen. *Diabetes Care* 1999; **22**(5): 667–673.

15. Wolever T, Hamad S, Chiasson J-L, Josse RG, Leiter LA, Rodger NW, et al. Day-to-day consistency in amount and source of carbohydrate intake associated with improved BG control in type 1 diabetes. *J Am Coll Nutr* 1999; **18**(3): 242–247.

16. Brand Miller J, Hayne S, Petrocs P, Colagiuri S. Low-glycaemic index diets in the management of diabetes — a meta-analysis of randomised controlled trials. *Diabetes Care* 2003; **26**: 2261–2267.

17. Thomas D, Elliott E. Low glycaemic index, or low glycaemic load, diets for diabetes mellitus. *Cochrane Database Syst Rev* 2009: CD006296.

18. Opperman A, Venter C, Oosthuizen W, Thompson R, Vorster H. Meta-analysis of health effects of using the glycaemic index in meal-planning. *Br J Nutr* 2004; **92**: 367–381.

19. Buyken A, Toeller M, Heitkamp G, Karamanos B, Rottiers R, Muggeo M, et al. Glycemic index in the diet of Eurpoean outpatients with Type 1 diabetes: relations to glycated haemoglobin and serum lipids. *Am J Clin Nutr* 2001; **73**: 574–581.

20. Kelley D. Sugars and starch in the nutritional management of diabetes mellitus. *Am J Clin Nutr* 2003; **78**(Suppl. 1): 858S–864S.

21. Tappy L, Le KA, Tran C, Paquot N. Fructose and metabolic diseases: new findings, new questions. *Nutrition* 2010; **26**: 1044–1049.

22. Livesey G. Health potential of polyols as a sugar replacer, with emphasis on low glycemic properties. *Nutr Res Rev* 2003; **16**: 163–191.

23. Quinn M, Ficociello L, Rosner B. Change in glycaemic control predicts change in weight in adolescent boys with Type 1 diabetes. *Pediatric Diabetes* 2003; **4**: 162–167.

24. Strychar I, Cohn JS, Renier G, Rivard M, Aris-Jilwan N, Beauregard H, et al. Effects of a diet higher in carbohydrate/lower in fat versus lower in carbohydrate/higher in monounsaturated fat on postmeal triglyceride concentrations and other cardiovascular risk factors in type 1 diabetes. *Diabetes Care* 2009; **32**(9): 1597–1599.

25. Kiehm T, Anderson J, Ward K. Beneficial effects of a high carbohydrate, high fiber diet on hyperglycaemic diabetic men. *Am J Clin Nutr* 1976; **29**: 895–899.

26. Simpson R, Mann J, Eaton J, Carter RD, Hockaday TD. High-carbohydrate diets and insulin-dependent diabetics. *BMJ* 1979; **2**: 523–525.

27. Hollenbeck C, Connor W, Riddle M, Alaupovic P, Leklem JE. The effects of a high-carbohydrate low-fat cholesterol-restricted diet on plasma lipid, lipoprotein, and apoprotein concentrations in insulin-dependent (Type 1) diabetes mellitus. *Metabolism* 1985; **34**(6): 559–566.

28. Buyken A, Toeller M, Heitkamp G, Vitelli F, Stehle P, Scherbaum WA, et al. Relation of fibre intake to HbA1c and the prevalence of severe ketoacidosis and severe hypoglycaemia. *Diabetologia* 1998; **41**: 882–890.

29. Giacco R, Parillo M, Rivellese A, Lasorella G, Giacco A, D'Episcopo L, et al. Long-term dietary

treatment with increased amounts of fiber-rich low–glycemic index natural foods improves BG control and reduces the number of hypoglycaemic events in type 1 diabetic patients. *Diabetes Care* 2000; **23**(10): 1461–1466.

30. UK Hypoglycaemia Study Group. Risk of hypoglycaemia in types 1 and 2 diabetes: effects of treatment modalities and their duration. *Diabetologia* 2007; **50**(6): 1140–1147.

31. Slama G, Traynard PY, Desplanque N, Pudar H, Dhunputh I, Letanoux M, et al. The search for an optimised treatment of hypoglycaemia. Carbohydrates in tablets, solution or gel for the correction of insulin reactions. *Arch Intern Med* 1990; **150**(3): 589–593.

32. International Diabetes Federation. Short-term complications. Module III-6. International Curriculum for Diabetes Health Professional Education. IDF, 2008.

Diet, education and behaviour in type 1 diabetes

Pamela Dyson

University of Oxford, Oxford Centre for Diabetes, Endocrinology and Metabolism, Churchill Hospital, Oxford, UK

3.4.1 Introduction

The effective management of type 1 diabetes imposes challenges for those living with the disease, requiring as it does self-management strategies, including blood glucose monitoring, insulin adjustment and administration, dietary adjustment, physical activity and hypoglycaemia management. The demands placed upon the individual are considerable and, despite clear evidence showing that optimal glycaemic control significantly reduces diabetes complications [1], it is estimated that 70–90% of people with diabetes have HbA1c levels above the recommended targets of 53 mmol/mol (7.0%) [1,2]. There are many reasons for this, one of which has been identified as the lack of education and skills to support effective management of type 1 diabetes [3]. The Global Partnership for Effective Diabetes Management (GPEDM) has outlined practical steps to improve management of type 1 diabetes and includes the recommendation that everyone should be provided with a structured education programme at initiation of insulin and thereafter, including education about prevention, recognition and treatment of hypoglycaemia [3]. There is growing evidence that diabetes education is effective in improving clinical outcomes and quality of life [4] and that it is cost-effective, as the benefits outweigh the costs associated with any intervention [5].

3.4.2 Education

Diabetes education is widely held to be an essential part of diabetes care, and the International Diabetes Federation (IDF) includes education provision in its framework for diabetes care. The IDF defines the aim of diabetes education as 'to provide information in an acceptable form in order that people with diabetes develop the knowledge and skills to self-manage and make informed choices' [6].

In the United Kingdom (UK), it is recommended that diabetes education should recognise that self-management is a fundamental part of diabetes care, and should provide lifestyle education as a package [7]. Furthermore, the criteria for structured education proposed by the Department of Health and Diabetes UK should be adopted. These criteria state that structured education programmes should be patient-centred and incorporate individual assessment, be reliable, valid, relevant and comprehensive, theory-driven and evidence-based, flexible and able to cope with diversity, able to utilise different teaching techniques, resource effective with supporting materials, written down (including philosophy, aims and objective, timetables and detailed content), delivered by trained educators, subject to quality assurance and, finally, that they should be subject to robust audit and evaluation [8].

Advanced Nutrition and Dietetics in Diabetes, First Edition. Edited by Louise Goff and Pamela Dyson.
© 2016 John Wiley & Sons, Ltd. Published 2016 by John Wiley & Sons, Ltd.

The UK recommendations also state that culturally appropriate education should be offered to all adults with type 1 diabetes after diagnosis, and offered according to need at annual review [9]. In the United States (US) and Canada, diabetes education is referred to specifically as diabetes self-management education (DSME) and recommendations state that it should be supplied at diagnosis and when needed thereafter [10,11].

Multidisciplinary teams

The American Diabetes Association (ADA) and the National Institute for Health and Clinical Excellence (NICE) both recommend that education is delivered by multidisciplinary teams (MDTs) [4,12] and these teams may include specialist nurses, dietitians, physicians, pharmacists, exercise physiologists, psychologists and podiatrists. In the US, there is evidence that DSME is more effective when delivered by a MDT [4].

Components of diabetes education

The key components of diabetes education have been summarised by NICE and state that diabetes education models should:

- Reflect established principles of adult learning
- Utilise a multidisciplinary group-based approach
- Be accessible to a broad range of people
- Use a variety of learning styles [7].

Principles of adult learning

Health education generally has been defined as 'any combination of learning experiences designed to facilitate voluntary actions conducive to health' [13]. Health education (including diabetes education) includes an implicit expectation that acquiring knowledge is not sufficient for improving health, and that some behaviour change is necessary to move the individual towards a state of optimal health. Traditionally, diabetes education has been delivered using a didactic, one-to-one model, but this model does not address principles of adult learning. Newer

theories and models underpinning health education and addressing behaviour change have been summarised by the National Institute for Health in the US [14] and include the following models: social cognitive (learning) theory, theory of reasoned action and planned behaviour, health belief model, transtheoretical model, relapse prevention model, social support and ecological approaches.

Social cognitive theory is the basis of most health education and has a central principle of self-efficacy. Self-efficacy reflects the estimate or personal judgement of an individual's ability and capacity to succeed in achieving specific goals. In addition, social cognitive theory includes the concepts of incentive and value from any health behaviour change.

The theory of reasoned action and planned behaviour depends upon the individual attitudes and the influence of the social environment and includes the concept of perceived behavioural control. This concept is similar to that of self-efficacy.

The health belief model takes into account perceptions, including perceptions of severity of any illness, individual susceptibility and the advantages and disadvantages of making a health behaviour change.

The transtheoretical model is probably the best-known theory and relates to readiness to change and embraces five key stages: precontemplation, contemplation, preparation, action and maintenance. The key to utilising this model effectively is matching the intervention to the stage of change.

Relapse prevention addresses the concept of adherence and examines the process of identifying high-risk situations and formulating solutions. It commonly involves four stages: identifying the specific problem, brainstorming all possible solutions, evaluating each solution and committing to action.

Social support and ecological approaches rely upon extrinsic models of health education and comprise the creation of supportive environments in both physical and emotional terms to support behaviour change.

These approaches have been developed to support the individual behaviour change process relying upon intrinsic theories such as self-efficacy.

Although there is insufficient evidence to identify the most effective model for diabetes education and behaviour change, it is assumed that behavioural interventions are likely to improve outcomes in type 1 diabetes as they do in type 2 diabetes (See Chapter 4.6).

Learning style

Four main categories of adult learning styles have been identified, and employing different learning styles increases engagement and learning.

The activist relies on concrete experience, and prefers doing and experimenting.
The reflector uses observation and reflection.
The theorist relies on abstract conceptualisation and wants to understand underlying concepts, reasons and relationships.
The pragmatist uses active experimentation and likes to try things out to see if they work.

In addition to matching education to learning styles, there is evidence that innovative approaches may be needed to deliver education to people with diabetes [7,15]. Patients with chronic disease, including diabetes, state that they would like information in as many formats as possible and as early as possible after diagnosis [16]. A variety of techniques have been suggested for providing health education for people with diabetes, including picture charts, video techniques, computer packages, text messaging and e-mail tailored to the group or individual. These techniques are useful to support diabetes education provided by health professionals, and are not necessarily designed as stand-alone programmes. Evidence is accumulating about the use of technology in delivering diabetes education and has shown that mobile phone interventions can reduce HbA1c by 6 mmol/mol (0.5%), although there is significantly greater reduction in people with type 2 diabetes compared to those with type 1 (9 vs 3 mmol/mol, 0.8 vs 0.3%, $p=0.02$) [17].

Evidence for type 1 diabetes education

There is wide recognition that education played a central role in the success of a landmark study designed to improve glycaemic control and reduce the risk of tissue damage in people with type 1 diabetes [18]. Although education is regarded as a cornerstone in self-management and is considered an integral part of treatment, there are few studies evaluating the overall effect of education, behavioural strategies and self-management programmes specifically for type 1 diabetes, although most report positive outcomes [12]. Education programmes incorporating carbohydrate assessment and insulin adjustment have been shown to be effective in improving glycaemia and quality of life, reducing hypoglycaemia and are cost-effective [19–21].

Accessibility

It is recommended that type 1 diabetes education is made available to a broad range of individuals including black and minority ethnic groups, and vulnerable adults such as those who live in institutional settings, such as prisons, hostels, nursing and residential homes.

Delivery of education programmes

There is insufficient evidence at present to recommend one method of education delivery for type 1 diabetes over another, and a lack of evidence for the setting and frequency of education sessions and whether group-based education or one-to-one is more effective [15]. However, most of the recent studies showing improvements in diabetes management have been based upon the model of structured group education and this is generally regarded as an effective model, although one-to-one education remains as an option [7].

Group education

Diabetes group education for type 1 diabetes is usually offered as a package, with integrated dietary advice and topics for education programmes for type 1 diabetes including [4]:

- Description of diabetes and treatment options
- Nutritional management
- Physical activity
- Insulin therapy
- Self-monitoring, including blood glucose monitoring
- Prevention, recognition and treatment of short-term complications
- Prevention, recognition and treatment of long-term complications
- Diabetes management during illness ('sick day rules')
- Psychosocial aspects of diabetes management.

In terms of the content of dietary education for people with type 1 diabetes, it is generally agreed that carbohydrate management and insulin adjustment are critical for achieving and maintaining glycaemic control and for increasing dietary flexibility, and education to support this strategy is recommended by most authorities, including Diabetes UK and the ADA [10,11,22]. Carbohydrate management for people with type 1 diabetes is discussed fully in Chapter 3.3.

However, although glycaemic control is the primary focus of dietary management of type 1 diabetes, there are other nutritional factors for consideration. People with type 1 diabetes are at increased risk of cardiovascular disease compared to those without diabetes, with men showing a 3.6-fold higher risk and women a 7.7-fold higher risk [23]. In addition, people with type 1 diabetes have been shown to consume a more atherogenic diet than those without diabetes [2,24]. As a result, it is recognised that lifestyle measures to address cardiovascular risk reduction may be an important component of dietary education. Cardiovascular risk reduction includes the concepts of weight management and dietary factors such as fat and fibre intake and is discussed more fully in Chapter 9.2.

One-to-one Education

A variety of strategies to induce behaviour change have been used in both group and one-to-one education, including goal-setting, problem-solving, identifying and reducing barriers to change, self-monitoring, using incentives or rewards and motivational interviewing [25].

Motivational interviewing (MI) has been proposed as a model for supporting self-management techniques and is promoted as a model for use in one-to-one consultations for people with diabetes [26]. It is a collaborative, guided approach to behaviour change, which seeks to identify and resolve the ambivalence that most people feel about making changes [27], and consists of five key principles:

- Expressing empathy through active listening
- Rolling with resistance
- Avoidance of confrontation or arguing with the individual with diabetes
- Resolving ambivalence
- Supporting self-efficacy and autonomy.

MI is a skill-based practice, and utilises four basic communication skills, often remembered by the mnemonic OARS:

Open questions
Affirmation
Reflection
Summarise

Motivational interviewing has been promoted as an effective strategy for diabetes, as many people find challenges associated with self-management in terms of blood glucose monitoring and lifestyle, and exploring the ambivalence around these challenges should improve management skills. However, a recent review suggests that MI cannot be recommended as an evidence-based strategy for diabetes self-management [28], although this conclusion was due to methodological issues with the studies reviewed rather than lack of effect, as 50% of the studies reported improvements in health-related behaviour, including smoking cessation and improvements in glycaemic control, diet and weight management.

3.4.3 Summary

Education to support self-management for people with type 1 diabetes has shown improved outcomes and evidence is accumulating for innovative approaches to the delivery of education aimed at both individuals and groups and encompassing new technologies.

Key points

- Diabetes education can support self-management in people with type 1 diabetes and is recommended by most authorities.
- Education should be delivered by multidisciplinary teams, use the principles of adult education, address difference learning styles and be adapted for use in different environments.
- Education can be delivered either in group or one-to-one settings.

References

1. Nathan DM, Zinman B, Cleary PA, Backlund JY, Genuth S, Miller R, et al. Modern-day clinical course of type 1 diabetes mellitus after 30 years' duration: the diabetes control and complications trial/epidemiology of diabetes interventions and complications and Pittsburgh epidemiology of diabetes complications experience (1983–2005). *Arch Intern Med* 2009; **169**(14): 1307–1316.
2. Calvert M, Shankar A, McManus RJ, Lester H, Freemantle N. Effect of the quality and outcomes framework on diabetes care in the United Kingdom: retrospective cohort study. *BMJ* 2009; **338**: b1870.
3. Aschner P, Horton E, Leiter LA, Munro N, Skyler JS; Global Partnership for Effective Diabetes Management. Practical steps to improving the management of type 1 diabetes: recommendations from the Global Partnership for Effective Diabetes Management. *Int J Clin Pract* 2010; **64**(3): 305–315.
4. Funnell MM, Brown TL, Childs BP, Haas LB, Hosey GM, Jensen B, et al. National Standards for diabetes self-management education. *Diabetes Care* 2011; **34**(Suppl 1): S89–S96.
5. Boren SA, Fitzner KA, Panhalkar PS, Specker JE. Costs and benefits associated with diabetes education: a review of the literature. *Diabetes Educator* 2009; **35**(1): 72–96.
6. IDF. IDF Position Statement: Self-management education. Brussels: International Diabetes Federation, 2011.
7. NICE. Guidance on the use of patient-education modules for diabetes. Technical Appraisal Guidance 60. London: National Institute of Clinical Excellence, 2003.
8. Diabetes UK. Structured Patient Education in Diabetes. London: Diabetes UK and Department of Health, 2005.
9. NICE. Diagnosis and management of type 1 diabetes in children, young people and adults. London: National Institute for Health and Clinical Excellence, 2004.
10. American Diabetes Association. Standards of medical care in diabetes – 2011. *Diabetes Care* 2011; **34**(Suppl. 1): S1–S61.
11. Canadian Diabetes Association. Canadian Diabetes Association 2008 clinical practice guidelines for the prevention and management of diabetes in Canada. *Can J Diabet* 2008; **32**(Suppl. 1): S1–S201.
12. NICE. Type 1 diabetes in adults: full guideline part 2. London: National Institute of Clinical Excellence, 2008.
13. Green LW, Kansler CC. The Professional and Scientific Literature on Patient Education. Detroit: Dale Research Co, 1980
14. NIH. Theory at a glance: A guide for health promotion practice. National Institute of Health, 2005.
15. NICE. Patient Education Models for Diabetes. London: National Institute for Clinical Excellence, 2002.
16. Corben S, Rosen R. Self-management for long-term conditions. London: King's Fund, 2005.
17. Liang X, Wang Q, Yang X, Cao J, Chen J, Mo X, et al. Effect of mobile phone intervention for diabetes on glycaemic control: a meta-analysis. *Diabet Med* 2011; **28**(4): 455–463.
18. DCCT Study Group. The effect of intensive treatment of diabetes on the development and progression of long-term complications in insulin-dependent diabetes mellitus. The Diabetes Control and Complications Trial Research Group. *N Engl J Med* 1993; **329**(14): 977–986.
19. DAFNE Study Group. Training in flexible, intensive insulin management to enable dietary freedom in people with type 1 diabetes: dose adjustment for normal eating (DAFNE) randomised controlled trial. *BMJ 2002*; **325**(7367): 746.
20. Sämann A, Mühlhauser I, Bender R, Kloos Ch, Müller UA. Glycaemic control and severe hypoglycaemia following training in flexible, intensive insulin therapy to enable dietary freedom in people with type 1 diabetes: a prospective implementation study. *Diabetologia* 2005; **48**(10): 1965–1970.
21. Shearer A, Bagust A, Sanderson D, Heller S, Roberts S. Cost-effectiveness of flexible intensive insulin management to enable dietary freedom in people with Type 1 diabetes in the UK. *Diabet Med* 2004; **21**(5): 460–467.
22. Dyson PA, Kelly T, Deakin T, Duncan A, Frost G, Harrison Z, et al.; Diabetes UK Nutrition Working Group. Diabetes UK evidence-based nutrition guidelines for the prevention and management of diabetes. *Diabet Med* 2011; **28**(11): 1282–1288.
23. Soedamah-Muthu SS, Fuller JH, Mulnier HE, Raleigh VS, Lawrenson RA, Colhoun HM. High risk of cardiovascular disease in patients with type 1 diabetes

in the U.K.: a cohort study using the general practice research database. *Diabetes Care* 2006; **29**(4): 798–804.

24. Snell-Bergeon JK, Chartier-Logan C, Maahs DM, Ogden LG, Hokanson JE, Kinney GL, et al. Adults with type 1 diabetes eat a high-fat atherogenic diet that is associated with coronary artery calcium. *Diabetologia* 2009; **52**(5): 801–809.

25. Peyrot R, Rubin RR. Behavioral and psychosocial interventions in diabetes: A conceptual review. *Diabetes Care* 2007; **30**(10): 2433–2440.

26. Christie D, Channon S. The potential for motivational interviewing to improve outcomes in the management of diabetes and obesity in paediatric and adult populations: a clinical review. *Diabetes Obes Metab* 2014; **16**(5): 381–387.

27. Rollnick S, Miller WR, Butler CC. Motivational Interviewing in Health Care. New York: The Guilford Press, 2008.

28. Clifford Mulimba A, Byron-Daniel J. Motivational interviewing-based interventions and diabetes mellitus. *Br J Nurs* 2014; **23**(1): 8–14.

Lifestyle issues and type 1 diabetes – physical activity, alcohol and recreational drugs

Elaine Hibbert-Jones
Royal Gwent Hospital, Newport, UK

3.5.1 Introduction

Recommendations for people with type 1 diabetes often emphasise management in terms of insulin administration and nutritional intake, but there are other lifestyle factors that have an impact on glycaemic control and quality of life. This chapter discusses the evidence relating to physical activity, alcohol and recreational drugs and provides guidelines for management.

3.5.2 Physical activity

All levels of physical activity, from leisure activities and recreational sport to competitive performance, can be undertaken by people with type 1 diabetes who do not have complications and are in good blood glucose control [1]. There are, however, some restrictions or outright bans on high risk sports, see Table 3.5.1.

Although physical activity is an important part of improving glycaemic control in the management of type 2 diabetes, in type 1 diabetes, exercise may actually worsen control unless care is taken to adjust carbohydrate intake and insulin dosage [2,3]. The advantages of exercise in type 1 diabetes relate more to its protective cardiovascular effects than to improved glycaemic control. The successful management of blood glucose levels during exercise poses a challenge for people with type 1 diabetes. The ability to adjust the therapeutic regimen to allow safe participation and high performance is an important management strategy. This means that careful consideration needs to be given to blood glucose levels, food intake and the insulin regimen.

People with type 1 diabetes have an important role in collecting information on the blood glucose response to different types of exercise and changes made to insulin or carbohydrate intake. They need the advice of experts to help interpret these data to help improve their sports performance. This is particularly important for those patients who take part in competitive sport [2]. A basic understanding of exercise physiology, energy sources and metabolism enable health professionals to advise the individual with type 1 diabetes.

Exercise physiology

Oxygen consumption

During exercise, whole-body oxygen consumption increases to supply adequate oxygen for the working muscles (VO_2). Oxygen uptake increases with exercise intensity until the maximum energy intensity is reached (VO_2 max). The intensity of any given exercise is measured as a percentage of an individual's maximum oxygen uptake (%VO_2 max) [4].

Table 3.5.1 Restrictions on sports for people with type 1 diabetes [2]

Banned sports	Restrictions
• Bobsleigh	• Gliding
• Boxing	• Motorcycle racing
• Paragliding	• Parachuting/
• Flying	Skydiving
• Horse racing	• Powerboat racing
• Motor racing	• SCUBA diving
	• Ballooning
	• Rowing

Further information can be obtained from the national sport's governing body.

Energy metabolism

The way energy is used during exercise affects blood glucose concentration. Factors affecting the overall demands of exercising muscles include speed of movement, the force produced and the length of any activity. This energy is provided by three energy systems that supply energy as ATP (adenosine triphosphate) [5,6].

(1) *ATP-CP system*   Also known as the 'phosphagen system'. This fuels short, intense activities for a few seconds. Creatine phosphate (CP) in muscles provides phosphate to convert ADP (adenosine diphosphate) to replenish ATP for the first 6–10 seconds of activity. This process does not require oxygen and therefore is described as *anaerobic*. This system is used for high-intensity, short duration activities, such as the clean and jerk in weight-lifting and the fast break in basketball.

(2) *Lactic acid system*   Also known as the 'anaerobic glycolytic system', this supplies energy for short intense activities lasting longer than 10 seconds but less than about 2–3 minutes. This system can produce energy anaerobically through the breakdown of muscle glycogen (glycogenolysis) followed by glycolysis, with lactic acid being formed as a by-product. As lactic acid builds up, the pH of the muscle drops, causing fatigue or 'burn'. This system only provides a small amount of ATP and is used in activities such as 200 m swimming events, 800 m runs

and stop–start activities such as hockey and basketball.

Neither of these anaerobic systems can provide sufficient ATP to sustain longer duration activities. Consequently, the oxidative pathway is utilised to fuel events lasting for more than 2–3 minutes.

(3) *Aerobic system*   Glycogen, in the presence of oxygen, produces much more ATP than anaerobic glycolysis. In addition, intramuscular and adipose tissue triglycerides are also used and, occasionally, small amounts of amino acids. This system, therefore, is essential for longer duration, moderate intensity activities, such as walking, running, swimming, cycling and rowing. Endurance events such as marathon running and long distance cycling also use this energy system. Multiple sprint sports, such as rugby, hockey, tennis and squash use a combination of aerobic and anaerobic systems [4]. This is important when considering the effect of this type of exercise on blood glucose concentrations.

Energy substrates

The two main factors that influence the energy substrate (carbohydrate, fat, protein) used for exercise are the intensity (VO_2 max) and duration of the exercise. The substrates used are a mixture of fat and carbohydrate. Protein tends only to be used for energy in extreme endurance exercise.

Exercise intensity

At rest in the fasting state, the main energy substrate used by the body are free fatty acids. During exercise, the body switches to using carbohydrate as the main energy substrate. This is derived first from glycogen stored in the muscle, then as plasma glucose from hepatic glycogenolysis, gluconeogenesis and intestinal absorption [7]. In high-intensity, anaerobic exercise (e.g. sprinting), the energy substrate is almost entirely carbohydrate but as the intensity decreases more energy is derived from free fatty acids from lipolysis and intramuscular triglycerides. Many sports have periods of low intensity exercise interspersed with periods of high-intensity activity (e.g. football, rugby, hockey, ice hockey, netball, some fitness classes). This is referred to as 'intermittent high-intensity' exercise.

Exercise duration

In longer duration, moderate intensity exercise, free fatty acids become the main energy substrate, which coincides with a decrease in glycogen stores in the muscles and liver [4,7], see Figure 3.5.1.

Fatigue and carbohydrate metabolism

As the glycogen stores are utilised during prolonged exercise, ATP resynthesis cannot supply the demand of the active muscles and the exercise intensity cannot be maintained. In a treadmill marathon race, carbohydrate oxidation gradually decreased, while fat oxidation increased. At the 35 km mark fat and carbohydrate made an equal contribution to energy metabolism and runners were forced to reduce their running speed due to the inability of the carbohydrate stores to continue to fuel sufficient ATP production [4]. This is known as 'hitting the wall'. Trained athletes can utilise energy substrates more efficiently and use a higher proportion of fatty acids, sparing their glycogen sources. For people with type 1 diabetes, this means that as a training regimen becomes established, insulin requirements will need to be reviewed as less glucose is metabolised.

Prior to a competition, glycogen stores can be enhanced by consuming a high carbohydrate diet and by tapering training for 3 to 4 days before the competition [4,8,9]. This is sometimes referred to as 'carbohydrate loading' and will require a further review of insulin requirements.

Glucose transporter proteins

Exercise stimulates the translocation of insulin-independent glucose transporter proteins (GLUT 4 transporters) that accelerate the transport of glucose into the muscle [4,8]. These proteins remain active after exercise has ceased and have an important role in glycogen resynthesis. Their release increases with training, which means that, in type 1 diabetes, less insulin will be required to maintain blood glucose levels and the insulin regimen will need to be altered as a regular exercise programme is established.

Adaptation of the endocrine system to exercise

Glycaemia is maintained during exercise by hormonal changes. At the start of exercise, insulin concentrations fall and glucagon concentrations increase, allowing hepatic glucose production to increase. As the exercise progresses, other counter-insulin hormones, such as catecholamines, are released [1], leading to

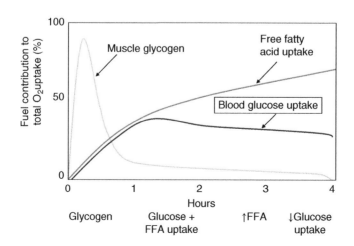

Figure 3.5.1 The contribution of energy sources used depending on the duration of the activity

an increase in glucose, from gluconeogenesis to supply the working muscles, and fatty acids from lipolysis.

Altered response to exercise in type 1 diabetes

The energy regulation described above is essentially lost in type 1 diabetes. If there is insufficient circulating insulin, there is an excessive release of counter-regulatory hormones which, together with hepatic glucose production in response to exercise, can further increase blood glucose, leading to hyperglycaemia. This is common following short duration, high-intensity exercise, in response to competition stress, heat stress, dehydration and arm exercises [7]. If ketones are present, exercise can lead to diabetic ketoacidosis (DKA).

If there is excessive circulating insulin, this can reduce or even prevent hepatic glucose production but increase muscle glucose utilisation, leading to hypoglycaemia. Therefore, the amount of insulin circulating before, during and after exercise is critical to exercise performance and prevention of fatigue, see Table 3.5.2. A summary of the implications of theses altered responses for individuals with type 1 diabetes undertaking different types of exercise is summarised in Table 3.5.3.

Variables that affect blood glucose response to exercise

There are a number of variables that can affect the blood glucose response to exercise that need to be taken into account when deciding on

a suitable treatment strategy to enable people with diabetes to exercise safely and to the best of their ability. These include type, duration and intensity of exercise, pre-exercise blood glucose concentration, fitness and training programme, environmental conditions (for example temperature, hydration, time of day when exercising), type and timing of insulin doses, injection site, timing and composition of previous meal, antecedent hypoglycaemia.

General exercise guidelines for people with type 1 diabetes

- The Association of British Clinical Diabetologists (ABCD) recommends that every patient with type 1 diabetes who wishes to start strenuous exercise should have a thorough medical examination [2].
- Patients at high risk of underlying cardiovascular disease may require a graded exercise test (see Chapter 4.7).
- Guidelines for blood glucose concentrations prior to starting exercise are given in Table 3.5.4
- Blood glucose should be monitored before, during and after exercise in order to identify when changes in insulin or food intake are necessary.
- Individuals should learn to identify their glycaemic response to different exercise conditions. This can be achieved by keeping a training diary that includes information on the effect of the variables described above on blood glucose, and can be used to plan any changes needed.

Table 3.5.2 Blood glucose response and circulating insulin levels

Status of plasma insulin	Hepatic glucose production	Muscle glucose utilisation	Blood glucose concentration
Normal or slightly diminished	⇑	⇑	→
Markedly diminished	⇑	↑	↑
Increased	↑	⇑	↓

Table 3.5.3 Activity type and implications for type 1 diabetes [7]

Exercise type	Implications for individuals with type 1 diabetes	Reason
Longer duration,	1. Predisposition to hypoglycaemia after 20–60 minutes	Insulin levels do not fall at the start of exercise leading to potential over-insulinisation. This can inhibit glucose production increasing the risk of hypoglycaemia as glycogen stores are depleted
	2. Predisposition to hypoglycaemia during and following endurance activities	The stimulation of GLUT 4 transporters increases the risk of hypoglycaemia, particularly during the post-exercise phase
	3. Increased risk of hypoglycaemia when exercising at around 70% maximal heart rate	Highest rates of aerobic glucose oxidation
	4. Increased risk of hyperglycaemia after several hours of exercise	Greater reliance on fat as an energy substrate and reduced activity of insulin due to time lapse from previous injection
Short duration, high intensity, anaerobic activity	Predisposition to hyperglycaemia	Increase in catecholamines that stimulates glucose production. Cannot compensate with increased endogenous insulin production
Intermittent, high-intensity exercise	Reduced risk of hypoglycaemia. May cause hyperglycaemia	Bursts of high-intensity exercise increase counter-regulatory hormones and stimulate glucose production. Likely to need less carbohydrate and smaller reductions in insulin to prevent hypoglycaemia

Table 3.5.4 General exercise guidelines for type 1 diabetes

Blood glucose concentration (mmol/l)	Action	Carbohydrate needed
Less than 4 No ketones	Avoid exercise. Treat hypoglycaemia	10–20 g for every 30 minutes of exercise. In addition to carbohydrate to treat hypoglycaemia
4–12 No ketones	Consider if additional carbohydrate needed, which will depend on type and duration of exercise	0–20 g for the first 30 minutes and 10–20 g for every 30 minutes of exercise thereafter
Greater than 12 No ketones	Exercise with caution and continue to monitor blood glucose	Generally not required until glucose level has fallen
Greater than 12 Ketones present	Avoid exercise	–

- Individuals should consume carbohydrate as needed to avoid hypoglycaemia and ensure suitable foods are readily available before, during and after exercise
- Individuals should ensure adequate hydration.

Weight training and glycaemia

The American College of Sports Medicine (ACSM) recommend muscle strengthening activity as a key part of an exercise regimen [10].

This is described further in Chapter 4.7. Weight training is one type of exercise used to develop muscle strength but there is little evidence-based information on the acute effects weight training has on glycaemia, and findings from a recent systematic review were inconclusive [11]. Studies included in the review were in subjects with good glycaemic control and showed weight training may increase, minimally affect or decrease post-exercise glycaemia, depending on the individual response. The authors found no data on the glycaemic effect in patients with poor glycaemic control (HbA1c >86 mmol/mol, >10%) and further research is required in this area.

Hypoglycaemia

Hypoglycaemia is a common complication of exercise. It can result in under-performance or prevent a person from completing an activity and prove to be life-threatening in some hazardous sports. The risk of hypoglycaemia during exercise is increased if the individual has had hypoglycaemia in the previous 24 hours (antecedent hypoglycaemia). This risk increases with increasing severity of the preceding hypoglycaemic episode [7].

Post-exercise hypoglycaemia

For individuals with type 1 diabetes, post-exercise hypoglycaemia can develop some hours after exercise. This is due to a combination of glycogen resynthesis, increased insulin sensitivity, augmented insulin absorption, impaired glucagon secretion and reduced catecholamine responses [8]. A combination of additional carbohydrate post-exercise and insulin reduction will reduce this risk and allow adequate restoration of glycogen stores between bouts of exercise.

Strategies to prevent exercise-induced hypoglycaemia

(1) *Reduction in insulin dose*   Any reductions in insulin dose will need to take into account the variables that can affect the blood glucose response to exercise. Normally it is the rapid acting insulin dose that is reduced

Table 3.5.5   General insulin dose reductions for endurance sports [5]

Duration (min)	Low intensity	Moderate intensity	High intensity
	Insulin reductions (%)		
15	None	5–10	0–15 [a]
30	None	10–20	10–30
45	5–15	15–30	20–45
60	10–20	20–40	30–60
90	15–30	30–55	45–75
120	20–40	40–70	60–90
180	30–60	60–90	75–100

[a]For very intense exercise, the insulin dose may need to increase, not decrease, to counter the glucose-raising effect of hormones released.

prior to exercise, see Table 3.5.5 [5,12]. It is also important to consider the time since the last pre-meal insulin bolus. If exercising soon after a dose, insulin activity will be higher and there may need to be an even greater reduction in the dose than if the exercise occurs some time after the last insulin dose.

There are concerns that large reductions in pre-exercise insulin may increase the risk of developing DKA. However, a recent study found that in individuals with type 1 diabetes, up to 75% reduction in the pre-exercise, rapid-acting insulin dose had little impact on ketogenesis following running [13].

Basal insulin can also be adjusted to prevent hypoglycaemia during and following exercise, which may reduce the need to consume additional carbohydrate, although this may cause hyperglycaemia [7,14].

People treated by pump therapy should be advised to adjust insulin doses 90 minutes before starting exercise. However, the flexibility of the pump allows for impromptu exercise and hypoglycaemia can be reduced with suspension of the usual basal rate during exercise [14]. There is an increased risk of hyperglycaemia post-exercise in people using insulin pump therapy unless managed appropriately.

(2) *Increase in carbohydrate*   Grimm et al. studied 67 patients with type 1 diabetes who

were allocated into 4 groups according to their normal treatment strategy to prevent hypoglycaemia: (i) reduction of insulin only; (ii) additional carbohydrate only; (iii) additional carbohydrate plus reduction in insulin and (iv) no changes to insulin or carbohydrate. The groups performed seven different sports at three different intensities. The results indicated that adequate carbohydrate replacement during and after exercise was the most effective measure to prevent hypoglycaemia [15]. The amount of carbohydrate required also depends on the timing of the last pre-meal insulin dose, with the longer the time since injection, the less additional carbohydrate needed to maintain euglycaemia [16].

(3) *Integration of a 10 second maximal sprint* In a study of individuals with type 1 diabetes, blood glucose concentrations fell significantly following 20 minutes of moderate intensity exercise with usual insulin dose and carbohydrate intake, and they continued to fall over the subsequent 120 minutes. However, a 10 second maximal sprint at the end of the exercise prevented a further fall in blood glucose. This was associated with an increase in the counter regulatory hormones [14,17].

(4) *Intermittent high-intensity exercise in the training programme* A recent study comparing the glycaemic changes following 45 minutes of continuous moderate-intensity exercise found there was less post-exercise hypoglycaemia and more post-exercise hyperglycaemia with the addition of intermittent high-intensity bouts of exercise (9 bouts of 15 seconds). There were more incidences of nocturnal hypoglycaemia following continuous exercise without the high-intensity bouts, despite the consumption of a bedtime carbohydrate snack [18].

Diet for exercise – carbohydrate

Carbohydrate is the most important substrate for exercising muscles. Approximately 50–60% of energy during 1–4 hours of continuous exercise at 70% of maximal heart rate is derived from carbohydrate [6]. Carbohydrate is stored in limited amounts in the muscles and liver and these stores can be rapidly depleted, particularly during high-intensity exercise and intermittent high-intensity exercise.

The amount of carbohydrate required depends on the total daily energy expenditure, type of sport, gender and environmental conditions, although athletes do not need to consume a diet that is substantially different from the dietary recommendations for the general population. Current recommendations are 6 to 10 g of carbohydrate/kg body weight/day [6].

How much extra carbohydrate is needed?

The amount of additional carbohydrate needed for exercise varies. For moderate intensity, aerobic exercise lasting longer than 20–30 minutes, a rough guide is 10–20 g carbohydrate per 30 minutes of activity. For longer duration, higher intensity exercise, this may increase to 30–60 g per hour. Guidance on the amounts of carbohydrate used by athletes with type 1 diabetes for different sports, dependent on body weight, are given by Grimm [3] and by exercise intensity, duration and pre-exercise blood glucose level by Colberg [5].

Carbohydrate requirements for training

As energy requirements increase, athletes should first aim to consume the maximum number of servings, appropriate to their needs, from the carbohydrate-based food groups. Athletes who have lower energy requirements will need to pay greater attention to choosing nutrient dense foods [6]. With regards to the timing of meals and snacks, consideration needs to be given to the athlete's gastrointestinal characteristics as well as to the duration and intensity of the exercise workout.

Prior to exercising eating can improve performance compared to exercising in the fasted state [6]. The meal should be low in fat and fibre to facilitate gastric emptying and minimise gastrointestinal discomfort.

There should be adequate carbohydrate to maintain blood glucose and maximise glycogen stores and it should contain moderate amounts of protein. There is no conclusive evidence to support a beneficial effect on performance based on the glycaemic index of the meal. It is sensible for athletes to try out new foods and beverages at practice sessions to see what works best for them. Additional carbohydrate *may* be needed 20–30 minutes before exercise, depending on the pre-exercise blood glucose concentration, the type and duration of exercise and the normal blood glucose response to exercise. This can be provided by fluid or food containing rapidly absorbed carbohydrate, such as isotonic sports drinks, low fat confectionery (e.g. jelly sweets), or less rapidly absorbed carbohydrate to provide glucose later on in the exercise (e.g. cereal bar, fruit).

During exercise lasting 1 hour or less, sports drinks containing 6–8% carbohydrate are suitable to provide both energy and fluid [19]. For longer periods of exercise, performance is enhanced by consuming 30–60 g/hour of carbohydrate (0.7 g/kg body weight) [6]. Ideally this should be taken at 15–20 minute intervals. When >70 g/hour of carbohydrate is required, a mixture of sources is recommended (i.e. 2:1 ratio of glucose and fructose results in a higher rate of carbohydrate oxidation) [8,9]. The carbohydrate can be provided as fluid, food or a carbohydrate gel plus water.

Following exercise, the timing and composition of the post-recovery meal or snack will depend on the intensity and duration of the exercise. For those people who are training daily, then it is more important to ensure they replenish their glycogen stores in time for the next bout of exercise compared to those who are exercising occasionally. The highest rates of glycogen repletion are within the first 2 hours after exercise. 1.0–1.5 g carbohydrate per kg within 30 minutes of exercise and then at 2 hour intervals for up to 6 hours is recommended for the former group [6]. The latter group need to ensure they have sufficient carbohydrate in the following 24 hours, both to replenish glycogen stores and prevent hypoglycaemia. Including some protein in the post-exercise meal may provide amino acids for muscle protein repair.

The ACSM reviewed 25 studies investigating the macronutrient composition of diets in the recovery period [6]. Nine studies reported increased muscle glycogen synthesis with high carbohydrate diets (0.8–1.0 g/kg body weight/hour), two studies reported no significant effect of meal timing on muscle glycogen synthesis, and studies focusing on carbohydrate consumption during recovery periods of 4 hours or more suggest improvements in performance.

Protein requirements and sport

There are many misconceptions about protein requirements and sport. An increasing number of athletes with type 1 diabetes are being recommended to consume a diet low in carbohydrate and high in protein, with some using protein supplements. In the United Kingdom (UK), the current reference nutrient intake (RNI) for protein in adults is 0.75 g/kg/day with a maximum of 1.5 g/kg/day [20], in the United States the recommended daily amount (RDA) is 0.8 g/kg body weight [21] and in Australia it is 0.84 g/kg/day [22].

There is little evidence that healthy adults require additional protein for endurance or resistance exercise, although nitrogen balance studies have shown that endurance athletes and strength athletes, particularly those in the early phase of training when muscle mass is being developed, require more protein than that recommended for the healthy population. The ACSM and the Australian Institute of Sport recommends protein intakes of 1.2–1.7 g/kg /day for endurance and strength trained athletes [6,23].

Proteins, such as whey, casein and soy, are effectively used for the maintenance, repair and synthesis of skeletal muscle in response to training. However, as their use has not been shown to positively affect athletic performance, it is more important to look at the individual's overall diet first [6]. In the majority of cases, the individual is consuming sufficient protein from their diet without needing additional supplements. In the recovery period, providing the carbohydrate intake is sufficient, there is no significant benefit of additional protein intake [6]. Competitive athletes should also be made aware that dietary supplements and ergogenic aids (nutritional products that enhance performance) may be contaminated with banned or nonpermissable substances.

Fluid requirements

Adequate hydration is essential for optimum exercise performance. High sweat losses, if not appropriately replaced, can result in water and electrolyte imbalances. Sweat losses in competitive individuals can be 0.5–2.0 litres/hour and sweat sodium concentration averages 35 mmol/l [19]. A loss of >2% body weight (dehydration) may impair mental/cognitive performance and aerobic exercise performance and dehydration is a risk factor for heat exhaustion and heat stroke. Dehydration (3–5% body weight) does not impair either anaerobic performance or muscular strength. Dehydration and sodium deficits are associated with skeletal muscle cramps and hyponatremia. Fluid consumption that exceeds sweating rate can lead to exercise-associated hyponatremia [19].

Body weight changes can be used to calculate individual fluid replacement needs; 1 kg of body weight loss is equivalent to 1000 ml of sweat loss. The ACSM make the following recommendations [19]:

- Start the exercise hydrated. If needed, prehydration should begin at least 4 hours before exercise by slowly drinking approximately 5–7 ml/kg of fluid. If this does not result in urine production or the urine is still dark, slowly drink 3–5 ml/kg 2 hours before exercise. Consuming drinks containing sodium or salty snacks can stimulate thirst and retain the consumed fluid.
- During exercise, drink to prevent dehydration and excessive changes in electrolyte balance to avoid compromised exercise performance.

If consuming drinks containing carbohydrate, the concentration should not exceed 8%, as high concentrations will reduce gastric emptying
- After exercise, if time permits, consuming normal meals and drinks will replace fluid and electrolyte losses. If dehydrated, aim for 1.5 l per kg weight loss. Water is not the ideal choice in this case and drinks such as sports drinks providing sodium are preferable [30]. As sports drinks contain carbohydrate, these may also prevent hypoglycaemia [7].
- Alcohol can act as a diuretic and should only be consumed in moderation, especially during the post exercise period when rehydration is needed and there is risk of exercise- induced hypoglycaemia.

Sports drinks

It is recommended that these contain approximately 20 mmol/l of sodium, 2–5 mmol/l potassium and 5–10% carbohydrate [19]. The need for these will depend on the intensity, duration of exercise and weather conditions. Caution is needed in type 1 diabetes because of the effect on blood glucose concentration. Consuming 150–200 ml of an isotonic sports drink, containing 6–8 g/100ml of carbohydrate, every 15–20 minutes will provide 30–60 g of carbohydrate and 450–800 ml /hour of fluid.

Summary

Managing type 1 diabetes with sport and exercise is challenging. Cooperation between the athlete with diabetes, the physician and dietitian is important in enabling the person with diabetes to exercise safely and to the best of their ability in their chosen sport.

3.5.3 Alcohol

Alcohol in moderate amounts can be enjoyed safely by most people with type 1 diabetes. Moderate intakes (1–2 units per day) confer similar benefits for people with diabetes, in terms of cardiovascular risk reduction and all-cause mortality, as for those without diabetes [24]. Alcohol can cause hypoglycaemia even with the ingestion of food [25], at relatively low levels and up to 12 hours after ingestion [26] by inhibiting gluconeogenesis and lipolysis, impairing glucose counter-regulation and blunting hypoglycaemic awareness.

A systematic review concluded that ingestion of moderate amounts of alcohol does not have an acute effect on glycaemic control [25]. A study using continuous glucose monitoring in adolescents after moderately heavy drinking (mean 9 drinks for males and 6.3 drinks for females) found that, compared to the same period when no alcohol was consumed, less time was spent with low glucose values but there was greater variation in the blood glucose levels [26]. The authors concluded that the higher blood glucose readings could be attributed to the individuals having a meal before going out and a snack before bed, most of the drinks were pre-mixed spirits and sweetened carbonated beverages and the majority of the study group did little activity.

Guidelines for alcohol consumption [24]

- Alcohol in moderate amounts can be enjoyed safely by most people with type 1 diabetes.
- The recommendations are no more than 2–3 units/day for women, 3–4 units per day for men with a maximum of 14 and 21 units per week, respectively.
- At higher intakes there is an increased risk of liver problems, reduced fertility, hypertension, some cancers and cardiovascular disease.
- Hypoglycaemia is a risk with alcohol consumption in people with type 1 diabetes and although there is no evidence for the most effective treatment to prevent it, a reduction in insulin dose, or additional carbohydrate or a combination of these is recommended.
- Alcohol should be avoided during pregnancy and in some medical conditions, for example hypertension, hypertryglyceridaemia, some neuropathies and retinopathy.

3.5.4 Recreational and prescription drug use

Little is known about the effects of recreational drug use in people with type 1 diabetes. It has been reported that drug use may coexist with other high risk behaviours, may indicate poor social support and a chaotic lifestyle [33].

One review reported lifetime prevalence of drug use was 5–25% in adolescents aged 12–20 years and 29% in young adults aged 16–30 years [27]. Two anonymous surveys reported 29–77% of respondents had used drugs at least once, 47% within the last year and 15–68% were poly-drug users [29,33]. Cannabis and stimulants were the most popular drugs used. In another study in which young adults presenting with DKA were questioned, 50% admitted to using drugs within the previous 48 hours, including cannabis, ecstasy, ketamine, benzodiazepines and heroin. 37% were poly-drug users [28].

In a report from the Yorkshire register of diabetes in children and young adults reporting on the causes of death in subjects diagnosed with type 1 diabetes before the age of 29 years, 16% of all deaths were related to drug misuse, including insulin, analgesics and opiates, with the highest number in the 20–29 year old age group [31]. The authors concluded that there may be an emerging trend for young people with type 1 diabetes to misuse recreational and prescription drugs.

Some drugs have effects including hallucinations, depression and dissociation. Little is known about the effects on glycaemia and metabolic complications in type 1 diabetes although HbA1c is reported to be higher in drug users [33]. This may be related to an effect on self-care behaviours, including blood testing, insulin administration and food intake, as many people with type 1 diabetes do not check blood glucose concentration before drug use, do not alter their insulin dose or omit insulin altogether [33]. Complications of the use of substances by people with type 1 diabetes are hyperglycaemia (particularly cannabis), DKA (from ketamine, opioids, e.g. heroin and cocaine), hyponatremia (particularly ecstasy), hyperglycaemic hyperosmolar state (cocaine), seizures and death [27].

Management should focus on harm minimisation rather than advocating abstinence, including alternative insulin regimens for social weekends and action plans based on blood glucose and ketones recorded during the night [27], eating low glycaemic index foods, wearing medic alert identification and blood glucose testing before and after drug use [29]. Young people who are leaving home to attend a university or college in another town should have a formal re-education session to remind them about the risks of hypoglycaemia and the potentially adverse effects of alcohol and drugs on diabetes control [32].

Key points

- People with type 1 diabetes can safely exercise, although management of blood glucose levels, food intake and insulin is key.
- Frequent blood glucose monitoring is recommended.
- Hypoglycaemia is common and can be managed with a combination of increased carbohydrate and reduced insulin dose.
- Adequate hydration is important during exercise.
- Alcohol can be consumed in moderation by people with type 1 diabetes; guidelines do not differ from those for the general public.
- Alcohol increases the risk of hypoglycaemia.
- Recreational drugs are used by people with type 1 diabetes and may interfere with self-care behaviours.

References

1. American Diabetes Association. Physical activity/exercise and diabetes mellitus. Position statement. *Diabetes Care* 2004; **27**: S58–S62.
2. Nagi D, Gallen I. ABCD position statement on physical activity and exercise in diabetes. *Practical Diabetes Int* 2010; **27**(4): 158–163
3. Grimm JJ. Exercise in type 1 diabetes. In Nagi D (ed.) *Exercise and Sport in Diabetes*, 2nd edn. London: John Wiley & Sons Ltd, 2005, pp. 25–43.
4. Williams C. Physiological responses to exercise. In Nagi D (ed.) *Exercise and Sport in Diabetes*, 2nd edn. London: John Wiley & Sons Ltd, 2005, pp.1–24.
5. Colberg SR (ed.) Diabetic Athlete's Handbook. Champaign, IL: Human Kinetics, 2009.
6. American Dietetic Association, Dietitians of Canada. Nutrition and athletic performance: joint position statement. *Med Sci Sports Exercise* 2009; **41**(3): 709–731.
7. Perry E, Gallen IW. Guidelines on the current best practice for the management of type 1 diabetes, sport and exercise. *Practical Diabetes Int* 2009; **26**(3): 116–123.
8. Gallen IW, Hume C, Lumb A. Fuelling the athlete with type 1 diabetes. *Diabetes Obes Metabolism* 2011; **13**: 130–136.
9. Jeukendrup A, Williams C. Carbohydrate. In Lanham-New SA, Stear SJ, Shirreffs SM, Collins AL (eds) on behalf of the Nutrition Society. Sport and Exercise Nutrition. Chichester: Wiley–Blackwell, 2011, pp. 31–40.
10. American College of Sports Medicine and the American Heart Association. Physical activity and public health: updated recommendation. *Med Sci Sports Exercise* 2007; **39**(8): 1423–1434.
11. Chisholm J, Kilbride L, Charlton J, McKnight J. Acute effects of weight training on glycaemia in type 1 diabetes. *Practical Diabetes* 2012; **294**(4): 155–159.
12. Rabasa-Lhoret R, Bourque J, Ducros F, Chiasson J-L. Guidelines for premeal insulin dose reduction for post-prandial exercise of different intensities and durations in type 1 diabetic subjects treated intensively with a basal-bolus insulin regimen. *Diabetes Care* 2001; **24**(4): 625–630.
13. Bracken RM, West DJ, Stephens JW, Kilduff LP, Luzio S, Bain SC. Impact of pre-exercise rapid-acting insulin reductions on ketogenesis following running in type 1 diabetes. *Diabet Med* 2011; **28**: 218–222.
14. Lumb AN, Gallen I. Diabetes management for intense exercise. *Curr Opin Endocrinol Diabetes Obes* 2009; **16**: 150–155.
15. Grimm JJ, Ybarra J, Berne C, Muchnick S, Golay A. A new table for the prevention of hypoglycaemia during physical activity in type 1 diabetic patients. *Diabetes Metab* 2004; **30**: 465–470.
16. Francescato MP, Geat M, Simonetta S, Stupar G, Noacco C, Cattin L. Carbohydrate requirement and insulin concentration during moderate exercise in type 1 diabetic patients. *Metabolism* 2004; **53**(9): 1126–1130.
17. Bussau V, Ferreira LD, Jones TW, Fournier PA. The 10-s maximal sprint. A novel approach to counter an exercise-mediated fall in glycaemia in individuals with type 1 diabetes. *Diabetes Care* 2006; **29**(3): 601–606.
18. Iscoe KE, Riddell MC. Continuous moderate-intensity exercise with or without intermittent high-intensity

work: effects on acute and late glycaemia in athletes with type 1 diabetes mellitus. *Diabet Med* 2011; **28**: 824–832.

19. American College of Sports Medicine. Position Stand. Exercise and fluid replacement. *Med Sci Sports Exercise* 2007; **39**(2): 377–390.

20. Department of Health Report on Health and Social subjects 41. Dietary reference values for food, energy, and nutrients for the United Kingdom. London: TSO (The Stationery Office), 1991.

21. United States Department of Health and Human Services and United States Department of Agriculture. Dietary guidelines for Americans. Washington, DC: US Government Printing Office, 1991.

22. National Health and Medical Research Council. Nutrient reference values for Australia and New Zealand. https://www.nhmrc.gov.au/_files_nhmrc/publications/attachments/n35.pdf. Accessed 9 June 2015

23. Burke L, Deakin V (eds). Clinical Sports Nutrition, 3rd edn. McGraw-Hill Australia Pty Ltd, 2006.

24. Diabetes UK Nutrition Working Group. Evidence-based nutrition guidelines for the prevention and management of diabetes. *Diabet Med* 2011; **28**(11): 1282–1288.

25. Howard AA, Arnsten J, Gourevitch MN. Effect of alcohol consumption on diabetes mellitus: a systematic review. *Ann Intern Med* 2004; **140**: 211–219.

26. Ismail D, Gebert R, Vuillermin PJ, Fraser L, McDonnell M, Donath SM, et al. Social consumption of alcohol in adolescents with type 1 diabetes is associated with increased glucose lability but not hypoglycaemia. *Diabet Med* 2006; **23**: 830–833.

27. Lee P, Greenfield JR, Campbell LV. Managing young people with type 1 diabetes in a 'rave' new world: metabolic complications of substance abuse in type 1 diabetes. *Diabet Med* 2009; **26**: 328–333.

28. Lee P, Greenfield JR, Campbell LV. "Mind the gap" when managing ketoacidosis in type 1 diabetes. *Diabetes Care* 2008; **31**(7): e58.

29. Ng RSH, Darko DA, Hillson RM. Street drug use among patients with type 1 diabetes in the UK. *Diab Med* 2003; **21**: 295–296.

30. Shirreffs SM. Fluids and electrolytes. In: Lanham-New SA, Stear SJ, Shirreffs SM, Collins AL (eds) on behalf of the Nutrition Society. *Sport and Exercise Nutrition*. Chichester: Wiley-Blackwell, 2011, pp. 59–65.

31. Feltbower RG, Bodansky HJ, Patterson CC, Parslow RC, Stephenson CR, Reynolds C, et al. Acute complications and drug misuse are important causes of death for children and young adults with type 1 diabetes. *Diabetes Care* 2008; **31**: 922–926.

32. Strachan MWJ, MacCuish AC, Frier BM. The care of students with insulin-treated diabetes mellitus living in university accommodation: scope for improvement? *Diabet Med* 2000; **17**: 70–73.

33. Lee P, Greenfield JR, Gilbert K, Campbell LV. Recreational drug use in type 1 diabetes: an invisible accomplice to poor glycaemic control? *Intern Med J* 2012; **42**(2): 198–202.

Useful websites

www.runsweet.com particularly useful for athletes with diabetes

www.sportsdietitians.org.uk

SECTION 4

Type 2 diabetes

Chapter 4.1

Epidemiology, aetiology and pathogenesis of type 2 diabetes

David R. Matthews

University of Oxford, Oxford Centre for Diabetes, Endocrinology and Metabolism, Oxford, UK

4.1.1 Epidemiology

Type 2 diabetes is now so widespread and so frequently found that it is truly pandemic. It is not a disease confined either to higher income or to low and middle-income countries, although the emerging nations seem especially susceptible [1]. This was not the case in the 1950s, but it is now. Sixty years ago, type 2 diabetes had a prevalence of less than 1% in almost all countries of the world, and indeed in some communities, for example in many parts of Africa, it was scarcely found at all [2].

The Pima Indian population of Arizona [3] attracted attention in the 1970s because the Pimas had been a fit hunter-gatherer nation overtaken by Westernisation. Their diet became high in fat, sugar and energy dense food, and their daily physical activity plummeted. This had a disastrous effect on their health, with progressive obesity and diabetes found in a large proportion of the population. It was then noted that this was not an isolated finding and the Polynesian populations – and notably that of Nauru – had a similar propensity [4]. At the time this seemed to be fascinating epidemiology about 'special' communities. But the Pima and Micronesian finding was soon to be replicated globally. As overweight and obesity became widespread, so in its wake came type 2 diabetes. In the subsequent decades the low prevalence of type 2 diabetes increased in the developed world: it is now 4% in the United Kingdom (UK) [5] and well in excess of 8% in most States of the United States (US) [6]. In the emergent economies prevalences range up to 50% (urban elderly) of the population [7]. In stark terms, this means that in the UK, 1 in 25 adults has diabetes, while in the US the figure is 1 in 12. The problem is even greater in the developing economies, with diabetes being found in 1 in 5 adults [1]. The increasing prevalence of type 2 diabetes is not restricted to adults; there is evidence that the incidence in children and young adults has increased in tandem with obesity. Incidence rates are now estimated to be 1–51/1000 depending on ethnic group, with the highest rates seen in Native American Indian, Hispanic, Black and South Asian communities [8].

The International Diabetes Federation (IDF) estimate that there are now 382 million people worldwide with diabetes, with estimates of 592 million by 2035 [1] (Figure 4.1.1).

The magnitude of the problem is so great that it is going to have profound economic consequences. Diabetes is associated with complications of blindness, renal failure, coronary artery disease, amputations and stroke. But it is also a chronic disease, with pathological processes unfolding over decades. As complications accumulate in any individual, the healthcare costs escalate, quality of life declines and capacity to work attenuates.

Advanced Nutrition and Dietetics in Diabetes, First Edition. Edited by Louise Goff and Pamela Dyson.
© 2016 John Wiley & Sons, Ltd. Published 2016 by John Wiley & Sons, Ltd.

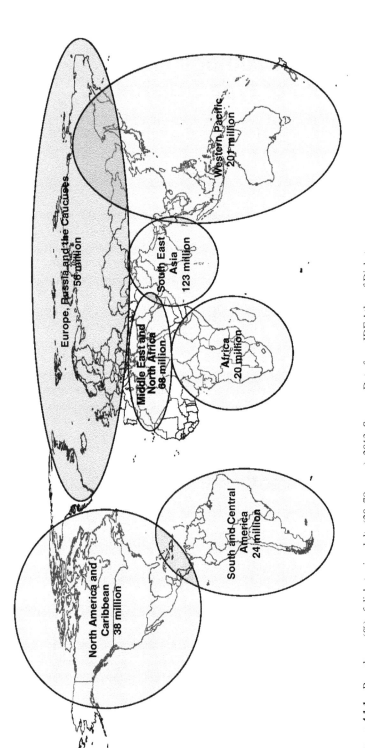

Figure 4.1.1 Prevalence (%) of diabetes in adults (20–79 years), 2013. Source: Data from IDF Atlas of Diabetes

4.1.2 Aetiology and pathogenesis

The aetiology (or cause) of type 2 diabetes is broadly understood, although the details of the pathological processes remain obscure. There are four mechanisms that can be regarded as having an influence on the emergence of the disease: genes, beta-cell failure, insulin resistance and the environment.

Genetic influences on type 2 diabetes

There are important genes causing diabetes, though none of them are responsible for the pandemic aspect or the huge increase in prevalence seen over the past few years. Genetic make-up cannot change in one generation – 30 years – although that is the time-frame for the emergence of type 2 diabetes as the most significant of all the non-communicable diseases.

There are certain sub-types of diabetes that appear early in life, and look similar to type 2 diabetes. These conditions have retained the old terminology of 'maturity onset diabetes' with the added phrase 'of the young', known by the acronym MODY. MODY, as a subset of type 2 diabetes, is important as treatment is dictated by the specific genetic mutation [9]. The condition is caused by single gene autosomal dominant mutation and gives rise to specific defects that are identifiable. MODY presents clinically as type 2 diabetes diagnosed in people who typically have early onset diabetes that is not insulin dependent, and where there is a strong family history of diabetes (from previous generations carrying the gene) [10]. Often the diagnosis can be deduced from a multi-generation family tree showing the affected members – the defect genes are autosomal (i.e. not-sex-linked) dominant, so there is 50% chance of transmission to offspring. There are several identified categories where the effect of the gene has been identified, and now these are generally identified with a postscript label to indicate the site of the pathology e.g. MODY glucokinase, MODY HNF1α [11]. MODY glucokinase itself is widely recognised as a problem that needs explicit diagnosis, this is the category where there is a

nonsense or missense mutation of the glucokinase gene and at least 21 of these have been identified [12]. Glucokinase is the enzyme sensor for glucose at the insulin-producing beta-cell. With half the coding for the correct enzyme synthesis missing there is only half the usual enzyme activity present. Reduction of activity leads to raised plasma glucose since there is insufficient insulin secretion, and small doses of sulfonylurea drugs can be all the treatment that is required [13]. This condition is not associated with progressive loss of beta-cell function. MODY has also been important as the clear proof that diabetes is heterogeneous. Even within the narrow category of the MODY defects, each family has its own particular mutation.

More germane to diabetes as a whole, there has been much research into genes for the common condition. This research over two decades has focused on the idea of genome-wide association studies (GWAS) to attempt to identify which genes were associated with the appearance of diabetes, and which were not. This search led to the recognition of a large number of genes found more often in those with diabetes than in those without [14]. Almost all of the genes seemed to be linked to aspects of beta-cell function though two, interestingly, were not. These were a PPARγ defect (a nuclear receptor involved in insulin resistance) and FTO, a gene linked with body weight. Subjects with homozygous FTO defects were likely to be 3 kg heavier than the control population [15].

Genes have been shown to be associated with diabetes by effects that are monogenic (single gene gives identified defect), pleotrophic (gene has lots of effects that can give clinical tendencies) or polygenic (many genes contribute). Combinatorial mathematics may show that clusters of small propensity genes contribute to the clinical syndrome, but such findings are unlikely to allow predictive genetic identification of those at risk. Nor are slightly increased genetic propensities likely to be an explanation of our current pandemic, although these may be an explanation for some aspects of high national or race-specific tendencies. Even if this were to be true, it has yet to be elucidated and, as yet, no Micronesian or Pima genes have been identified, even as combinatorial risks.

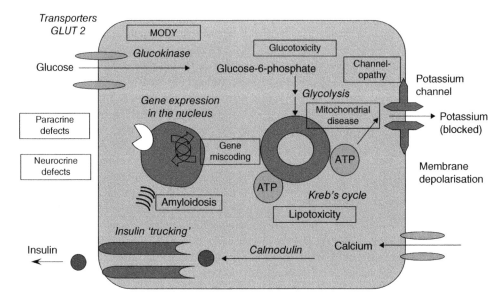

Figure 4.1.2 Dynamic systems in the beta-cell. The boxed items are pathological mechanisms variously proposed to explain the beta-cell dysfunction

Beta-cell failure

All diabetes is associated with some level of beta-cell deficiency. This can be absolute, as in the case of type 1 diabetes where auto-immune destruction of the beta-cells causes the near-total loss of insulin secretory capacity, or it can be partial, where gradual failure of secretion leads to slowly progressive hyperglycaemia. The understanding of beta-cell failure has been crucial in the development of new drugs and therapies for diabetes. The molecular mechanism within the beta-cell is understood in considerable detail (Figure 4.1.2). Metabolism of glucose is the crucial engine producing high energy adenosine triphosphate (ATP), and ATP, in turn, switches the electrical activity of the cell and mobilises the trucking of insulin to the vesicles that merge with the cell membrane to allow insulin release. Mechanisms are known to modulate the early signal, to change the metabolism, to alter the electrical activating channels, to activate modulating receptors and to alter the activity of other cells in the islets of Langerhans, of which beta-cells are a component part.

Yet despite all this understanding, the main aetiological process – that of declining beta-cell function – remains elusive. Some authors have maintained that beta-cell mass declines in type 2 diabetes, but this is disputed, and does not sit well with the observations of recovery of function demonstrated in a wide variety of therapeutic approaches [16]. In particular, the observation that diabetes resolves rapidly after some bariatric bypass surgery suggests that beta-cell function can be reactivated over very short periods of time [17], and this effect has been replicated in studies using very low calorie liquid diets [18]. The challenge is to find that mechanism.

Beta-cell failure can be addressed in a variety of directed therapies. Sulfonylurea drugs mimic ATP in blocking so-called Kir channels (inwardly rectifying potassium channels), and cause cell depolarisation and insulin secretion. Glucagon-like peptide-1 (GLP-1) agonists mimic the endocrine signal that is triggered by food in the gut, and dipepdidyl peptidase 4 (DPP4) inhibitors block the enzymes that destroy the naturally occurring GLP-1.

Insulin resistance

Insulin resistance (IR) was at one time thought to be the primary aetiology of diabetes [19]. It was characterised by the demonstration that insulin concentrations in early type 2 diabetes were high, rather than low, although since the glucose is raised they are relatively low. Relatively, here, means that normal subjects whose blood glucose is raised to mimic that found in diabetes have even higher insulin concentrations. Infusing insulin is a better demonstration of the IR phenomenon, where it can be demonstrated, in control and diabetes subjects with identical plasma concentrations of insulin, that the control subjects clear glucose faster and in greater amount than the diabetes patients.

Insulin resistance is universally found in diabetic states – and more so in type 2 diabetes than in type 1. But enthusiasm for thinking that it was central to the aetiopathology of diabetes has waned over the years. The reason is that IR is found in many non-diabetic states, of which the most common is obesity. Yet obesity can persist for many years without diabetes supervening, so diabetes is by no means an inevitable sequel, but obesity is a major risk. This leaves the question of whether IR in diabetes is a cause, or just an associated finding. On the basis that it might be a cause, two decades ago the pharmaceutical companies searched for agents that might reduce IR, and produced agonists of identified IR-associated nuclear receptors called peroxisome proliferator-activated receptors gamma (PPARγ) [20]. The thiazolidinedione (TZD) drugs, troglitazone, rosiglitazone and pioglitazone, were identified as high affinity ligands for these receptors. Troglitazone emerged, in clinical practice, to be hepatotoxic [21], and rosiglitazone increased the likelihood of cardiac failure without a proven benefit on longevity or cardiovascular disease [22]. Both drugs were discontinued. Pioglitazone continues to be prescribed and certainly reduces IR (and has good trial outcomes in cardiovascular disease [23]), but the chequered history of the PPARγ agonists reopened the debate as to whether modulating IR is wise.

The toxic environment

One important aspect of any epidemic is the recognition that there must be environmental as well as genetic aetiology, and new triggers to explain the increase in caseload. Although genes may alter population susceptibilities, and individual risks may have a genetic component, the epidemic causation will always be based on exposure to transmittable, toxic or environmental pathogens. A second important feature relates to prevention. If the problem did not exist 60 years ago and it now does, it also follows that we could potentially move back to the pre-existing prevalence if the pathophysiology can be identified and risk factors eliminated or minimised.

The most apparent risk of diabetes is overweight and obesity. Figure 4.1.2 shows the extent to which obesity and the single most important gene affecting obesity (FTO) contribute to the risk of getting diabetes. It is immediately apparent that environment-induced obesity is the overwhelming risk factor, and the logical conclusion is that we need to address the obesity epidemic – the prodrome to type 2 diabetes.

The size of the epidemic increase over the last four decades has been startling in its geographical extent and unprecedented in its scale. Developed and developing countries have been afflicted, though the greatest extent of the problem is seem in the lower and middle income countries. For example, although the USA now has in excess of 9% of its adult population with type 2 diabetes (1 in 11 of all its adults), Sri Lanka has over twice the prevalence with 18.9% of the population afflicted [24].

This pandemic has such grave consequences that it has been likened to the Black Death of the 14th century [25]. The speed and the characteristics of the epidemic strongly suggest a change in environment and/or behaviour that has supervened in the last half century. This environment has been termed the 'toxic environment' and is associated with the increasing availability of energy-dense foods and low levels of physical activity [26]. The role of individual responsibility has long been debated, and what populations eat and do may, at a micro level, be a matter of personal choice, but at an environmental and national level are clearly matters of food availability, appropriate taxation, cost and environment encouragement or discouragement for physical activity [27].

The question then arises as to whether the epidemic could be addressed by case-finding of

- Food labelling – cost to
  public purse is ZERO

- Eating less – the cost to the
  individual is NEGATIVE

- Using stairs instead of lifts/
  walking to work rather than
  using a car – the cost is
  NEGATIVE and it saves the
  planet's resources

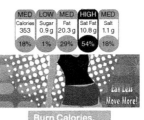
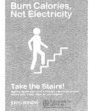

Figure 4.1.3 Community interventions can be cost saving. Labelling, advertising and prompts all help to reduce the risks of diabetes

those at highest risk. Such individuals (middle-aged, overweight, with a family history of diabetes and sedentary lifestyle) are certainly in need of advice and help, but by the time they have become middle-aged, overweight and sedentary the opportunity for health persisting into old age may have been lost. Since diabetes is now so common, a whole community approach to prevention should be adopted [28]. Prevention of diabetes will involve a significant shift in managing the toxic environment, and multiple stakeholder interventions are needed to address it. In practice this means community interventions for health [29] where permutations of many encouragements to a better living environment can be advocated and enacted. Such activity could, for example include:

Taxation of high sugar drinks
Subsidy (from such taxation) for healthy foods
Limitation of advertising unhealthy food to
  children
Limiting energy content of snacks at cinemas,
  sports events and public arenas
Legislation for healthy meals at schools
Labelling of energy in readable text on all food-
  stuffs
Labelling of energy content in restaurants and
  other food outlets
Making healthy-choice literature widely
  available

Health education for parents about effects of
  obesity on their children
Promoting physical activity
Campaigning against closure of playing fields
  and encouraging schools to embed physical
  activity in their curriculum
Using prompts to encourage the use of stairs
Encouraging architects to design new public
  buildings with accessible stairs to all floors.

These steps are seen as an encouragement to make the healthy choice the easy choice by modifying the environment to reduce obesity and improve the health of all, whether they are at risk of diabetes or not. Case-finding for those at risk of diabetes is inappropriate when the whole of society is exposed to the predisposing unhealthy choices. Nor should interventions be regarded as necessarily being expensive, Figure 4.1.3 demonstrates cost-savings for various interventions.

4.1.3 Conclusion

In conclusion, type 2 diabetes is caused at the molecular and physiological level by genes, by beta-cell failure and by insulin resistance. But much more importantly, it is caused by our world pandemic of obesity, in turn predicated on low levels of physical activity and consuming too much energy. Community interventions to reduce risk and improve health at the population level are needed.

Key points

- The prevalence of type 2 diabetes is increasing around the world.
- Type 2 diabetes is associated with modifiable lifestyle factors including obesity, physical inactivity and unhealthy diets.
- It most commonly diagnosed in adults and the elderly, but can occur at any age.
- Genetic factors, beta-cell failure, insulin resistance and the toxic environment all contribute to the aetiology of type 2 diabetes.

References

1. International Diabetes Federation. Diabetes Atlas, 6th edn. Brussels, Belgium: IDF, 2013. Available from: http://www.idf.org/diabetesatlas.

2. Herman WH, Zimmet P. Type 2 diabetes: an epidemic requiring global attention and urgent action. *Diabetes Care* 2012; **35**(5): 943–944.

3. Bennett PH, Burch TA, Miller M. Diabetes mellitus in American (Pima) Indians. *Lancet* 1971; **2**(7716): 125–128.

4. King H, Zimmet P, Raper LR, Balkau B. The natural history of impaired glucose tolerance in the Micronesian population of Nauru: a six-year follow-up study. *Diabetologia* 1984; **26**(1): 39–43.

5. Morgan CL, Peters JR, Currie CJ. The changing prevalence of diagnosed diabetes and its associated vascular complications in a large region of the UK. *Diabet Med* 2010; **27**(6): 673–678.

6. Centers for Disease Control and Prevention: National Diabetes Surveillance System. Available online at: http://www.cdc.gov/diabetes/statistics/index.htm., 2010.

7. Katulanda P, Sheriff MH, Matthews DR. The diabetes epidemic in Sri Lanka - a growing problem. *Ceylon Med J* 2006; **51**(1): 26–28.

8. Pulgaron ER, Delamater AM. Obesity and type 2 diabetes in children: epidemiology and treatment. *Curr Diab Rep* 2014; **14**(8): 508.

9. Hattersley A. Can molecular genetics help in the clinic? *Diabet Med* 1999; **16**(9): 788–791

10. Velho G, Robert JJ. Maturity-onset diabetes of the young (MODY): genetic and clinical characteristics. *Horm Res* 2002; **57**(Suppl. 1): 29–33.

11. Winckler W, Weedon MN, Graham RR, McCarroll SA, Purcell S, Almgren P, et al. Evaluation of common variants in the six known maturity-onset diabetes of the young (MODY) genes for association with type 2 diabetes. *Diabetes* 2007; **56**(3): 685–693.

12. Thomson KL, Gloyn AL, Colclough K, Batten M, Allen LI, Beards F, et al. Identification of 21 novel glucokinase (GCK) mutations in UK and European Caucasians with maturity-onset diabetes of the young (MODY). *Hum Mutat* 2003; **22**(5): 417.

13. Hattersley AT. Molecular genetics goes to the diabetes clinic. *Clin Med* 2005; **5**(5): 476–481.

14. Morris AP, Voight BF, Teslovich TM, Ferreira T, Segré AV, Steinthorsdottir V, et al. Large-scale association analysis provides insights into the genetic architecture and pathophysiology of type 2 diabetes. *Nat Genet* 2012; **44**(9): 981–990.

15. Frayling TM, Timpson NJ, Weedon MN, Zeggini E, Freathy RM, Lindgren CM, et al. A common variant in the FTO gene is associated with body mass index and predisposes to childhood and adult obesity. *Science* 2007; **316**(5826): 889–894.

16. Meier JJ, Bonadonna RC. Role of reduced β-cell mass versus impaired β-cell function in the pathogenesis of type 2 diabetes. *Diabetes Care* 2013; **36** (Suppl. 2): S113–S119.

17. Salehi M, D'Alessio DA. Going with the flow: adaptation of β-cell function to glucose fluxes after bariatric surgery. *Diabetes* 2013; **62**(11): 3671–3673.

18. Lim EL, Hollingsworth KG, Aribisala BS, Chen MJ, Mathers JC, Taylor R. Reversal of type 2 diabetes: normalisation of beta cell function in association with decreased pancreas and liver triacylglycerol. *Diabetologia* 2011; **54**(10): 2506–2514.

19. Himsworth H, Kerr R. Insulin-sensitive and insulin insensitive types of diabetes mellitus. *Cin Sci* 1939; **4**: 119–152.

20. Sakamoto J, Kimura H, Moriyama S, Odaka H, Momose Y, Sugiyama Y, et al. Activation of human peroxisome proliferator-activated receptor (PPAR) subtypes by pioglitazone. *Biochem Biophys Res Commun* 2000; **278**(3): 704–711.

21. Lee WM. Drug-induced hepatotoxicity. *N Engl J Med* 2003; **349**(5): 474–485.

22. Kung J, Henry RR. Thiazolidinedione safety. *Expert Opin Drug Saf* 2012; **11**(4): 565–579.

23. Dormandy JA, Charbonnel B, Eckland DJ, Erdmann E, Massi-Benedetti M, Moules IK, et al. Secondary prevention of macrovascular events in patients with type 2 diabetes in the PROactive Study (PROspective pioglitAzone Clinical Trial In macroVascular Events): a randomised controlled trial. *Lancet* 2005; **366**(9493): 1279–1289.

24. Katulanda P, Constantine GR, Mahesh JG, Sheriff R, Seneviratne RD, Wijeratne S, et al. Prevalence and projections of diabetes and pre-diabetes in adults in Sri Lanka–Sri Lanka Diabetes, Cardiovascular Study (SLDCS). *Diabet Med* 2008; **9**: 1062–1069.

25. Matthews DR, Matthews PC. Banting Memorial Lecture 2010. Type 2 diabetes as an 'infectious' disease: is this the Black Death of the 21st century? *Diabet Med* 2011; **28**(1): 2–9.

26. Wadden TA, Brownell KD, Foster GD, Obesity: responding to the global epidemic. *J Consult Clin Psychol* 2002; **70**(3): 510–525.

27. Brownell KD, Kersh R, Ludwig DS, Post RC, Puhl RM, Schwartz MB, et al. Personal responsibility and obesity: a constructive approach to a controversial issue. *Health Affairs* 2010; **29**(3): 379–387.

28. World Health Organization. Global action plan for the prevention and control of noncommunicable diseases 2013–2020. Geneva: WHO, 2012.

29. O'Connor Duffany K, Finegood D, Matthews DR, McKee M, Venkat Narayan KM, Puska P, et al. Community Interventions for Health (CIH): A novel approach to tackling the worldwide epidemic of chronic diseases, *CVD Prev Control* 2011; **6**(2): 47–56.

Chapter 4.2

Clinical management of hyperglycaemia in type 2 diabetes

David R. Matthews

University of Oxford, Oxford Centre for Diabetes, Endocrinology and Metabolism, Oxford, UK

4.2.1 Introduction

Type 2 diabetes is a multisystem disease. It often begins insidiously without any overt symptoms, but can progress to devastating clinical problems related to high glucose levels and tissue damage to both large and small blood vessels. These latter are designated macrovascular disease and microvascular disease, respectively, and each have three broad categories of pathology (see Table 4.2.1)

4.2.2 Multiple-risk-factor approach to treatment

Pharmacological management of type 2 diabetes involves agents that treat hyperglycaemia (anti-hyperglycaemic agents) and agents that are specifically directed to complications. It is known, for example, that lowering cholesterol with statins and treating hypertension are fundamental adjuncts to glycaemic management in diabetes [1]. Smoking, with or without diabetes, kills 50% of those who indulge [2]. Here, however, only the current approaches to the treatment of glycaemia are considered.

4.2.3 Treatment of hyperglycaemia

The treatment of hyperglycaemia in diabetes can be addressed by both lifestyle adjustments and a wide array of available pharmacological agents. A number of guidelines have been produced [3–5], though here we refer primarily to the International ADA/EASD position statement [6]. The primary thrust of this paper was in the direction of patient-centred care – by which is meant that the choice of agent for any individual is dependent on a wide array of characteristics of that patient, including, for example, age, duration of diabetes and capacity for self-care. These are illustrated in Figure 4.2.1, where an example line has been drawn on each characteristic to indicate that there is not usually a 'right' answer to the glycaemic goal, and pragmatic adjustment is based on such criteria. Figure 4.2.2 illustrates the various treatment alogrithms for individuals with type 2 diabetes.

Glycaemic targets are discussed widely within the academic and clinical community, and these are most commonly assessed as HbA1c values (a useful measure of average glycaemic exposure). Low targets (e.g. 6.0–6.5% [42–48 mmol/mol]) might be considered in selected patients where no

Advanced Nutrition and Dietetics in Diabetes, First Edition. Edited by Louise Goff and Pamela Dyson.
© 2016 John Wiley & Sons, Ltd. Published 2016 by John Wiley & Sons, Ltd.

Table 4.2.1 Type 2 diabetes. The symptoms and conditions that need preventing, addressing and, if necessary, treating

Early symptoms (entirely reversible on treatment)	Related to hyperglycaemia	Excess urine (polyuria), often disturbing rest at night (nocturia) Thirst Tiredness Susceptibility to infection (urinary tract, thrush)
Late symptoms (essentially irreversible, though treatable)	Related to blood vessel disease	Macrovascular disease Microvascular disease
	Macrovascular disease	
	Coronary artery disease	Angina, myocardial infarction
	Cerebro-vascular disease	Stroke, ischaemic attacks
	Peripheral vascular disease	Claudication (pain in the legs with walking) Foot ulceration
	Microvascular disease	
	Retinopathy	Eye disease, and potential blindness
	Neuropathy	Loss of sensation in the feet and then susceptible to foot ulceration and amputation
	Nephropathy	Renal failure, anaemia

comorbidities exist and when this can be achieved without significant hypoglycaemia [6]. By contrast, less stringent HbA1c goals (e.g. 7.5–8.0% [58–64 mmol/mol]) are appropriate for patients with a history of severe hypoglycaemia, and/or comorbid conditions. It is clear from the evidence that lower glycaemia prevents the *development* of complications in both type 1 and type 2 diabetes [7,8]. But once complications have developed, lowering glycaemia to tight control targets may well increase the overall mortality [9].

Hyperglycaemia contributes unequivocally to the risk of complications. This has been demonstrated in both type 1 and type 2 diabetes, and the evidence is strongly in favour of good control early in the disease process [10,11]. In type 2 diabetes this is for both microvascular and macrovascular disease [12].

Type 2 diabetes is characterised by progressive failure of the insulin-producing cells in the islets of the pancreas (β-cells) [13]. This means that therapeutically there needs to be regular surveillance of the effects of any agent, and often a necessity of combining agents in established diabetes [14].

Lifestyle approaches

Type 2 diabetes is often related to becoming overweight, and this in turn is consequent on excess energy intake (usually over many years) and low physical activity. Both of these precipitating features can be addressed, and very low calorie diets may temporarily abolish hyperglycaemia altogether [15], though the sustainability of such an approach has yet to be tested. Ultimately, it is patients who make the final decisions regarding their lifestyle choices, but consistent encouragement by healthcare professionals can pay dividends in terms of the intensity of other treatment likely to be needed. Overweight and obesity are strongly related to insulin resistance (where insulin function is reduced) [16], and reversing any of this with weight loss is advantageous.

Weight reduction in people with type 2 diabetes, achieved through dietary means alone or with adjunctive medical or surgical intervention, improves glycaemic control and other cardiovascular risk factors [17,18]. Modest weight loss

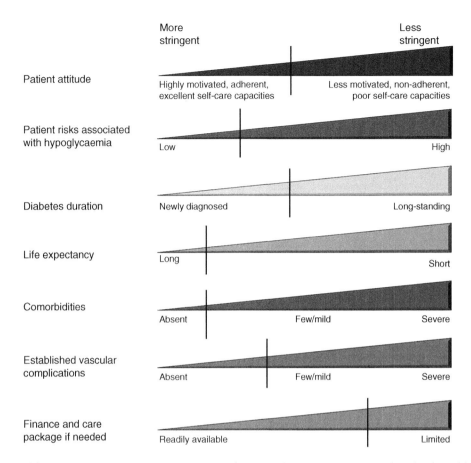

Figure 4.2.1 Glycaemic goals need to be personalised for each patient. A young, highly motivated patient with no comorbidity should have stringent goals. By contrast, an elderly patient with low life expectancy and poor health-care support may need less stringent control. The lines on each triangle show how each of these characteristics may have an influence on where the final target is set (Source: Adapted from Inzucchi, 2012 [6])

(5–10%) contributes meaningfully to achieving improved glucose control. Accordingly, establishing a goal of weight reduction, or at least weight maintenance, is recommended.

Dietary advice should be personalised. Patients should be encouraged to eat healthy foods that are consistent with the prevailing population-wide dietary recommendations and with an individual's preferences and culture. Foods high in fibre (such as vegetables, fruits, wholegrains and legumes), low-fat dairy products and fresh fish should be emphasised. High-energy foods, including those rich in saturated fats, and sweet desserts and snacks should be eaten less frequently and in lower amounts. Patients may have cycles of weight loss and relapse. The healthcare team should remain non-judgmental but persistent, re-visiting and encouraging therapeutic lifestyle changes frequently, if needed.

As much physical activity as possible should be promoted, ideally aiming for at least 150 minutes/ week of moderate activity, including aerobic, resistance and flexibility training [19]. In older individuals or those with mobility challenges any increase in activity level is advantageous (if this is tolerated from a cardiovascular standpoint).

Metformin

Metformin, a biguanide, remains the most widely used first-line type 2 diabetes drug; its mechanism of action remains obscure, but it

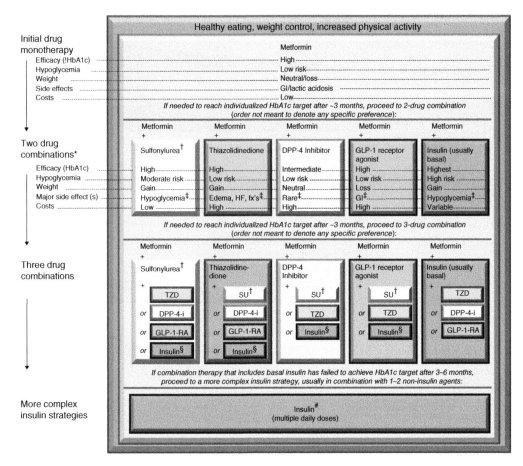

Figure 4.2.2 Therapy of type 2 diabetes is based on a background of healthy eating, weight control and increased physical activity. Beyond this, metformin is usually the first line agent and two-drug combinations or three-drug combinations can be used. When β-cell failure becomes severe, insulin is the only option (Source: Adapted from Inzucchi, 2012 [6])

probably has most of its effect on the gut [20]. It is given in large doses (1–2.5 g), and the tablets are therefore large. About 15% of patients are intolerant of its use, mainly from gastrointestinal side-effects, but it is cheap and it does have a good evidence base [21,22]. It is generally considered weight neutral with chronic use and does not increase the risk of hypoglycaemia.

Sulfonylureas

The first discovered oral agents for treating the hyperglycaemia of diabetes were the sulfonylureas. Long after their discovery it was established that they function through increasing insulin release from β-cells [23]. This secretion is only partially glucose dependent so, while they are effective in controlling glucose levels, their use is associated with modest weight gain of approximately 3 kg and risk of hypoglycaemia [24]. Some of the sulfonylureas may cause more rapid β-cell failure than metformin alone [25]. Nevertheless, they are cheap, widely available and have a good evidence base [7].

A subgroup of sulfonylurea-like agents, the meglitinides, are short-acting and are taken with meals. They are not widely used.

Thiazolidinediones

Thiazolidinediones (TZDs) are agents that improve insulin sensitivity in skeletal muscle and reduce hepatic glucose production [26]. They do not increase the risk of hypoglycaemia and may be more durable in their effectiveness than sulfonylureas and metformin [24]. Pioglitazone had benefit on cardiovascular events as a secondary outcome in one large trial involving patients with overt macrovascular disease [27]. Rosiglitazone is no longer available in Europe after concerns of increased myocardial infarction risk [28]. Recognised side-effects of thiazolidinediones include weight gain, fluid retention leading to oedema and/or heart failure in predisposed individuals and some increased risk of bone fractures. Pioglitazone can be used in combination with metformin and sulfonylureas, and there is no contraindication to its use with insulin, though this is commoner in the USA than in Europe.

Incretin-axis agents

GLP-1 agonists

Glucagon-like peptide 1 (GLP-1) is a hormone produced by the gut, and signals directly to the β-cell of the pancreas, as well as to other tissues [29]. GLP-1 secretion is a major part of the so-called 'incretin axis', which is the name given to the observed phenomenon that glucose delivered to the gut causes a much greater insulin secretion than the equivalent glucose stimulus delivered intravenously. This incretin effect has a major advantage over direct pharmacological stimulus of the β-cell in that it is glucose dependent. This means that GLP-1 has an excellent stimulating effect when the glucose is high, but as the glucose reaches normal concentration the effect switches off. So GLP-1 agents are not, of themselves, associated with the side-effect of hypoglycaemia. GLP-1 also has direct effects on slowing gastric emptying, on reducing glucagon secretion and on the brain to reduce appetite. This latter effect seems to be the primary cause of the weight loss of approximately 2.5 kg associated with GLP-1 agonists, itself a very useful effect in the management of diabetes [30].

GLP-1 is a peptide with a very short half-life in the plasma. The therapeutic GLP-1 agents are, therefore, analogues or homologues of the native hormone and, because the hormone is a peptide, they have to be injected. (Peptides are digested very rapidly if they are given orally). The major side-effects of GLP-1 agents are some early nausea, and occasional vomiting, but in general this settles over a few weeks. The weight loss observed is related to decreased food intake and it may be that careful dietetic instruction about eating less would counter some of the nausea. The commonest agents used in the United Kingdom (UK) are liraglutide (injected daily) and exendin-4 (injected twice daily). Agents are in development with longer half-lives and similarly good therapeutic effects and which can be administered once weekly. GLP-1 agents can be used with metformin or thiazolidinediones. They are expensive.

DPP4-inhibitors

The oral dipeptidyl dipeptidase 4 (DPP-4) inhibitors enhance circulating concentrations of active GLP-1 [31] by reducing the extent to which GLP-1 is degraded. They therefore allow a greater effect of endogenously produced GLP-1 and other incretin hormones but clearly cannot mimic the pharmacological doses administered by the agonists. However, because the inhibitors are not peptides, they can be given by mouth. They have very few side-effects. They are weight neutral and weaker in effect than GLP-1 agonists. They do not cause hypoglycaemia because they act through the glucose-dependent incretin system. Agents available include alogliptin, saxagliptin, sitagliptin, linagliptin and vildagliptin. They can be used alone or in combination with metformin and with sulfonylureas, though hypoglycaemia can occur when the latter combination is used. There is little logic in using them with the GLP-1 agonists. Once weekly DPP-4 inhibitors are currently undergoing trials.

α-Glucosidase inhibitors

α-Glucosidase inhibitors retard gut carbohydrate absorption [32]. The result of this is that more sugars are delivered to the colon and this can cause wind and occasional diarrhoea. The effects are relatively weak. They are not widely prescribed in the UK, but are more widely used in countries with a traditionally high carbohydrate diet, such as China [33].

SGLT-2 inhibitors

Sodium glucose transporter 2 (SGLT-2) inhibitors are agents that act directly on the kidney to cause glycosuria – glucose loss into the urine [34]. This mechanism seems counter-intuitive in that normally glycosuria is a sign of diabetes out of control. This is because the renal threshold – the glucose level above which glucose is lost into the urine – is normally about 12 mmol/l. So glycosuria was a marker of high glucose. However, with SGLT-2 inhibitors, glucose loss into the urine occurs at much lower levels - typically at about 6 mmol/l, and so up to 100 g of glucose (about 400 kcal) per day can be lost. This lowers plasma glucose and helps weight loss. However, because of the glucose in the urine, thrush is commoner in women and occasional balanitis is observed in men. Agents available in the UK include dapagliflozin and canagliflozin. The agents can be combined with many other treatments, including most oral agents and, indeed, with insulin. They are new agents, however, and caution should moderate enthusiasm until more trial data are published [35].

Insulin

Until the 1980s, insulin was only available by extraction and purification from the pancreas of cattle and pigs. This animal insulin is still in use but has been largely replaced by human insulin that is engineered genetically in laboratories. Newer analogue insulin has been introduced over the past few years in an attempt to replicate the action of naturally produced insulin in the body. Table 4.2.2 summarises the different preparations of insulin available to treat diabetes.

Side-effects of insulin treatment include weight gain of approximately 6 kg, and hypoglycaemia [7]. Weight gain is variable and depends on both the amount and type of insulin used; use of an intensive prandial regime was associated with higher weight gain (6.4 kg) compared to biphasic regimens (5.7 kg) and a once-daily basal insulin (3.6 kg) in the 4-T study [36], although there is limited evidence that dietary education and support can ameliorate weight gain [37]. Ideally, an insulin treatment programme should be designed specifically for an individual patient, to match the supply of insulin to his or her dietary/exercise habits and prevailing glucose trends, as revealed through self-monitoring. Anticipated glucose-lowering effects should be balanced with the convenience

Table 4.2.2 Characteristics of insulin preparations to treat diabetes

Type of insulin	Onset of action (min)	Peak action	Duration (h)	Comments
Rapid-acting analogues	5–10	90 min	3	Taken with, or directly after, food
Short-acting human insulin	20–30	2 h	4–8	Taken 2–30 min before eating
Medium-/long-acting insulin	90	4–12 h	12–24	Taken once or twice a day
Long-acting analogues	Flat profile	Flat profile	18–24	Taken once a day, and takes up to 3 days for full effect
Mixed insulin	30	2–8 h	16–20	Mixture of short-acting and medium- or long-acting, taken twice daily
Mixed analogues	5–10	90	16–20	Mixture of rapid-acting and long-acting analogues, taken twice daily

of the regimen, in the context of an individual's specific therapy goals.

Proper patient education regarding glucose monitoring, insulin injection technique, insulin storage, recognition/treatment of hypoglycaemia, and 'sick day' rules is imperative. Where available, certified diabetes educators can be invaluable in guiding the patient through this process.

Combination agents

Some new interesting combinations of peptide agents are under close scrutiny. Using insulin combined with liraglutide (IDeg-Lira) may be advantageous in terms of combining two agents that would otherwise need separate injections [38].

Single, fixed dose combinations (often metformin + other active agents) may have a role, and there are certainly many possible combinations that could be appropriately combined [39]. Compliance is likely to be greater with such agents.

4.2.4 Implementation strategies

It is generally agreed that metformin, if not contraindicated and if tolerated, is the preferred and most cost-effective first agent [6]. It is initiated at, or soon after, diagnosis, especially in patients in whom lifestyle intervention alone has not achieved, or is unlikely to achieve, HbA1c goals. Because of frequent gastrointestinal side-effects, it should be started at a low dose with gradual titration.

If metformin cannot be used, another oral agent could be chosen, such as a sulfonylurea, pioglitazone or a DPP-4 inhibitor; in occasional cases where weight loss is seen as an essential aspect of therapy, initial therapy with a GLP-1 receptor agonist might be useful.

Beyond monotherapy there are a number of options. Many agents can be usefully combined and most treatments will involve more than one oral agent before therapy is moved to insulin. Ultimately, because of β-cell failure, most patients beyond a decade of type 2 diabetes will need insulin – and some considerably earlier.

4.2.5 Hypoglycaemia

Hypoglycaemia in type 2 diabetes was long thought to be a trivial issue, as it occurs less commonly than in type 1 diabetes, although emerging evidence suggests duration of insulin treatment is associated with increased risk of severe hypoglycaemia [40]. However, there is emerging concern, based mainly on the results of recent clinical trials and some cross-sectional evidence, of increased risk of brain dysfunction in those with repeated episodes. In the ACCORD trial, high levels of both minor and major hypoglycaemia occurred in intensively managed patients [9]. Hypoglycaemia is more dangerous in the elderly and occurs consistently more often as glycaemic targets are lowered. Perhaps just as importantly, additional consequences of frequent hypoglycaemia include work disability and erosion of the confidence of the patient (and that of family or caregivers) to live independently. Accordingly, in at-risk individuals, drug selection should favour agents that do not precipitate such events and, in general, blood glucose targets may need to be moderated.

4.2.6 Conclusions

Managing hyperglycaemia is an art more than a science. It is essential to lower the HbA1c to as near normal as possible within the constraints of patient enthusiasm and adherence, realistic goals, collaborative working towards such goals, avoidance of hypoglycaemia and due regard for social and work circumstances. A laissez-faire attitude to hyperglycaemia will increase the later burden of micro- and macrovascular disease. The overall aim of treating hyperglycaemia is to avoid acute symptoms in the short term (polyuria, thirst, blurring of vision and tiredness), and tissue complications in the long term. In this regard concentration on the glycaemic goals alone is inappropriate – diet, exercise, lipids and smoking habits all need to be addressed.

Key points

- Clinical management of type 2 diabetes should address glycaemic control and cardiovascular risk using a patient-centred approach.
- The aim of glycaemic control is to lower HbA1c levels in order to reduce the risk of long-term complications.
- The choice of pharmacological agent depends upon many factors, including age, weight, gender, ethnicity and comorbidities.
- Beta-cell failure is a feature of type 2 diabetes and most people will have to use combination therapies to control blood glucose levels.

References

1. Gaede P, Vedel P, Parving HH, Pedersen O. Intensified multifactorial intervention in patients with type 2 diabetes mellitus and microalbuminuria: the Steno type 2 randomised study. *Lancet* 1999; **353**(9153): 617–622.
2. Doll R, Peto R, Boreham J, Sutherland I. Mortality in relation to smoking: 50 years' observations on male British doctors. *BMJ* 2004; **328**(7455): 1519–1528.
3. IDF Clinical Guidelines Task Force. Global Guideline for Type 2 Diabetes. Brussels, Belgium: International Diabetes Federation, 2012.
4. Canadian Diabetes Association Clinical Practice Guidelines Expert Committee. Canadian Diabetes Association 2013 Clinical Practice Guidelines for the Prevention and Management of Diabetes in Canada. *Can J Diabetes* 2013; **37**(Suppl. 1): S1–S212.
5. NICE. Type 2 Diabetes: The Management of Type 2 Diabetes: NICE Clinical Guideline 87. National Institute for Health and Clinical Excellence, 2009.
6. Inzucchi SE, Bergenstal RM, Buse JB, Diamant M, Ferrannini E, Nauck M, et al. Management of hyperglycaemia in type 2 diabetes: a patient-centered approach. Position statement of the American Diabetes Association (ADA) and the European Association for the Study of Diabetes (EASD). *Diabetologia* 2012; **55**(6): 1577–1596.
7. UKPDS Group. Intensive blood-glucose control with sulphonylureas or insulin compared with conventional treatment and risk of complications in patients with type 2 diabetes (UKPDS 33). UK Prospective Diabetes Study (UKPDS) Group. *Lancet* 1998; **352**(9131): 837–853.
8. DCCT study group. The effect of intensive treatment of diabetes on the development and progression of long-term complications in insulin-dependent diabetes mellitus. The Diabetes Control and Complications Trial Research Group. *N Engl J Med* 1993; **329**(14): 977–986.
9. Gerstein HC, Miller ME, Byington RP, Goff DC, Jr., Bigger JT, Buse JB, et al. Effects of intensive glucose lowering in type 2 diabetes. *N Engl J Med* 2008; **358**(24): 2545–2559.
10. Stratton IM, Adler AI, Neil HA, Matthews DR, Manley SE, Cull CA, et al. Association of glycaemia with macrovascular and microvascular complications of type 2 diabetes (UKPDS 35): prospective observational study. *BMJ* 2000; **321**(7258): 405–412.
11. DCCT/EDIC Writing Group. Sustained effect of intensive treatment of type 1 diabetes mellitus on development and progression of diabetic nephropathy: the Epidemiology of Diabetes Interventions and Complications (EDIC) study. *JAMA* 2003; **290**(16): 2159–2167.
12. Holman RR, Paul SK, Bethel MA, Matthews DR, Neil HA. 10-year follow-up of intensive glucose control in type 2 diabetes. *N Engl J Med* 2008; **359**(15): 1577–1589.
13. Ferrannini E, Gastaldelli A, Miyazaki Y, Matsuda M, Mari A, DeFronzo RA. Beta- cell function in subjects spanning the range from normal glucose tolerance to overt diabetes: a new analysis. *J Clin Endocrinol Metab* 2005; **90**: 493–500.
14. Nyenwe EA, Jerkins TW, Umpierrez GE, Kitabchi AE. Management of type 2 diabetes: evolving strategies for the treatment of patients with type 2 diabetes. *Metabolism* 2011; **60**: 1–23.
15. Lim EF, Hollingsworth KG, Aribisala BS, Chen MJ, Mathers JC, Taylor R. Reversal of type 2 diabetes: normalisation of beta cell function in association with decreased pancreas and liver triacylglycerol. *Diabetologia* 2011; **54**(10): 2506–2514.
16. Kahn BB, Flier JS. Obesity and insulin resistance. *J Clin Invest* 2000; **106**(4): 473–481.
17. Dyson PA, Kelly T, Deakin T, Duncan A, Frost G, Harrison Z, et al.; Diabetes UK Nutrition Working Group. Diabetes UK evidence-based nutrition guidelines for the prevention and management of diabetes. *Diabet Med* 2011; **28**(11): 1282–1288.
18. Evert AB, Boucher JL, Cypress M, Dunbar SA, Franz MJ, Mayer-Davis EJ, et al.; American Diabetes Association. Nutrition therapy recommendations for the management of adults with diabetes. *Diabetes Care* 2013; **36**(11): 3821–3842.
19. Boule NG, Haddad E, Kenny GP, Wells GA, Sigal RJ. Effects of exercise on glycemic control and body mass in type 2 diabetes mellitus: a meta-analysis of controlled clinical trials. *JAMA* 2001; **286**(10): 1218–1227.
20. Bailey CJ, Turner RC. Metformin. *N Engl J Med* 1996; **334**: 574–579.
21. UKPDS Group. Effect of intensive blood-glucose control with metformin on complications in overweight patients with type 2 diabetes (UKPDS 34). UK Prospective Diabetes Study (UKPDS) Group. *Lancet* 1998; **352**(9131): 854–865.

22. Lamanna C, Monami M, Marchionni N, Mannucci E. Effect of metformin on cardiovascular events and mortality: a meta-analysis of randomized clinical trials. *Diabetes Obes Metab* 2011; **13**: 221–228.

23. Bryan J, Crane A, Vila-Carriles WH, Babenko AP, Aguilar-Bryan L. Insulin secretagogues, sulfonylurea receptors and K(ATP) channels. *Curr Pharm Des* 2005; **11**: 2699–2716.

24. De Fronzo RA. Pharmacological therapy for type 2 diabetes. *Ann Intern Med* 1999; **131**: 281–303.

25. Kahn SE, Haffner SM, Heise MA, Herman WH, Holman RR, Jones NP, et al. Glycemic durability of rosiglitazone, metformin, or glyburide monotherapy. *N Engl J Med* 2006; **355**(23): 2427–2443.

26. Yki-Järvinen H. Thiazolidinediones. *N Engl J Med* 2004; **351**: 1106–1118.

27. Dormandy JA, Charbonnel B, Eckland DJ, Erdmann E, Massi-Benedetti M, Moules IK, et al. Secondary prevention of macrovascular events in patients with type 2 diabetes in the PROactive Study (PROspective pioglitAzone Clinical Trial In macroVascular Events): a randomised controlled trial. *Lancet* 2005; **366**(9493): 1279–1289.

28. Nissen SE, Wolski K. Rosiglitazone revisited: an updated meta-analysis of risk for myocardial infarction and cardiovascular mortality. *Arch Intern Med* 2010; **170**(14): 1191–1201.

29. Drucker DJ, Nauck MA. The incretin system: glucagon-like peptide-1 receptor agonists and dipeptidyl peptidase-4 inhibitors in type 2 diabetes. *Lancet* 2006; **368**(9548): 1696–1705.

30. Amori RE, Lau J, Pittas AG. Efficacy and safety of incretin therapy in type 2 diabetes: systematic review and meta-analysis. *JAMA* 2007; **298**(2): 194–206.

31. Deacon CF. Dipeptidyl peptidase-4 inhibitors in the treatment of type 2 diabetes: a comparative review. *Diabetes Obes Metab* 2011; **13**(1): 7–18.

32. Van de Laar FA, Lucassen PL, Akkermans RP, Van de Lisdonk EH, Rutten GE, Van Weel C. Alpha-glucosidase inhibitors for type 2 diabetes mellitus. *Cochrane Database Syst Rev* 2005; (2): CD003639.

33. Weng J, Soegondo S, Schnell O, Sheu WH, Grzeszczak W, Watada H, et al.; Acarbose pooled Database Integrated Analysis-Non-Interventional Studies (AcarDIA-NIS) project. Efficacy of acarbose in different geographical regions of the world: analysis of a real-life database. *Diabetes Metab Res Rev* 2014. doi: 10.1002/dmrr.2576.

34. Nair S, Wilding JP. Sodium glucose cotransporter 2 inhibitors as a new treatment for diabetes mellitus. *J Clin Endocrinol Metab* 2010; **95**(1): 34–42.

35. Cefalu WT, Buse JB, Del Prato S, Home PD, LeRoith D, Nauck MA, et al. Beyond metformin: safety considerations in the decision-making process for selecting a second medication for type 2 diabetes management: reflections from a diabetes care editors' expert forum. *Diabetes Care* 2014; **37**(9): 2647–2659.

36. Holman RR, Farmer AJ, Davies MJ, Levy JC, Darbyshire JL, Keenan JF, et al.; 4-T Study Group. Three-year efficacy of complex insulin regimens in type 2 diabetes. *N Engl J Med* 2009; **361**(18): 1736–1747.

37. Barratt R, Frost G, Millward DJ, Truby H. A randomised controlled trial investigating the effect of an intensive lifestyle intervention v. standard care in adults with type 2 diabetes immediately after initiating insulin therapy. *Br J Nutr* 2008; **99**(5): 1025–1031.

38. Gough SC, Bode B, Woo V, Rodbard HW, Linjawi S, Poulsen P, et al.; NN9068-3697 (DUAL-I) trial investigators. Efficacy and safety of a fixed-ratio combination of insulin degludec and liraglutide (IDegLira) compared with its components given alone: results of a phase 3, open-label, randomised, 26-week, treat-to-target trial in insulin-naive patients with type 2 diabetes. *Lancet Diabetes Endocrinol* 2014; **2**(11): 885–893.

39. Bell DS, Dharmalingam M, Kumar S, Sawakhande RB. Triple oral fixed-dose diabetes polypill versus insulin plus metformin efficacy demonstration study in the treatment of advanced type 2 diabetes (TrIED study-II). *Diabetes Obes Metab* 2011 Sep; **13**(9): 800–805.

40. Heller SR. Hypoglycaemia in Type 2 diabetes. *Diabetes Res Clin Pract* 2008; **82**(Suppl. 2): S108–S111.

Chapter 4.3

Nutritional management of glycaemia in Type 2 diabetes

Pamela Dyson

University of Oxford, Oxford Centre for Diabetes, Endocrinology and Metabolism, Churchill Hospital, Oxford, UK

4.3.1 Introduction

There is strong evidence that improvements in glycaemic control in people with Type 2 diabetes are associated with significant reductions in risk from both microvascular and macrovascular disease. The United Kingdom Prospective Diabetes Study (UKPDS) reported that a reduction in HbA1c of 10 mmol/mol (0.9%) over median 10 years was associated with a 12% reduction in risk from any diabetes-related end-point, a 25% reduction in risk from microvascular disease and a 16% trend to reduced risk from myocardial infarction [1], and that these benefits were sustained long-term [2]. There is robust evidence that nutritional therapy is effective in reducing HbA1c [3–6], and meta-analyses of both randomised controlled trials (RCT) and observational cohort studies have indicated that dietary advice can reduce HbA1c by 3–30 mmol/mol (0.25–2.9%) [7], with the greatest reduction seen in those newly diagnosed with type 2 diabetes [8]. Despite this strong evidence for the overall beneficial effects of nutritional interventions, evidence for the effects of specific dietary strategies on glycaemic control is somewhat contradictory.

The majority of published guidelines emphasise the importance of weight loss for the 90% of those with type 2 diabetes who are overweight or obese, and of the three macronutrients (carbohydrate, fat and protein), carbohydrate management has also been identified as a key strategy for blood glucose control [3–6].

4.3.2 Weight management and glycaemic control

Type 2 diabetes is associated with an increased prevalence of overweight and obesity. In the UK and the US, studies suggest that approximately 90% of people with type 2 diabetes are overweight (BMI >25 kg/m^2) and 50% are obese (BMI >30 kg/m^2) [9,10]. Weight reduction is recommended as a primary strategy and has been shown to improve glycaemic control, quality of life, mobility, sleep apnoea, sexual function and bring reductions in depression and cardiovascular (CVD) risk factors [11]. However, due to a variety of factors outlined below, not all studies have shown significant associations between weight loss and HbA1c reduction.

Length of follow-up

The majority of published dietary studies are short-term (<12 months), and often report highly significant reductions in both body weight and HbA1c at three and six-month follow-up. It is widely recognised that maintaining weight loss is challenging for those with type 2 diabetes, and some weight regain is typically seen at 12-months follow-up and beyond [12]. Despite this, most dietary studies in people with diabetes report that the majority do not regain all the weight lost, and at 4–5 years follow-up have sustained a non-significantly lower body weight than at baseline. In the Look-AHEAD trial which investigated

Advanced Nutrition and Dietetics in Diabetes, First Edition. Edited by Louise Goff and Pamela Dyson.

intensive lifestyle therapy in a sample of 5154 people with established type 2 diabetes, a significant weight loss of 6% was sustained in the intervention group over 9.6 years follow-up [13].

Amount of weight lost

It has been widely reported that modest weight loss (<10%) has beneficial effects on insulin resistance and glycaemic control in people with type 2 diabetes [14]. It now appears that weight losses of at least 5% are necessary for significant improvements in glycaemic control over the longer-term; a recent meta-analysis stated that studies reporting <5% weight loss showed a non-significant reduction in HbA1c of 0.2% at 12 months follow-up [12]. The Look-AHEAD trial reported a decrease in HbA1c of 0.6% associated with a weight loss of 8.6% [13], and a Mediterranean-style dietary intervention in newly diagnosed subjects reported a decrease of 1.2% in HbA1c with mean weight losses of 7.2% [15].

Duration of diabetes

Larger reductions in HbA1c are commonly seen in those newly diagnosed with type 2 diabetes, however, for those who have established disease the degree of weight loss is not necessarily related to improvements in glycaemic control [12]. In newly diagnosed people in the UKPDS study, where the only intervention in the first three months was dietary therapy, mean weight losses of 4.5 kg were associated with a reduction in HbA1c of 2.0% [16], and a Mediterranean-style diet study showed similar, sustained reductions in both HbA1c and weight at one year's follow-up after diagnosis [15].

Strategies for weight reduction

There has been much discussion, and many studies, about the most effective way to lose weight and improve glycaemic control in people with type 2 diabetes [14]. A healthful diet, including largely unprocessed foods, such as fruit and vegetables, wholegrain carbohydrate foods, fish and seafood, yogurt, pulses, legumes and nuts and vegetable oil, and lower in red and processed meat, refined carbohydrate foods and added sugars, is recommended by most authorities [3–6], but there are few head-to-head studies evaluating this strategy for weight reduction against other approaches. Evidence suggests that a variety of dietary interventions are effective for weight loss and improving glycaemic control [17] including energy-restricted diets [18], Mediterranean-style diets [19], high protein diets [20], low carbohydrate diets [21], very low energy liquid diets [22] and meal replacements [23]. Overall, successful weight reduction appears to be determined by adherence to a chosen dietary strategy that achieves energy restriction long-term, rather than by a specific diet, and this approach is recommended by most dietary guidelines [3–6].

4.3.3 Macronutrients and glycaemic control

There is no conclusive evidence for the ideal macronutrient content of the diet to improve outcomes in people with type 2 diabetes, whether for improving glycaemic control, promoting weight loss or reducing CVD risk. This is because most meta-analyses include studies in which the intervention diet achieved greater weight loss than the comparator diet, making it difficult to draw firm conclusions about the effect of different dietary components independent of weight loss [24]. In addition, other confounding factors such as changes in medication are often not fully reported. Two systematic reviews and meta-analyses have attempted to answer this question. One identified that Mediterranean-style diets, low GI diets, low carbohydrate diets and high protein diets were all associated with improvements in glycaemic control [25], and the other that many different strategies were associated with improved outcomes [26]. However, neither analysis corrected for differences in weight loss, and a more recent systematic review that only included studies where there were no differences in weight change concluded that there was insufficient evidence to recommend a particular diet or macronutrient [24]. As a result, the majority of national and international dietary guidelines do not make a specific recommendation for carbohydrate, fat and protein in terms of glycaemic control, but emphasise the importance of individualised nutritional goals.

4.3.4 Carbohydrate and glycaemic control

Carbohydrate has long been a focus for attention as this nutrient has the most direct effect on blood glucose levels after eating. Research studies have investigated the effects of both the quantity and quality of dietary carbohydrate, and as no clear message has emerged most authorities now recommend an individualised approach to carbohydrate management in people with type 2 diabetes (Table 4.3.1).

Quantity of carbohydrate

Globally, carbohydrate provides approximately 40–80% of total energy intake amongst adults [27], and there is limited evidence showing that people with diabetes obtain 45% of total energy requirements from carbohydrate [26].

The majority of studies investigating the effect of high carbohydrate diets have failed to show superiority for people with diabetes [26], although this may be explained by confounding factors such as decreases in fat and protein intake and the type of carbohydrate consumed. High carbohydrate diets including processed high GI carbohydrates do not appear to improve glycaemic control, whereas high carbohydrate diets which are rich in dietary fibre and low in fat and which include unprocessed carbohydrates have been shown to improve glycaemic control and serum lipid concentrations [28].

The role of low carbohydrate diets in the treatment of type 2 diabetes has long been controversial. In the early part of the 20th century, low carbohydrate, relatively high fat diets were recommended for diabetes, but this underwent radical change in the 1980s in light of research suggesting that high intakes of saturated fat and low intakes of dietary fibre were associated with increased risk of CVD [28]. As a result, most authorities then recommended high carbohydrate, low fat diets for the management of diabetes. However, as carbohydrate is the nutrient most strongly associated with postprandial hyperglycaemia, there is a renewed interest in low carbohydrate diets, including calls for carbohydrate restriction as first-line nutritional therapy for people with diabetes [29].

Table 4.3.1 Key recommendations for carbohydrate intake and glycaemic control in type 2 diabetes

Recommendation	Diabetes UK [3]	American Diabetes Association [4]	Canadian Diabetes Association [5]	European Association [6]
Total daily intake of carbohydrate	Individual goals: No specific recommendation	Individual goals: No specific recommendation	45–60% of total energy intake stressing individualization	45–60% of total energy intake
Total free sugars	Reduce dietary sugar: No specific recommendation	Can be included, but care taken to avoid excessive intake	≤10% of total energy intake	≤10% of total energy intake
Glycaemic index/ load (GI/GL)	Low GI diets may offer additional modest improvements in glycaemic control	Substituting low GI foods may modestly improve glycaemic control	Replace high GI foods with low GI foods	Low GI foods should be encouraged in those with high carbohydrate intake
Dietary fibre	Recommendations similar to those for the general public (30g/day) [34]	Recommendations similar to those for the general public (14g/1,000kcal/ day) [35]	15–25g/1,000kcal/ day	>40g/day (or 20g/1,000kcal/ day)

A meta-analysis of early studies in people with type 2 diabetes suggested that low carbohydrate diets showed beneficial effects on glycaemic control, although there was no evidence of a beneficial effect on weight loss and insufficient evidence of CVD risk reduction [30]. This was supported by further meta-analysis that showed significant beneficial effects of low carbohydrate diets on both glycaemic control and body weight [20]. More recent meta-analyses and systematic reviews including more studies have failed to confirm these findings, reporting that although there may be some evidence of short-term improvements in glycaemic control, these are not sustained over the longer term [31–33]. In summary, although low carbohydrate diets may be effective for improving glycaemic control in people with type 2 diabetes, they do not demonstrate superiority over other dietary approaches, and uncertainty about long-term side effects remains.

There may be little evidence to support a defined amount of carbohydrate in the diet, but most recommendations acknowledge the importance of monitoring and controlling carbohydrate intake [3–6].

Quality of carbohydrate

Traditionally, people with diabetes were advised to avoid large amounts of sugar and sugary foods and to base their carbohydrate intake on 'starchy' carbohydrates. Recent evidence suggests that foods containing processed or rapidly digested starches e.g. potatoes, white rice and white bread may have adverse effects on both glycaemic control and general health and that unprocessed and wholegrain carbohydrates should be recommended as primary carbohydrate sources both for those with diabetes [17,28] and the general population [35].

It has been recommended that the term 'free sugars' be adopted to include all mono and disaccharides added to foods during manufacture, cooking or consumption together with any sugars naturally present in honey, syrups and unsweetened fruit juices and concentrates [36]. There is growing evidence that free sugars, and in particular sugar-sweetened beverages (SSB), may increase the risk of both obesity and type 2 diabetes [37,38], but there is little evidence of

the role of free sugars in glycaemic control in people with diagnosed type 2 diabetes. Short-term studies investigating sucrose intake in people with diabetes have shown that the total amount of carbohydrate, rather than the type, predicts postprandial blood glucose concentrations and that sucrose intakes of 10–35% of total energy intake do not have a negative effect on glycaemic control when compared to isocaloric amounts of starch [39]. In terms of general health, recent guidelines have recommended that free sugars should contribute no more than 5–10% of total daily energy intake [34–36], and it is probably prudent to recommend this to people with type 2 diabetes.

Diets high in dietary fibre are associated with improvements in glycaemic control [28]. A meta-analysis reported that diets containing fibre-rich foods or fibre supplements providing 37.4–42.6 g/day of fibre were associated with a 0.55% reduction in Hba1c [40]. Soluble fibre appears to have a greater effect on glycaemic control than the insoluble fibre found in wholegrains and some fruit and vegetables [41]. Recommendations for fibre intake for people with diabetes are generally similar to those for the general population.

Low GI diets have been reported to improve glycaemic control and reduce HbA1c by 0.14–0.5% [20,42]. There has been a suggestion that the benefit of low GI diets may be due partly to the effect of dietary fibre as low GI foods tend to be higher in soluble fibre [17]. Recommendations for GI are shown in Table 4.3.1.

4.3.5 Fat and glycaemic control

The majority of recommendations about dietary fat and type 2 diabetes relate to CVD risk reduction rather than the relationship with glycaemic control. A comprehensive systematic review concluded that total fat intakes and type of fat were not associated with blood glucose concentrations, although the beneficial effects of monounsaturated fat (MUFA) on both insulin sensitivity and fasting insulin concentrations were considered as probable [43]. This is supported by a study showing that substituting

MUFA for saturated fat (SFA) as part of a Mediterranean-style diet improved glycaemic control at 2 years follow-up [44].

4.3.6 Protein and glycaemic control

Early metabolic studies showed that dietary protein had little immediate effect on postprandial blood glucose concentrations in people with type 2 diabetes, but that it reduced glucose concentrations two hours after ingestion [45]. Further work indicated that when dietary protein is ingested with glucose, it acts to increase insulin secretion and decrease blood glucose concentrations [46], suggesting that high protein diets may be useful in regulating glycaemic control. These findings have not been replicated in dietary intervention studies [39] and concerns about the relationship between high protein intakes and risk of renal disease have resulted in recommendations that people with diabetes should eat moderate amounts of protein at amounts similar to the general population (15–20% of total energy intake). There is little evidence that low protein intakes are protective for renal disease in people with type 2 diabetes [47].

In summary, guidelines for people with type 2 diabetes state that a moderate protein intake similar to the general population should be recommended. Protein has been shown to increase insulin response after eating and for this reason it is recommended that that protein-containing foods are not used to treat hypoglycaemia [3,4].

4.3.7 Foods versus nutrients

Recent publications have emphasised the benefits of food, rather than nutrient, based approaches to nutritional recommendations for general health and to reduce the risk of non-communicable diseases (NCD) including type 2 diabetes [35,48,49]. Healthful dietary patterns include largely unprocessed foods, such as fruit and vegetables, whole grains, pulses and legumes, seafood, yogurt and vegetable oils and less red and processed meat, refined grains and

sugar and sugary foods, particularly SSB. These dietary patterns are naturally rich sources of dietary fibre, minerals and vitamins and unsaturated fats and contain less sugar, saturated fat and salt and have a lower glycaemic load. There are a variety of dietary patterns that conform to this style of eating, including conventional low fat, high fibre 'healthy eating' diets, Mediterranean-style diets, the DASH diet and vegetarian and vegan diets, and all these have been shown to improve outcomes in people with diabetes [47]. However, dietary advice should also include the concepts of overall portion control and carbohydrate management.

4.3.8 Conclusions

For the majority of people with type 2 diabetes, weight management is a key priority and this can be achieved by a variety of strategies with little evidence of superiority of any particular approach. Weight loss is more effective in improving glycaemic control in those newly diagnosed with type 2 diabetes. There is no evidence supporting specific amounts of fat, protein or carbohydrate in the diet for improving glycaemic control and an individualised approach is key [50]. Healthful eating patterns have been shown to improve both glycaemic and cardiovascular outcomes and these can be combined with carbohydrate monitoring and control to maximise benefit.

Key points

- Weight management is a key strategy for those with type 2 diabetes
- A variety of weight management strategies are effective
- The ideal amount of macronutrients is unknown
- Carbohydrate management can improve glycaemic control
- A variety of dietary patterns are associated with improved outcomes and individualised advice is recommended

References

1. UKPDS Group. Intensive blood-glucose control with sulphonylureas or insulin compared with conventional treatment and risk of complications in patients with type 2 diabetes (UKPDS 33). UK Prospective Diabetes Study (UKPDS) Group. *Lancet* 1998; **352**(9131): 837–853.

2. Holman RR, Paul SK, Bethel MA, Matthews DR, Neil HA. 10-year follow-up of intensive glucose control in type 2 diabetes. *N Engl J Med* 2008; **359**(15): 1577–1589.

3. Dyson PA, Kelly T, Deakin T, Duncan A, Frost G, Harrison Z, Khatri D, Kunka D, McArdle P, Mellor D, Oliver L, Worth J; on behalf of Diabetes UK Nutrition Working Group. Diabetes UK evidence-based nutrition guidelines for the prevention and management of diabetes. *Diabet Med* 2011; 28(11): 1282–1288.

4. Evert AB, Boucher JL, Cypress M, Dunbar SA, Franz MJ et al. Nutrition therapy recommendations for the management of adults with diabetes. *Diabetes Care* 2014; 37(Suppl 1): S120–143.

5. Canadian Diabetes Association Clinical Practice Guidelines Expert Committee, Dworatzek PD, Arcudi K, Gougeon R, Husein N, Sievenpiper JL, Williams SL. Nutrition therapy. *Can J Diabetes*. 2013; 37(Suppl 1): S45–55.

6. Mann JI, De Leeuw I, Hermansen K, Karamanos B, Karlström B et al; Diabetes and Nutrition Study Group (DNSG) of the European Association. Evidence-based nutritional approaches to the treatment and prevention of diabetes mellitus. *Nutr Metab Cardiovasc Dis* 2004; **14**(6): 373–394.

7. Pastors JG, Warshaw H, Daly A, Franz M, Kulkarni K. The evidence for the effectiveness of medical nutrition therapy in diabetes management. *Diabetes Care* 2002; **25**(3): 608–613.

8. Wilding J. The importance of weight management in type 2 diabetes mellitus. Int J clin Pract 2014; **68**(6): 682–691.

9. Public Health England. *Adult Obesity and Type 2 Diabetes.* PHE, London; 2014.

10. Tobias DK, Pan A, Jackson CL, O'Reilly EJ, Ding EL et al. Body-mass index and mortality among adults with incident type 2 diabetes. *N Engl J Med* 2014; **370**(3): 233–244.

11. Wing RR; Look AHEAD Research Group. Implications of Look AHEAD for clinical trials and clinical practice. *Diabetes Obes Metab* 2014; 16(12): 1183–1191.

12. Mann J. Nutrition recommendations for the treatment and prevention of type 2 diabetes and the metabolic syndrome: an evidenced-based review. *Nutr Rev* 2006; **64**(9): 422–427.

13. Look AHEAD Research Group, Wing RR, Bolin P, Brancati FL, Bray GA, Clark JM et al. Cardiovascular effects of intensive lifestyle intervention in type 2 diabetes. *N Engl J Med* 2013; **369**(2): 145–154.

14. Franz MJ, Boucher JL, Rutten-Ramos S, VanWormer JJ. Lifestyle weight-loss intervention outcomes in overweight and obese adults with type 2 diabetes: a systematic review and meta-analysis of randomized clinical trials. J Acad Nutr Diet 2015; **115**(9): 1447–1463.

15. K. Esposito, M.I. Maiorino, M. Ciotola, Di Palo C, Scognamiglio P et al. Effects of a Mediterranean-style diet on the need for antihyperglycemic drug therapy in patients with newly diagnosed type 2 diabetes: A randomized trial. *Ann Intern Med* 2009; **151**(5): 306–314.

16. Manley SE, Stratton IM, Cull CA, Frighi V, Eeley EA et al. United Kingdom Prospective Diabetes Study Group. Effects of three months' diet after diagnosis of Type 2 diabetes on plasma lipids and lipoproteins (UKPDS 45). UK Prospective Diabetes Study Group. *Diabet Med* 2000; **17**(7): 518–523.

17. Ley SH, Hamdy O, Mohan V, Hu FB. Prevention and management of type 2 diabetes: dietary components and nutritional strategies. *Lancet* 2014; **383**(9933): 1999–2007.

18. Hensrud DD. Dietary treatment and long-term weight loss and maintenance in type 2 diabetes. *Obes Res* 2001; **9** (Suppl 4):348S–353S.

19. Esposito K, Giugliano D. Mediterranean diet and type 2 diabetes. *Diabetes Metab Res Rev* 2014; **30** (Suppl 1): 34–40.

20. Ajala O, English P, Pinkney J. Systematic review and meta-analysis of different dietary approaches to the management of type 2 diabetes. *Am J Clin Nutr* 2013; 97: 505–516.

21. van Wyk HJ, Davis RE, Davies JS. A critical review of low-carbohydrate diets in people with Type 2 diabetes. *Diabet Med* 2016; 33(2): 148–157.

22. Leeds AR. Formula food-reducing diets: A new evidence-based addition to the weight management tool box. *Nutr Bull* 2014; **39**(3): 238–2246.

23. Hamdy O, Zwiefelhofer D. Weight management using a meal replacement strategy in type 2 diabetes. *Curr Diab Rep* 2010; **10**(2): 159–164.

24. Emadian A, Andrews RC, England CY, Wallace V, Thompson JL. The effect of macronutrients on glycaemic control: a systematic review of dietary randomised controlled trials in overweight and obese adults with type 2 diabetes in which there was no difference in weight loss between treatment groups. *Br J Nutr* 2015; **114**(10): 1656–1666.

25. Ajala O, English P, Pinkney J. Systematic review and meta-analysis of different dietary approaches to the management of type 2 diabetes. *Am J Clin Nutr* 2013; **97**(3): 505–516.

26. Wheeler ML, Dunbar SA, Jaacks LM, Karmally W, Mayer-Davis EJ et al. Macronutrients, food groups, and eating patterns in the management of diabetes: a systematic review of the literature, 2010. *Diabetes Care* 2012; **35**(2): 434–445.

27. Food and Agriculture Organisation/World Health Organisation. *Carbohydrates in Human Nutrition.* FAO, Rome; 1998.

28. Mann J, Morenga LT. Carbohydrates in the treatment and prevention of type 2 diabetes. Diabet Med 2015; **32**(5): 572–575.

29. Feinman RD, Pogozelski WK, Astrup A, Bernstein RK, Fine EJ et al. Dietary carbohydrate restriction as the first approach in diabetes management: critical review and evidence base. *Nutrition* 2015; **31**(1): 1–13.

30. Kirk JK, Graves DE, Craven TE, Lipkin EW, Austin M, Margolis KL. Restricted-carbohydrate diets in patients with type 2 diabetes: a meta-analysis. *J Am Diet Assoc* 2008; **108**(1): 91–100.

31. Castañeda-González LM, Bacardí Gascón M, Jiménez Cruz A. Effects of low carbohydrate diets on weight and glycemic control among type 2 diabetes individuals: a systemic review of RCT greater than 12 weeks. *Nutr Hosp* 2011; **26**:1270–1276.

32. Dyson P. Low carbohydrate diets and type 2 diabetes: What's the latest evidence? *Diabetes Ther* 2015; **6**(4): 411–424.

33. van Wyk HJ, Davis RE, Davies JS. A critical review of low-carbohydrate diets in people with Type 2 diabetes. *Diabet Med* 2016; **33**(2): 148–157.

34. Scientific Advisory Committee on Nutrition. *Carbohydrates and Health.* TSO, London; 2015.

35. U.S. Department of Health and Human Services and U.S. Department of Agriculture. *Dietary Guidelines for Americans, 2015-2020.* Available at: http://health.gov/dietaryguidelines/2015/. Accessed 8 February 2016.

36. World Health Organization. *Guideline Sugar Intakes for Adults and Children.* WHO, Geneva 2015.

37. Malik VS, Pan A, Willett WC, Hu FB. Sugar-sweetened beverages and weight gain in children and adults: a systematic review and meta-analysis. Am J Clin Nutr 2013; **98**(4): 1084–1102.

38. Malik VS, Popkin BM, Bray GA, Després JP, Willett WC, Hu FB. Sugar-sweetened beverages and risk of metabolic syndrome and type 2 diabetes: a meta-analysis. *Diabetes Care* 2010; **33**(11): 2477–2483.

39. Franz MJ, Powers MA, Leontos C, Holzmeister LA, Kulkarni K, Monk A, Wedel N, Gradwell E. The evidence for medical nutrition therapy for type 1 and type 2 diabetes in adults. *J Am Diet Assoc.* 2010; **110**(12): 1852–1889.

40. Silva FM, Kramer CK, de Almeida JC, Steemburgo T, Gross JL et al. Fiber intake and glycemic control in patients with type 2 diabetes mellitus: a systematic review with meta-analysis of randomized controlled trials. *Nutr Rev* 2013; **71**(12): 790–801.

41. Venn BJ, Mann JI. Cereal grains, legumes and diabetes. *Eur J Clin Nutr* 2004; **58**(11): 1443–1461.

42. Colagiuri S. Health potential of a low glycaemic index diet. *BMJ* 2015; **350**: h2267.

43. Schwab U, Lauritzen L, Tholstrup T, Haldorssoni T, Riserus U et al.. Effect of the amount and type of dietary fat on cardiometabolic risk factors and risk of developing type 2 diabetes, cardiovascular diseases, and cancer: a systematic review. *Food Nutr Res* 2014; **10**: 58.

44. Shai I, Schwarzfuchs D, Henkin Y, Shahar DR, Witkow S et al. Dietary Intervention Randomized Controlled Trial (DIRECT) Group. Weight loss with a low-carbohydrate, Mediterranean, or low-fat diet. *N Engl J Med* 2008; **359**(3): 229–241.

45. Hamdy O, Horton ES. Protein content in diabetes nutrition plan. *Curr Diab Rep* 2011; **11**(2): 111–119.

46. Gannon MC, Nuttall FQ Saeed A, Jordan K, Hoover K. An increase in dietary protein improves the blood glucose response in people with type 2 diabetes. *Am J Clin Nutr* 2003; **78**: 734–741.

47. Pan Y, Guo LL, Jin HM. Low-protein diet for diabetic nephropathy: a meta-analysis of randomized controlled trials. *Am J Clin Nutr* 2008; **88**(3): 660–666.

48. Sievenpiper JL, Dworatzek PD. Food and dietary pattern-based recommendations: an emerging approach to clinical practice guidelines for nutrition therapy in diabetes. *Can J Diabetes* 2013; **37**(1): 51–57.

49. Mozaffarian D. Dietary and policy priorites for cardiovascular disease, diabetes and obesity: a comprehensive review. *Circulation* 2016; Jan 8. pii: CIRCULATIONAHA.115.018585. [Epub ahead of print].

50. Franz MJ, Boucher JL, Evert AB. Evidence-based diabetes nutrition therapy recommendations are effective: the key is individualization. *Diabetes Metab Syndr Obes* 2014; **7**: 65–72.

Chapter 4.4

Obesity and cardiovascular risk in type 2 diabetes

Catherine Whitmore and John Wilding
University of Liverpool, Liverpool, UK

4.4.1 Introduction

It is well established that people with type 2 diabetes are at high risk of developing cardiovascular disease (CVD) and that risk factor control is integral to diabetes care to reduce this risk. Overweight and obesity are highly prevalent among this population and obesity is known to be an independent risk factor for CVD in the general population. Large scale epidemiological studies such as the Framingham Heart Study [1], The Nurses' Health Study [2] and the Interheart Study [3] have documented the association between overweight and obesity and increased risk of CVD.

Whilst Body Mass Index (BMI) is the most commonly used tool to define obesity, it does not distinguish between adipose and lean tissue or different fat depots such as visceral fat. As intra-abdominal, particularly visceral obesity, has been demonstrated to be of greater importance to health risk than total adiposity, the usefulness of BMI has been challenged. In recent years there has been a shift towards waist measurement or waist/hip ratio as more reliable indicators of cardiovascular (CV) risk.

In addition to increased risk driven by metabolic abnormalities associated with obesity, there are also adverse effects on the structure, function and haemodynamics of the cardiovascular system. Left and right ventricular hypertrophy (LVH and RVH), heart failure and arrhythmias have been linked with obesity [4,5].

4.4.2 Structural changes to the heart in obesity

The effects of obesity on the structure, geometry and function of the heart have been the subject of much research. Potential associations are complicated by the fact that many obesity-associated conditions, such as hypertension and diabetes, also affect the heart. However, it is now established that LVH is independently linked with obesity. The Cardiovascular Health Study [6] found that increased left ventricular mass was significantly related to incident coronary heart disease (CHD), congestive heart failure (CHF) and stroke, and all cause mortality, even after adjustment for traditional risk factors.

Effects of systemic adiposity

The increase in adipose tissue mass in obesity requires greater blood supply leading to an increased total blood volume proportionate to weight. The persistent rise in stroke volume induces a rise in cardiac output that, coupled with decreased peripheral resistance common in obesity [5], contributes to the development of hypertension [7]. This in turn causes increased stress to the left ventricular wall, resulting in ventricular dilation and subsequent compensatory eccentric hypertrophy of the left ventricular wall [5]. This may be referred to as cardiomyopathy of obesity. In a recent study using cardiovascular magnetic resonance (CMR) Rider et al. [8]

Advanced Nutrition and Dietetics in Diabetes, First Edition. Edited by Louise Goff and Pamela Dyson.
© 2016 John Wiley & Sons, Ltd. Published 2016 by John Wiley & Sons, Ltd.

challenged this traditional view of the process when they found significant LVH without the associated ventricular cavity dilatation and excess hypertrophic response was not associated with end diastolic volume changes in a group of otherwise healthy overweight and obese patients compared to normal weight. Significant hypertrophy of the right ventricle was also observed in the obese and morbidly obese group. They suggest that increased levels of the hormone leptin rather than ventricular dilatation may be responsible for the hypertrophic changes seen.

The atria are also affected in obesity; progressive enlargement of the diameter of the left atria in proportion to BMI has been observed [9,10]. Dublin's group [9] also found increased incidence of left atrial dilation in overweight and obese subjects with atrial fibrillation (AF) (78%) compared with normal weight controls with AF (51%).

Cardiac adiposity

The role of cardiac adiposity in the development of CVD is becoming of increasing interest. In the normal heart, epicardial fat covers around 80% of the surface, accounting for around 20% of the heart's total weight [11]. Despite the difficulty in reliably imaging severely obese patients, previous studies have demonstrated a direct relationship between total adiposity and amount of epicardial and myocardial fat [11–13]. One small study demonstrated obese subjects had a three-fold increase in myocardial fat and epicardial fat and circulating free fatty acid (FFA) levels twice as high as the lean subjects [12]. Gaborit [13] found that epicardial fat volume and myocardial triglycerides were increased in obese subjects compared to lean controls but were also higher in obese subjects with metabolic syndrome and type 2 diabetes than in uncomplicated obesity. Epicardial fat functions as a physical buffer but is also metabolically active, being an important source of (FFAs) [11], which in health are the main energy substrate for the myocardium but, when present in excess may also trigger arrhythmias [5].

Cardiac adipose tissue is also an important source of pro-inflammatory adipokines (TNF-α, IL-1, IL-6 and nerve growth factor) and of the anti-inflammatory protein adiponectin [5]. The pro-inflammatory adipokines are strongly linked to CVD with significantly higher levels seen in patients with coronary artery disease [11] and are powerful predictors for the development of type 2 diabetes [4]. Adiponectin levels are reduced in obesity and have been found to be lower in individuals with CHD [14,15], which may contribute to CHD and coronary plaque instability.

4.4.3 Obesity and dysrhythmias

Obesity, cardiomyopathy and LVH have been associated with cardiac dysrhythmias. Changes in echo-cardiogram tracings in obese subjects are characterised by leftward shifts in P, QRS and T-wave axes, low QRS voltage, T-wave flattening in the inferior and lateral leads, left atrial abnormalities and prolongation of the QTc interval [16]. Obesity has been shown to be a risk factor for AF. A meta-analysis of 16 studies that enrolled a total of 123 349 participants with average follow up of 4.7–25.2 years showed a 49% increase in the risk of AF in obese individuals when compared to non-obese [17]. Large-scale epidemiological studies have indicated that for every 1 unit increase in BMI the risk of developing AF increased between 4 and 8% [10,18]. The incidence of premature ventricular contraction in obese individuals increases 10-fold compared to lean controls and when eccentric LVH is present with obesity this increases to a 30-fold risk [19].

In some studies obesity has been associated with sudden cardiac death in adults, for example in 579 cases of non-ischaemic sudden cardiac death, 23.7% were associated with obesity [20]. The mechanisms of the effect obesity has on causing dysrhythmias are not entirely clear, possible explanations proposed include disturbances of intracellular current flow and depolarisation by the enlarged myocytes, mechanical stretching of ventricular myocytes increasing the excitability threshold or increased cardiac workload in obesity increasing myocardial oxygen demand that may then lead to subendocardial ischaemia and increased ventricular ectopy [16].

4.4.4 Obesity and hypertension

Large-scale population-based studies have consistently demonstrated a link between an increase in body weight and increased blood pressure. The Framingham study showed a 20–30% increase in the odds of hypertension with a 5% weight increase [21]. Obese people are at a 3.5 fold risk of developing hypertension [22]. The degree of overweight increases the risk of developing hypertension; the odds ratio is 1.7 for overweight compared with normal weight individuals, 2.6 for class 1 obesity (BMI 30–34.9), 3.7 for class 2 obesity (BMI 35–39.9), and 4.8 for class 3 obesity (BMI > 40) [23]. Systolic and diastolic blood pressure was found to be 9 mmHg and 7 mmHg higher in obese men and 11 mmHg and 6 mmHg higher in obese women than in their normal weight counterparts [24]. Weight gain of 1 kg/m^2 is associated with an approximate 1 mmHg rise in both systolic and diastolic blood pressure [25].

The mechanisms by which increased fat mass raises blood pressure are not yet fully understood but several mechanisms have been proposed, in addition to the mechanical effects of increased adipose tissue mass and increased peripheral vascular resistance described earlier, including the effect of insulin resistance and hyperinsulinaemia on the renal tubules thus increasing sodium re-absorption [4], the overproduction of inflammatory adipokines and underproduction of adiponectin by the dysfunctional adipose tissue in obesity that have a blunting effect on vasodilatation and cause endothelial dysfunction including decreased response to nitric oxide [22]. All components of the renin–angiotensin-aldosterone system are elevated in obesity, further augmenting sodium re-absorption [26].

4.4.5 Obesity and dyslipidemia

Adipose tissue plays a direct role in the regulation of plasma lipids through the release of adipose-derived FFAs and the uptake of plasma triglycerides [27]. Dyslipidemia in obesity is characterised by increased total cholesterol, triglycerides, low density lipoprotein cholesterol (LDLc), very low density lipoprotein cholesterol (VLDL) and reduced levels of high density lipoprotein cholesterol (HDLc) [4] – termed atherogenic dyslipidemia.

Lipolysis is increased in obesity, especially where there is increased visceral adiposity. The increased influx of FFAs from the adipose tissue to the liver promote an increase in triglyceride synthesis that then leads to an overproduction of VLDL; the insulin resistance present in obesity is associated with impaired adipocyte FFA trapping, excessive lipolysis and increased ApoCIII; a protein that blocks the re-uptake of remnant lipoprotein particles, both of which increase circulating FFAs [27].

4.4.6 Obesity insulin resistance and inflammation

The metabolic syndrome (or syndrome X) was coined by Reaven in 1988 and was used to describe a cluster of cardiovascular risk factors, including central obesity, hypertension, and dyslipidemia with insulin resistance [28]. Although different definitions have been used, the metabolic syndrome is present in about 5% of normal weight, 22% of overweight and 60% of obese subjects [29]. The features of metabolic syndrome are presented in Box 4.4.1. In addition to CVD, metabolic syndrome is associated with a variety of other diseases, including polycystic ovarian syndrome, non-alcoholic fatty liver disease, non-alcoholic steatohepatitis, gallstones and neurodegenerative disease [27].

There are a variety of factors contributing to insulin resistance in obesity, including the distribution of adiposity, the role of FFAs, adipokines and inflammatory mediators and genetic factors [4]. The increased rate of lipolysis associated

> **Box 4.4.1** Metabolic syndrome
>
> Central obesity (defined as waist circumference*
> ≥ 94 cm for Europid men and ≥ 80 cm for Europid
> women, with ethnicity specific values for other
> groups)
> *plus any two* of the following four factors:
>
> - Raised TG level: ≥ 150 mg/dL (1.7 mmol/L), or
>   specific treatment for this lipid abnormality
> - Reduced HDL cholesterol: < 40 mg/dL (1.03
>   mmol/L) in males and < 50 mg/dL (1.29 mmol/L)
>   in females, or specific treatment for this lipid
>   abnormality
> - Raised blood pressure: systolic BP ≥ 130 or
>   diastolic BP ≥ 85 mm Hg, or treatment of previ-
>   ously diagnosed hypertension
> - Raised fasting plasma glucose (FPG) ≥ 100 mg/dL
>   (5.6 mmol/L), or previously diagnosed type 2
>   diabetes. If above 5.6 mmol/L or 100 mg/dL, an
>   oral glucose tolerance test (OGTT) is strongly
>   recommended but is not necessary to define
>   presence of the syndrome
>
> *If BMI is >30 kg/m^2, central obesity can be
> assumed and waist circumference does not need to
> be measured.
> Source: Ref. [31]

with increased fat mass leads to an increase in FFAs. Increased FFA delivery to the liver is implicated in the inhibition of hepatic gluconeo-genesis and increased secretion of VLDL and triglycerides in the liver, leading to fatty change and worsening hepatic insulin resistance. Increased pro-inflammatory cytokines, such as TNFα, IL-1, IL-6, IL-1β and PAI-1, contribute to chronic inflammation and appear to worsen CV risk and insulin resistance, PAI-1 is a pro-coagu-lant enhancing the risk of thrombosis and arterial disease. Whilst there is increased release of pro-inflammatory adipokines, levels of adiponectin, which promotes insulin sensitivity and clear deposits of triglycerides from the tissues, fall [5].

Reaven originally postulated that insulin resistance was the primary defect and played a central role in the development of metabolic syndrome [28]. However, despite the strong asso-ciation, insulin resistance is only one of multiple intricately linked derangements occurring in the metabolic syndrome, making it difficult to study them in isolation so it still is not clear whether

insulin resistance plays a causal role or not [27]. The insulin resistance results in hyperinsulinae-mia as the body compensates. However, not all overweight and obese people will go on to develop diabetes. There is always a degree of insulin resistance present in obesity but it can only develop into type 2 diabetes when insulin secretion is also impaired [30].

4.4.7 Effects of weight loss on CV risk

Weight control is an important factor in the man-agement of CV risk and weight loss in the over-weight or obese person can help reduce the risk of CVD. Weight loss has been shown to lower blood pressure, improve lipid profile, reduce insulin resistance and have beneficial effects on the cardiac remodelling that takes place in obe-sity. Small-scale studies on obese and morbidly obese patients after short term (≤6 months) very low calorie diets (VLCDs) showed significant decreases (−32%) in epicardial fat [32], myocar-dial mass (−7%), myocardial triglyceride uptake (−26%) and cardiac workload (−26%) [33]. A meta-analysis showed a reduction in systolic and diastolic blood pressure of ~1 mmHg per 1 kg reduction in weight [34]. Fogari was able to demonstrate a reduction of 4.2 mmHg systolic pressure and 3.3 mmHg diastolic pressure accompanied by a decrease in fasting plasma glucose, fasting plasma insulin, leptin, aldoster-one and renin levels with a mean weight loss of 8.1 kg in overweight treatment naïve patients with stage 1 hypertension [35]. Furthermore, in this study almost half of the patients who were able to achieve a normalised weight (BMI <25 kg/m^2) also normalised blood pressure. The Swedish Obesity Study found plasma glucose and insulin levels significantly improved at 2 and 10 years post intervention in the bariatric surgical intervention group (who had lost, on average, 23% of initial weight at 2 years and between 21 and 38% of initial weight depending on the type of surgical intervention) whereas levels increased in the control (conventional therapy) group who had gained 1.6% starting weight at 10 years [36]. In a recent update of this study despite some weight regain at 15 years follow up, bariatric surgery reduced the long term incidence of type 2 diabetes by 78% in obese patients and reduced the risk by 87% in obese patients with impaired fasting glucose [37]. In a group of morbidly obese patients who underwent a roux-en-y gastric bypass and achieved an average 30% weight loss, significant reductions in glucose metabolism, blood pressure, LDLc, total cholesterol, triglycerides and C-reactive protein, combined with an increase in HDLc and adiponectin, were observed, significant reductions were also noted in the control group who received intensive lifestyle intervention and lost on average 8% of starting weight [38]. Although both groups experienced a reduction in CV risk factors the reduction was significantly greater in the surgical group, who lost more than 3× the weight of the control group, indicating that benefit is proportional to the amount of weight loss.

4.4.8 Obesity paradox

The obesity paradox is that whilst obesity contributes to the risk and development of CVD, however, once CHD (in particular heart failure) has developed, overweight and obese people appear to have a better prognosis than their underweight or normal weight counterparts [39]. The mechanisms for this are unclear but may include increased metabolic reserve, lower levels of brain natriuretic peptides, increased production of TNF-α receptors, neutralising some of the adverse effects of TNF-α in overweight and obese patients [40]. Whilst it is generally agreed that weight reduction advice should always be given to morbidly obese patients, the benefit of advising overweight to moderately obese people with heart failure to lose weight divides opinion [41], and a definitive clinical trial is needed.

4.4.9 What is the best dietary composition for the prevention of CVD?

Nutritional therapy is an essential component in the management of obesity, CV risk, the metabolic syndrome and type 2 diabetes. Even a moderate weight loss of 5–10% has been shown to be beneficial. To achieve weight loss, an energy deficit must occur, 500–1000 kcal/day less than is required for weight maintenance is recommended [42]. In the United Kingdom (UK) NICE recommends a 600 kcal/day deficit [43]. Weight management is a highly complex area and the optimum macronutrient composition and dietary pattern for weight loss has yet to be established [44], if indeed it exists. Traditionally, international advice from professional diabetes associations was to recommend higher carbohydrate content (45–60% dietary energy) and reduced total and saturated fat for weight management in patients with type 2 diabetes [45]. Then, in 2008, the American Diabetes Association updated its standards of care to include the use of low carbohydrate diets for up to a year [46].

There has been a great deal of debate around the use of high protein/low or moderate carbohydrate diets over the last few years. The role of protein in weight control includes enhanced satiety, enhanced thermogenesis and lean tissue conservation [47]. Evidence tends to suggest that increasing the protein component in a mixed meal increases satiety both between meals and over the 24 hour period although this is not consistently the case and the satiating effects of increased protein load may diminish over the long term [47,48]. The thermogenic effect of food refers to the increase in energy expenditure after ingestion; the thermogenic response of protein is around 20–30% of ingested energy, compared with 5–10% for carbohydrate and <5% for lipids; the mechanism for this is thought to be due to the more complex process of digesting and absorbing protein and subsequent substantial post-prandial changes in amino acid metabolism [49]. The effect of increased protein ratio on body composition and lean body mass is debatable. In a systematic review [48], although the majority of the ten studies demonstrated greater fat loss with high protein diets compared to low protein, the difference was only significant in three. A recent study of 130 obese people prescribed either a high protein (1.6 g/kg/d) or low protein (0.8 g/kg/d) energy restricted diet found no difference in weight loss at 12 months but weight loss derived from fat was greater in the high protein group (77% men and 67% women) than in the low protein group (63% and 57% for men and women respectively) and more fat relative to lean body mass was lost by both sexes in the high protein group [50].

Concerns over dyslipidemia and renal function, as well as long term safety, have been raised over high protein/reduced carbohydrate diets. Although limiting protein intake in populations with established renal disease may slow disease progression it is not clear whether high protein diets adversely affect renal function in healthy populations [48]. In a review, no clear evidence to suggest a high protein diet had adverse event on kidney function was found, however, further long term study was recommended [51]. The strongest evidence supporting the recommendation that protein consumption should not exceed 20% of total energy intake for people with diabetes came from the EURODIAB IDDM study [52] that was a multicentre European study involving 2696 patients with type 1 diabetes that found that increased (>20%) protein intake was associated with an increase in mean albumin excretion rate (AER). However Hamdy [53] argues that, on careful reading of the study, this effect was not seen in patients with controlled diabetes or in normotensive patients regardless of diabetes control and that it was hypertension, particularly in conjunction with poorly controlled diabetes, and not protein intake that was responsible for the increase in AER. Studies of the use of high protein diets in patients with type 2 diabetes without impaired renal function also show no clear evidence to suggest an adverse effect on kidney function [53,54]. A study by Larsen et al. showed a significantly higher 24-hour urea excretion in participants with type 2 diabetes on a high protein/moderate carbohydrate diet but this was not significant at 12 months [54].

The concern that high protein diets worsened dyslipidemia and CV risk has now been challenged. Many studies have actually shown a high protein/reduced carbohydrate diet to have a beneficial effect. In the short term ($\leq$6 months) significant decreases in TC, LDL, VLDL, triglycerides and triacylglycerols and increases in HDL were seen in high protein/reduced

carbohydrate diets more often than in high carbohydrate/low fat diets [54–58] although Larsen [54] and McCall [58] did find that in their studies the high carbohydrate/low fat groups decreased LDL more than the high protein groups. However, in all of the studies with more than 12 months follow up the gap closes and there are no really significant differences in lipid profile between high protein/low-moderate carbohydrate and high carbohydrate/low fat after 1 year [54,55,57] apart from a persistent increase in HDL in high protein groups after 1 year [55,57]. Both high protein/low-moderate carbohydrate and high carbohydrate/low fat demonstrated reductions in blood pressure, for most studies this was not significant between groups although two studies found significant difference in favour of high protein/low–moderate carbohydrate in reducing systolic BP at 6, 12, and 17 months [55] and in lower diastolic at 3,6 and 24 months [57]. This demonstrates the benefit of weight loss on CV risk whichever approach is used and also demonstrates the non-inferiority of using an increased protein/moderate carbohydrate plan.

4.4.10 Mediterranean diet

The Mediterranean diet (MedDiet) has been held up over the last decade as an example of a good diet that reduces the risk of CVD. Numerous large-scale studies [59] have found adherence to the MedDiet to be associated with reduced risk of CVD. There are nine widely accepted components of the MedDiet (see Box 4.4.2). There may be concern surrounding recommending increasing dietary fat (and hence energy) in someone who is already obese. In a reduced energy, moderate fat diet high in monounsaturated fatty acids (MUFAs) reductions in body weight, BMI, percentage body fat and waist circumference were greater than the reduction seen in the low fat comparator group [60]. In this study dropout rate for the moderate fat arm was less than half of that in the low fat arm, when both arms received the same support and interventions, suggesting that a reduced energy but moderate fat diet may be easier to comply with. The PREDIMED study that compared an ad lib. MedDiet with a low fat diet showed a lack of weight gain in any of the groups at 3 months, even in patients who were already obese [61].

A meta-analysis [62] showed a −1.7 mmHg systolic and −1.5 mmHg greater reduction in blood pressure on the MedDiet than on low fat and a slightly more favourable change in triglycerides and total cholesterol, although at 0.19 mmol/L this is unlikely to be clinically significant. There is some evidence that the phenolic compounds and healthy fatty acids in virgin olive oil (MUFAs) and nuts (polyunsaturated fatty acids – PUFAs) have an anti-inflammatory action [63]. The PREDIMED study demonstrated a reduction in CRP, IL-6, TNF60 and TNF80 and other endothelial and monocytary adhesion molecules and chemokines that cause circulating monocytes and lymphocytes to adhere to the endothelial cells during inflammation contributing to the development of atherosclerosis. Interestingly in the same study concentrations of these inflammatory markers and molecules were found to increase in patients following the low fat diet [64].

4.4.11 Summary

The mechanisms by which obesity increases the risk of CVD are not yet fully understood. It is understood that people with diabetes are at increased risk of CVD and the presence of obesity increases that risk. Obesity is a complex condition and patients are often ill-served by simplistic "eat less move more" messages. The

causes and effects of obesity are complex and multifactorial, spanning from a societal level right down to a molecular level. Dietary intervention is crucial to the management of obesity and it is becoming better understood how nutrition can be manipulated, for example with the addition of MUFAs and PUFAs or manipulations of macronutrients to address some of the factors exacerbating obesity and CV risk. More long-term research is needed but it may be time to explore the options outside the traditional advice as obesity, CVD and type 2 diabetes continue to increase.

Key points

- People with type 2 diabetes are at increased risk of CVD.
- Obesity is a well-established risk factor and is associated with insulin resistance, hypertension, dyslipidaemia, inflammation and cardiac dysrhythmia.
- Weight loss improves CV risk.
- There is little evidence for the most effective diet for weight loss and reducing CV risk, although there is now emerging evidence for the Mediterranean diet.

References

1. Hubert HB, Feinleib M, McNamara PM, Castelli WP. Obesity as an independent risk factor for cardiovascular disease: a 26-year follow-up of participants in the Framingham Heart Study. *Circulation* 1983; **67**(5): 968–977.
2. Willett WC, Manson JE, Stampfer MJ, Colditz GA, Rosner B, Speizer FE, et al. Weight, weight change, and coronary heart disease in women. Risk within the 'normal' weight range. *JAMA* 1995; **273**(6): 461–465.
3. Yusuf S, Hawken S, Ôunpuu S, Bautista L, Franzosi MG, Commerford P, et al. Obesity and the risk of myocardial infarction in 27000 participants from 52 countries: a case-control study. *Lancet* 2005; **366**(9497): 1640–1649.
4. Barnett AH, Kumar S, eds. *Obesity and Diabetes*. Chichester: Wiley, 2004.
5. Williams G, Fruhbeck G, eds. *Obesity: Science to Practice*. Oxford: Wiley-Blackwell, 2008.
6. Gardin JM, McClelland R, Kitzman D, Lima JAC, Bommer W, Klopfenstein HS, et al. M-Mode

echocardiographic predictors of six- to seven-year incidence of coronary heart disease, stroke, congestive heart failure, and mortality in an elderly cohort (the cardiovascular health study). *Am J Cardiol* 2001; **87**(9): 1051–1057.

7. Ashrafian H, Athanasiou T, le Roux CW. Heart remodelling and obesity: the complexities and variation of cardiac geometry. *Heart* 2011; **97**(3): 171–172.

8. Rider OJ, Petersen SE, Francis JM, Ali MK, Hudsmith LE, Robinson MR, et al. Ventricular hypertrophy and cavity dilatation in relation to body mass index in women with uncomplicated obesity. *Heart* 2011; **97**(3): 203–208.

9. Dublin S, French B, Glazer NL, Wiggins KL, Lumley T, Psaty BM, et al. RIsk of new-onset atrial fibrillation in relation to body mass index. *Arch Intern Med* 2006; **166**(21): 2322–2328.

10. Wang TJ, Parise H, Levy D, D'Agostino RB, Sr., Wolf PA, Vasan RS, et al. Obesity and the risk of new-onset atrial fibrillation. *JAMA* 2004; **292**(20): 2471–2477.

11. Rabkin SW. Epicardial fat: properties, function and relationship to obesity. *Obes Rev* 2007; **8**(3): 253–261.

12. Kankaanpää M, Lehto H-R, Pärkkä JP, Komu M, Viljanen A, Ferrannini E, et al. Myocardial triglyceride content and epicardial fat mass in human obesity: relationship to left ventricular function and serum free fatty acid levels. *J Clin Endocrinol Metabol* 2006; **91**(11): 4689–4695.

13. Gaborit B, Kober F, Jacquier A, Moro PJ, Cuisset T, Boullu S, et al. Assessment of epicardial fat volume and myocardial triglyceride content in severely obese subjects: relationship to metabolic profile, cardiac function and visceral fat. *Int J Obes* 2012; **36**(3): 422–430.

14. Iacobellis G, Pistilli D, Gucciardo M, Leonetti F, Miraldi F, Brancaccio G, et al. Adiponectin expression in human epicardial adipose tissue in vivo is lower in patients with coronary artery disease. *Cytokine* 2005; **29**(6): 251–255.

15. Broedl UC, Lebherz C, Lehrke M, Stark R, Greif M, Becker A, et al. Low Adiponectin Levels Are an Independent Predictor of Mixed and Non-Calcified Coronary Atherosclerotic Plaques. *PloS One* 2009; **4**(3): e4733.

16. Anand RG, Peters RW, Donahue TP. Obesity and Dysrhythmias. *J Cardiometab Syndr* 2008; **3**(3): 149–154.

17. Wanahita N, Messerli FH, Bangalore S, Gami AS, Somers VK, Steinberg JS. Atrial fibrillation and obesity—results of a meta-analysis. *Am Heart J* 2008; **155**(2): 310.

18. Frost L, Hune LJ, Vestergaard P. Overweight and obesity as risk factors for atrial fibrillation or flutter: the Danish Diet, Cancer, and Health Study. *Am J Med* 2005; **118**(5): 489–495.

19. Messerli FH. Cardiovascular effects of obesity and hypertension. *Lancet* 1982; **1**(8282): 1165.

20. Hookana E, Junttila MJ, Puurunen V-P, Tikkanen JT, Kaikkonen KS, Kortelainen M-L, et al. Causes of nonischemic sudden cardiac death in the current era. *Heart Rhythm* 2011; **8**(10): 1570–1575.

21. Vasan RS, Larson MG, Leip EP, Kannel WB, Levy D. Assessment of frequency of progression to hypertension in non-hypertensive participants in the Framingham Heart Study: a cohort study. *Lancet* 2001; **358**(9294): 1682–1686.

22. Kotchen TA. Obesity-related hypertension: epidemiology, pathophysiology, and clinical management. *Am J Hypertens* 2010; **23**(11): 1170–1178.

23. Nguyen NT, Magno CP, Lane KT, Hinojosa MW, Lane JS. Association of Hypertension, Diabetes, Dyslipidemia, and Metabolic Syndrome with Obesity: Findings from the National Health and Nutrition Examination Survey, 1999 to 2004. *J Am Coll Surgeons* 2008; **207**(6): 928–934.

24. Brown CD, Higgins M, Donato KA, Rohde FC, Garrison R, Obarzanek E, et al. Body mass index and the prevalence of hypertension and dyslipidemia. *Obes Res* 2000; **8**(9): 605–619.

25. Bovet P, Ross AG, Gervasoni J-P, Mkamba M, Mtasiwa DM, Lengeler C, et al. Distribution of blood pressure, body mass index and smoking habits in the urban population of Dar es Salaam, Tanzania, and associations with socioeconomic status. *Int J Epidemiol* 2002; **31**(1): 240–247.

26. Dorresteijn JAN, Visseren FLJ, Spiering W. Mechanisms linking obesity to hypertension. *Obes Rev* 2012; **13**(1): 17–26.

27. Ahima RS. *Metabolic Basis of Obesity*. Springer, 2010.

28. Reaven GM. Role of insulin resistance in human disease (syndrome X): an expanded definition. *Ann Rev Med* 1993; **44**: 121–131.

29. Park YW, Zhu S, Palaniappan L, Heshka S, Carnethon MR, Heymsfield SB. The metabolic syndrome: prevalence and associated risk factor findings in the US population from the Third National Health and Nutrition Examination Survey, 1988-1994. *Arch Intern Med* 2003; **163**(4): 427–436.

30. Kopelmann P, ed. *Obesity in Adults and Children*, 2nd edn. Oxford: Blackwell Publishing, 2005.

31. International Diabetes Federation. The IDF consensus worldwide definition of the metabolic syndrome. Brussels, Belgium, 2006.

32. Iacobellis G, Singh N, Wharton S, Sharma AM. Substantial changes in epicardial fat thickness after weight loss in severely obese subjects. *Obesity (Silver Spring)* 2008; **16**(7): 1693–1697.

33. Viljanen APM, Karmi A, Borra R, Pärkkä JP, Lepomäki V, Parkkola R, et al. Effect of caloric restriction on myocardial fatty acid uptake, left ventricular mass, and cardiac work in obese adults. *Am J Cardiol* 2009; **103**(12): 1721–1726.

34. Neter JE, Stam BE, Kok FJ, Grobbee DE, Geleijnse JM. Influence of Weight Reduction on Blood Pressure: A Meta-Analysis of Randomized Controlled Trials. *Hypertension* 2003; **42**(5): 878–884.

35. Fogari R, Zoppi A, Corradi L, Preti P, Mugellini A, Lazzari P, et al. Effect of body weight loss and normalization on blood pressure in overweight non-obese patients with stage 1 hypertension. *Hypertension Res* 2010; **33**(3): 236.

36. Sjöström L, Lindroos A-K, Peltonen M, Torgerson J, Bouchard C, Carlsson B, et al. Lifestyle, diabetes, and cardiovascular risk factors 10 years after bariatric surgery. *N Eng J Med* 2004; **351**(26): 2683–2693.

37. Sjöström L. Review of the key results from the Swedish Obese Subjects (SOS) trial - a prospective controlled intervention study of bariatric surgery. *J Intern Med* 2013; **273**(3): 219–234.

38. Hofsø D, Nordstrand N, Johnson LK, Karlsen TI, Hager H, Jenssen T, et al. Obesity-related cardiovascular risk factors after weight loss: a clinical trial comparing gastric bypass surgery and intensive lifestyle intervention. *Eur J Endocrinol* 2010; **163**(5): 735–745.

39. Lavie CJ, Milani RV, Ventura HO. The 'obesity paradox' in coronary heart disease. *Am J Cardiol* 2010; **106**(11): 1673.

40. Todd Miller M, Lavie CJ, White CJ. Impact of obesity on the pathogenesis and prognosis of coronary heart disease. *J Cardiometab Syndr* 2008; **3**(3): 162–167.

41. Anker SD, von Haehling S. The obesity paradox in heart failure: accepting reality and making rational decisions. *Clin Pharmacol Ther* 2011; **90**(1): 188–190.

42. Summerbell C. Dietary Management and Obesity. Association for the study of obesity; 2011. Factsheet.

43. National Institute for Health and Clinical Excellence. NICE clinical guideline 43 Obesity: guidance on the prevention, identification, assessment and management of overweight and obesity in adults and children. National Institute for Health and Clinical Excellence; 2006; Available from: https://www.nice.org.uk/guidance/cg43/resources/guidance-obesity-pdf. Accessed 16 June 2015.

44. ADA. Standards of Medical Care in Diabetes—2012. *Diabetes Care* 2012; **35**(Suppl. 1): S11–S63.

45. Arathuzik GG, Goebel-Fabbri AE. Nutrition therapy and the management of obesity and diabetes: an update. *Curr Diab Rep* 2011; **11**(2): 106–110.

46. American Diabetes Association Summary of Revisions for the 2008 Clinical Practice Recommendations. *Diabetes Care* 2008; **31**(Suppl. 1): S3–S4.

47. Mela DJ. *Food, Diet and Obesity*. CRC Press, 2005.

48. Halton TL, Hu FB. The Effects of High Protein Diets on Thermogenesis, Satiety and Weight Loss: A Critical Review. *J Am Coll Nutr* 2004; **23**(5): 373–385.

49. Mancini M, Ordovas J, Riccardi G, Rubba P, Strazzullo P. Nutritional and Metabolic Bases of Cardiovascular Disease. John Wiley & Sons, 2011.

50. Evans EM, Mojtahedi MC, Thorpe MP, Valentine RJ, Kris-Etheron PM, Layman DK. Effects of protein intake and gender on body composition changes: a randomized clinical weight loss trial. *Nutr Metabol* 2012; **9**(1): 55–63.

51. Eisenstein J, Roberts SB, Dallal G, Saltzman E. High-protein Weight-loss Diets: Are They Safe and Do They Work? A Review of the Experimental and Epidemiologic Data. *Nutr Rev* 2002; **60**(7): 189–200.

52. Toeller M, Buyken A, Heitkamp G, Brämswig S, Mann J, Milne R, et al. Protein intake and urinary albumin excretion rates in the EURODIAB IDDM Complications Study. *Diabetologia* 1997; **40**(10): 1219–1226.

53. Hamdy O, Horton E. Protein Content in Diabetes Nutrition Plan. *Curr Diab Rep* 2011; **11**(2): 111–119.

54. Larsen R, Mann N, Maclean E, Shaw J. The effect of high-protein, low-carbohydrate diets in the treatment of type 2 diabetes: a 12 month randomised controlled trial. *Diabetologia* 2011; **54**(4): 731–740.

55. Hession M, Rolland C, Kulkarni U, Wise A, Broom J. Systematic review of randomized controlled trials of low-carbohydrate vs. low-fat/low-calorie diets in the management of obesity and its comorbidities. *Obes Rev* 2009; **10**(1): 36–50.

56. Hamdy O, Carver C. The why WAIT program: Improving clinical outcomes through weight management in type 2 diabetes. *Curr Diab Rep* 2008; **8**(5): 413–420.

57. Foster GD, Wyatt HR, Hill JO, Makris AP, Rosenbaum DL, Brill C, et al. Weight and metabolic outcomes after 2 years on a low-carbohydrate versus low-fat diet: a randomized trial. *Ann Intern Med* 2010; **153**(3): 147–157.

58. McCall AL. Is there a magic diet? Studying the balance of macronutrients needed for best weight loss. *Curr Diab Rep* 2010; **10**(3): 165–169.

59. Trichopoulou A, Bamia C, Trichopoulos D. Anatomy of health effects of Mediterranean diet: Greek EPIC prospective cohort study. *BMJ* 2009; **338**: b2337.

60. McManus K, Antinoro L, Sacks F. A randomized controlled trial of a moderate-fat, low-energy diet compared with a low fat, low-energy diet for weight loss in overweight adults. *Int J Obes Relat Metab Disord* 2001; **25**(10): 1503–1511.

61. Estruch R, Martínez-González MA, Corella D, Salas-Salvadó J, Ruiz-Gutiérrez V, Covas MI, et al.; PREDIMED Study Investigators. Effects of a Mediterranean-style diet on cardiovascular risk factors: a randomized trial. *Ann Intern Med* 2006; **145**(1): 1–11.

62. Nordmann AJ, Suter-Zimmermann K, Bucher HC, Shai I, Tuttle KR, Estruch R, et al. Meta-analysis comparing Mediterranean to low-fat diets for modification of cardiovascular risk factors. *Am J Med* 2011; **124**(9): 841–851.

63. Perez-Martinez P, Garcia-Quintana JM, Yubero-Serrano EM, Tasset-Cuevas I, Tunez I, Garcia-Rios A, et al. Postprandial oxidative stress is modified by dietary fat: evidence from a human intervention study. *Clin Sci (Lond)* 2010; **119**(6): 251–261.

64. Urpi-Sarda M, Casas R, Chiva-Blanch G, Romero-Mamani ES, Valderas-Martinez P, Arranz S, et al. Virgin olive oil and nuts as key foods of the Mediterranean diet effects on inflammatory biomakers related to atherosclerosis. *Pharmacol Res* 2012; **65**(6): 577–583. Epub 2012/03/28.

Chapter 4.5

Diet, education and behaviour in type 2 diabetes

Trudi Deakin
X-PERT Health Charity, Hebden Bridge, UK

4.5.1 Diet and behaviour education

People living with diabetes have a crucial role in managing their condition on a day-to-day basis, and supporting self-care via patient education using effective behavioural strategies and resources should be central to any dietary intervention. The aim of patient education is for people with diabetes to improve their knowledge, skills and confidence, enabling them to take increasing control of their own condition and integrate effective self-management into their daily lives.

All people diagnosed with diabetes should receive individualised and ongoing nutritional advice from a registered dietitian with specific expertise and competence in nutrition [1,2]. In the United Kingdom (UK) it is recommended that there are four whole-time equivalent diabetes specialist dietitians per 250 000 population [3]. The International Diabetes Federation (IDF) global guidelines for type 2 diabetes state that there should be access to a dietitian or other healthcare professional trained in the principles of nutrition, at or around the time of diagnosis, offering one initial consultation with two or three follow-up sessions, individually or in groups [4].

Structured patient education is the term frequently used in the UK, and this has been defined as "*a planned and graded programme that is comprehensive in scope, flexible in content, responsive to an individual's clinical and psychological needs, and adaptable to his or her educational and cultural background*" [5].

In the United States (US), patient education is called diabetes self-management education (DSME) and is defined as "*the on-going process of facilitating the knowledge, skill and ability necessary for diabetes self-care*". The overall objectives of DSME are to support informed decision-making, self-care behaviours, problem-solving and active collaboration with the healthcare team and to improve clinical outcomes, health status and quality of life [6].

4.5.2 One-to-one education

Although individualised nutrition therapy has been shown to be an effective strategy in reaching treatment goals for glycaemia, lipids and blood pressure [7,8], Cochrane systematic reviews have concluded that there are no high quality data on the efficacy of the dietary treatment of type 2 diabetes [9] and that individual patient education only improves glycaemic control in sub-groups with a baseline glycated haemoglobin (HbA1c) greater than 64 mmol/mol (8%) [10]. However, more recent good quality, randomised controlled trials assessing the efficacy of intensive nutrition education do not support previous systematic review evidence and instead demonstrate that intensive nutrition education is effective in achieving weight loss, improving glycaemic control and reducing cardiovascular disease risk factors [11–13].

Advanced Nutrition and Dietetics in Diabetes, First Edition. Edited by Louise Goff and Pamela Dyson.
© 2016 John Wiley & Sons, Ltd. Published 2016 by John Wiley & Sons, Ltd.

A possible explanation for this controversy is that the systematic reviews included studies where the control and intervention groups received similar treatments. Another explanation could be that the studies implemented traditional, well-intentioned nutritional advice, which attempted to define an "ideal" nutrition prescription applicable to everyone with diabetes. People commonly found such didactic information difficult to understand and incorporate into their lives [14]. In contrast, the recent studies recognise that healthcare providers need to assess the person's readiness to change and facilitate joint decision-making by matching therapeutic recommendations to personal preferences. Further clinical trials are required to confirm recent findings before systematic reviews and meta-analyses are updated to reflect the evidence base and provide international guidance regarding individualised nutritional education.

4.5.3 Group-based education

Systematic reviews of group-based education have demonstrated a profound effect on clinical outcomes, quality of life and treatment satisfaction [5,15,16]. Evidence demonstrates that group education is effective by:

(1) Improving HbA1c and diabetes knowledge
(2) Reducing blood pressure, body mass index (BMI), waist circumference and requirement for prescribed diabetes medication
(3) Increasing consumption of fruit and vegetables, enjoyment of food, self-empowerment, self-management skills and treatment satisfaction [17,18].

A programme for newly-diagnosed diabetes has demonstrated improvements in weight loss and smoking cessation and positive improvements in beliefs about the condition [19].

Group education delivered by a team, with some degree of reinforcement made at additional points of contact, may provide the best opportunity for improvements in patient outcomes [5]. Introducing group education in primary care is feasible and effective [20], and improvement at

12 months can be sustained at three years [21]. Culturally-appropriate health education is more effective for people with diabetes from ethnic minority groups [22].

It is therefore suggested that all people with diabetes and/or their carers should receive structured education at the time of diagnosis, with annual reinforcement and review [23]. Key criteria for structured patient education should be met [24] and standards for DSME implemented [25]. Therapeutic patient education using the empowerment and patient-centred approach to diabetes treatment and management should be employed [26].

Implementation of group education is a complex intervention and it is difficult to identify the components that are most effective. It has evolved from primarily didactic presentations to more theoretically-based empowerment models and programmes incorporating behavioural and psychosocial strategies [17,19,26]. There is some evidence that ongoing support is critical in order to sustain progress made by participants [27], and that behavioural goal-setting is an effective strategy to support self-management behaviours [17], but further research is required to confirm these findings. Supplementary investigations are also needed to explore the most efficient strategies to address other factors, such as staging of information provision, meeting special and cultural needs, the ideal number of sessions, the best group size and reinforcement techniques. It has been suggested that group education may halt the progression of type 2 diabetes and reduce the requirement for prescribed medication [12,13,18]. Further research is required to confirm these findings.

4.5.4 Interventions that support behaviour change

There is evidence that education that incorporates behavioural strategies is more effective than the prescription of nutritional therapy alone [5]. Health-related behaviour change is a complex process involving many psychological, social and environmental factors. Models of behaviour change are derived from theory and attempt to provide an explanation of behaviour change. They provide frameworks to simplify the theory and to enable it to be put to practical use.

The models and theories of health behaviour represent a significant step towards an understanding of why some people actively and successfully self-manage their diabetes and others do not. However, interventions before consultations designed to help people address their information needs within consultations produce limited benefits to patients [28]. Thus, there are two main drawbacks to reliance upon models of behaviour change. First, the theories assume that people think about risks in a detailed, rational fashion, whereas in fact behaviour is driven by feelings, values and beliefs and people may modify their behaviour for vague and illogical reasons. Secondly, with the various reformations of the models and theories, the distinction between many of them has become blurred [29]. This is an under-researched area and although research does support the use of behavioural strategies, more diabetes-specific research is needed to predict, explain and support health behaviour change.

A number of psychosocial theories have been developed to predict, explain, and change health behaviours. These theories can be divided into two main groups, which are commonly referred to as 'social cognition models' and 'stage models', respectively. The term social cognition models refers to a group of similar theories each of which specifies a small number of cognitive and affective factors (beliefs and attitudes) as main drivers of behaviour. The five models that have been used most widely by health behaviour researchers in recent years are: the health belief model, protection motivation theory, self-efficacy theory, the theory of reasoned action and the theory of planned behaviour. Stage models use similar concepts but organise them in a different way. They involve movement through a sequence of discrete, qualitatively distinct stages. The dominant stage model of health behaviour is the transtheoretical model.

Whilst it is not possible to identify one theoretical model as being more effective in explaining behaviour change, the following behavioural strategies have been shown to be effective in supporting self-management: self-directed behavioural goal setting, problem solving, social support, patient-centred communication and exploration of feelings [30]. The successful tools incorporated within these strategies are: keeping diary logs for physical activity, weight and diet intake; taking small steps for behavioural change; learning through observation (demonstrations, shopping trips); identification of barriers to change; learning to deal with relapse; increasing confidence to change (self-efficacy) and progressive increases in the volume and frequency of physical activity behaviours [31].

Implementation of a model for goal-setting consisting of five steps [31] has been shown to result in positive health and quality of life outcomes [17,26] and an initiative that supports joint decision-making in developing individual care plans has been shown to improve patient experience and sense of control and to lead to positive behaviour change [31].

Behavioural change interventions should be dynamic, evidence-based and flexible to the needs of the individual and users should be involved in their ongoing development [32]. Behavioural strategies should support self-management attitudes, beliefs, knowledge and skills for the learner, their family and their carers [6].

An individual assessment and education plan should be developed collaboratively by the person with diabetes and the health provider to direct the selection of appropriate behavioural and self-management support strategies [33]. This assessment, education plan, intervention and outcomes should be documented in the education record [24].

4.5.5 Resources that support behaviour change

Traditional care relied on verbal advice backed up with written literature but person-centred education should incorporate the assessment of individual learning needs and be flexible, able to cope with diversity, use different teaching media, be resource effective and have supporting materials to meet these needs [24].

It has been demonstrated that the use of educational visual aids is an effective strategy to support the development of knowledge, skills and confidence for diabetes self-management [17]. This is a particularly useful approach when educating individuals whose first language is not English and for those with sub-optimal literacy skills, as vision is a common language understandable to the majority of people. A brief video intervention has been shown to increase diabetes knowledge amongst those newly diagnosed with type 2 diabetes and may comprise an effective way of directing education to such individuals [34].

Telemedicine is a relatively new resource that involves transmitting test results and using video technology for long-distance consultations or education. Although telemedicine has been shown to be acceptable and feasible, there is not yet enough evidence to show the effects on health outcomes or costs of many expensive uses of technology [35,36]. A study that investigated telephone-based education and support from non-medically-trained tele-carers concluded that tele-carers need to adopt a patient-centred approach, be flexible and recognise that patients vary in their knowledge, skills and psychological adaption to diabetes [37].

A variety of educational visual aids and resources have been shown to assist in the learning process but further research is required to provide a stronger evidence base to support the universal use of these educational aids. Telemedicine should be used with caution as current evidence suggests little clinical benefit [37].

4.5.6 Healthcare professional communication skills that support behaviour change

Healthcare professionals working in diabetes care should obtain relevant competences, not only in the treatment and management of diabetes, but also in effective healthcare delivery to fully support diabetes self-management [38].

Healthcare professional communication skills are vital as the presentation of information, and the way it is perceived, are important determinants of the person's view of their diabetes with the initial effects of the education process at diagnosis persisting two years later [39]. Health professionals tend to talk to patients about their disease rather than to train them in the daily management of their condition, and although competent in the medical treatment, they have not always had the opportunity to develop skills to address the educational, social and psychological aspects of the condition [40]. Therapeutic patient education, an empowering patient-centred approach, focuses on individual needs, resources, values and strategies. Unlike the traditional approach, empowerment is not something one does to patients. Rather, empowerment begins when healthcare professionals acknowledge that patients are in control of their daily diabetes care by making autonomous, informed decisions about their diabetes self-management and becoming active partners in their own treatment [41]. In order for the patient-centred approach to be universally accepted, healthcare providers need to be trained in the management of long-term conditions and therapeutic patient education [38]. It has been suggested that performance measures should be included to support the practice of therapeutic patient education [42]. Healthcare professionals trained in motivational interviewing and cognitive-behavioural approaches have been shown to facilitate both the preparation and support of individuals to make informed decisions and take charge of their diabetes [43].

Thus, collaborative diabetes care requires a new "empowerment" paradigm that involves a fundamental redefinition of roles and relationships of healthcare professionals and patients [44]. Relevant competences for the facilitation of diabetes self-management have been developed [45] and further research is required to ascertain whether healthcare provider training in patient-centeredness and cultural competence will improve communication with patients, enable clarification of patients' concerns in consultations and improve satisfaction with care [46,47]. Patient-centred approaches, such as consultation style, developing empathy and identifying and handling emotional problems,

Table 4.5.1 Comparison of diet and behaviour interventions

Study	Description	Improvements in outcomes[a]								
		HbA1c	Body weight	Waist circumference	Blood pressure (mmHg)	Total cholesterol	Triglycerides	Percentage participants who reduced diabetes medication from baseline	Lifestyle (diet / physical activity/ smoking cessation)	Psychosocial
	All interventions delivered diabetes education to people with type 2 diabetes.									Not reported
Look Ahead 1 year [50] Over 4 years (averaged) [11]	RCT evaluating the effects of an intensive lifestyle intervention (1-to-1 and group education). 5,145 participants aged 45–74 years with BMI > 25 kg/m².	−8 mmol/mol [−0.7%] −4 mmol/mol [−0.36%]	−8.6% −6.2%	Not reported Not reported	−6.8/ −3.0 −5.3/ −2.9	Not reported Not reported	−1.68 mmol/l −1.42 mmol/l	7.8% 9.4%	Fitness increased 20.9% Fitness increased 12.4%	
LOAAD 6 months [12]	RCT. Intensive individualised dietary advice for six months (1-to-1 and group education). 93 participants, <70 years with a HbA1c >53 mmol/mol	−5.5 mmol/mol [−0.5%]	−2.1 kg	−2.5 cm	NS	NS	NS	13%	Decrease in saturated fat and increase in protein	Not reported
Early ACTID [13] 6 months 12 months	RCT. Intensive diet intervention within 5–8 months from diagnosis (dietary consultation every 3 months with monthly nurse support). 593 participants aged 30–80 years.	−0.8 mmol/mol [−0.07%] −1 mmol/mol [−0.09%]	−1.7 kg −1.5 kg	−2 cm −2 cm	NS NS	NS NS	−0.04 mmol/l NS	35% less likely to increase diabetes medication at 12 months	Decreased insulin resistance at 6 and 12 months	Not reported

(Continued)

Table 4.5.1 (Continued)

Study	Description	Improvements in outcomes[a]								
X-PERT										
4 months [17]	RCT. Structured group education, 6 × 2½ hour sessions delivered over 6 consecutive weeks. 314 participants aged 30–85, mean duration of living with diabetes 7 years (range 0–36 years).	−4 mmol/mol [−0.4%]	−0.3 kg	−2 cm (F) −1 cm (M)	NS	−0.2 mmol/l	−0.2 mmol/	At 12 months 25% less likely to increase diabetes medication and 15% more likely to reduce it	Increased physical activity levels. Increased consumption of fruit and vegetables. Increased foot care.	At 4 and 14 months: Increased empowerment. Increased treatment satisfaction. Improved food-related quality of life
14 months [17]		−8 mmol/mol [0.7%]	−0.5 kg	−4 cm (F) −2 cm (M)	NS	−0.3 mmol/l	−0.3 mmol/l			
2 years [18]		−5.5 mmol/mol [−0.5%]	−1.2 kg	−4.3 cm (F) NS (M)	−2.5/ −0.7	−0.3 mmol/l	−0.1 mmol/l			
DESMOND										
4 months [19]	RCT. A structured group education programme for six hours delivered in the community by two trained healthcare professional educators. 824 adults, mean age 59.5 years. All newly diagnosed with type 2 diabetes.	NS	−2.84 kg	Not reported	NS	Not reported	Not reported	Not reported	Increase in physical activity only significant at 4 months. Smoking cessation significant up to 12 months.	NS improvement in QoL. Lower depression score at 12 months and positive improvements in beliefs about Illness.
8 months [19]		NS	NS −2.98 kg	NS	NS	NS	−0.57 mmol/l			
1 year [19]		NS	NS	NS	NS	NS	NS	NS		
3 years [49]		NS	NS	NS	NS	NS	NS	NS		

[a] Only outcomes reporting an improvement with a statistically significant level of $P \geq 0.05$ are shown.

RCT: randomised controlled trial. NS: not significant. F: female. M: male. QoL: quality of life.

are increasingly being incorporated into training for providers, although 'patient-centredness' is hard to define or measure [48]. Further diabetes-specific research is required to determine whether this training will make a difference to the use of healthcare and health and quality of life outcomes.

A comparison some of the recent interventions that incorporate diet and behaviour education can be seen in Table 4.5.1.

Key points

- Diabetes education can support self-management in people with type 2 diabetes and is recommended by most authorities.
- There is strong evidence of efficacy for group-based structured education.
- Strategies including self-directed behavioural goal setting, problem solving, social support, patient-centred communication and exploration of feelings show evidence of effect.
- Health professionals' communication skills are key.

References

1. Franz MJ, Powers MA, Leontos C, Holzmeister LA, Kulkarni K, Monk A, et al. The evidence for medical nutrition therapy for type 1 and type 2 diabetes in adults. *J Am Diet Assoc* 2010; **110**: 1852–1889.
2. Dyson PA, Kelly T, Deakin TA, Duncan A, Frost G, Harrison Z, et al.; Diabetes UK Nutrition Working Group. Evidence-based nutrition guidelines for the prevention and management of diabetes. *Diabet Med* 2011; **28**(11): 1282–1288.
3. Diabetes UK Task and Finish Group. Commissioning Specialist Diabetes Services for Adults with Diabetes. London: Diabetes UK, 2010.
4. International Diabetes Federation (IDF). Global Guideline for Type 2 diabetes. Brussels: IDF, 2005.
5. Loveman E, Frampton GK, Clegg AJ. The clinical effectiveness of diabetes education models for Type 2 diabetes: a systematic review. *Health Technol Assess* 2008; **12**(9): 1–150.
6. Funnell MM, Brown TL, Childs BP, Haas LB, Hosey GM, Jensen B, et al. National standards for diabetes self-management education. *Diabetes Care* 2011; **34**(Suppl. 1): S89–S96.
7. Pastors JG, Warshaw H, Daly A, Franz M, Kulkarni K. The evidence for the effectiveness of medical nutrition therapy in diabetes management. *Diabetes Care* 2002; **25**: 608–613.
8. Franz MJ. Evidence-Based Medical Nutrition Therapy for Diabetes. *Nutr Clin Pract* 2004; **19**: 137–144.
9. Nield L, Moore H, Hooper L, Cruickshank K, Vyas A, Whittaker V, et al. Dietary advice for treatment of type 2 diabetes mellitus in adults. *Cochrane Database Syst Rev* 2007; (3): CD004097.
10. Duke SAS, Colagiuri S, Colagiuri R. Individual patient education for people with type 2 diabetes mellitus. *Cochrane Database Syst Rev* 2009; (1): CD005268.
11. Look AHEAD Research Group, Wing RR. Long-term effects of a lifestyle intervention on weight and cardiovascular risk factors in individuals with type 2 diabetes mellitus: four-year results of the Look AHEAD trial. *Arch Intern Med* 2010; **170** (17):1566–1575.
12. Coppell KJ, Kataoka M, Williams SM, Chisholm AW, Vorgers SM, Mann JI. Nutritional intervention in patients with type 2 diabetes who are hyperglycaemic despite optimised drug treatment - Lifestyle Over and Above Drugs in Diabetes (LOADD) study: randomised controlled trial. *BMJ* 2010; **341**: c3337.
13. Andrews RC, Cooper AR, Montgomery AA, Norcross AJ, Peters TJ, Sharp DJ, et al. Diet or diet plus physical activity versus usual care in patients with newly diagnosed type 2 diabetes: the Early ACTID randomised controlled trial. *Lancet* 2011; **378**: 129–123.
14. Anderson RM, Funnell M. Compliance and adherence are dysfunctional concepts in diabetes care. *Diabetes Educ* 2000; **26**(4): 597–604.
15. Norris SL, Engelgau MM, Venkat Narayan KM. Effectiveness of self-management training in type 2 diabetes: a systematic review of randomised controlled trials. *Diabetes Care* 2001; **24**: 561–587.
16. Deakin TA, McShane CT, Cade JE, Williams DDR. Group based self-management strategies in people with type 2 diabetes mellitus (Review). Cochrane Metabolic and Endocrine Group. *Cochrane Database Syst Rev* 2005; (2): CD003417.
17. Deakin TA, Cade JE, Williams R, Greenwood DC. Structured patient education: the diabetes X-PERT Programme makes a difference. *Diabet Med* 2006; **23**: 944–954.
18. Deakin TA. The diabetes pandemic: is structured education the solution or an unnecessary expense? *Pract Diabetes* 2011; **28**: 1–14.
19. Davies MJ, Heller S, Skinner TC, Campbell MJ, Carey ME, Cradock S, et al. Effectiveness of the diabetes education for ongoing and newly diagnosed (DESMOND) programme for people with newly diagnosed type 2 diabetes: cluster randomised controlled trial. *BMJ* 2008; **336**(7642): 491–495.

20. Bastiaens H, Sunaert P, Wens J, Sabbe B, Jenkins L, Nobels F, et al. Supporting diabetes self-management in primary care: pilot-study of a group-based programme focusing on diet and exercise. *Prim Care Diabetes* 2009; **3**(2): 103–109.

21. Piatt GA, Anderson RM, Brooks MM, Songer T, Siminerio LM, Korytkowski MM, et al. 3-year follow-up of clinical and behavioral improvements following a multifaceted diabetes care intervention: results of a randomized controlled trial. *Diabetes Educ* 2010; **36**(2): 301–309.

22. Hawthorne K, Robles Y, Cannings-John R, Edwards AG. Culturally appropriate health education for Type 2 diabetes in ethnic minority groups: a systematic and narrative review of randomized controlled trials. *Diabet Med* 2010; **27**(6): 613–623.

23. National Institute for Health and Clinical Excellence (NICE). Diabetes in adults quality standard. March 2011. Internet http://www.nice.org.uk/guidance/qualitystandards/diabetesinadults/diabetesinadults qualitystandard.jsp (accessed 18 August 2011).

24. Department of Health & Diabetes UK. Structured Patient Education in Diabetes: Report from the Patient Education Working Group. London: Department of Health; Gateway Reference: 4982, 2005.

25. Golay A, Lagger G, Chambouleyron M, Carrard I, Lasserre-Moutet A. Therapeutic education of diabetic patients. *Diabetes Metab Res Rev* 2008; **24**(3): 192–196.

26. Anderson RM, Funnell MM, Aikens JE, Krein SL, Fitzgerald JT, Nwankwo R, et al. Evaluating the efficacy of an empowerment-based self-management consultant intervention: results of a two-year randomized controlled trial. *Patient Educ* 2009; **1**(1): 3–11.

27. Bajardi M, Borgo E, Cavallo F, Passera P, Porta M, Tomalino M, et al. A 5-Year Randomized Controlled Study of Learning, Problem Solving Ability, and Quality of Life Modifications in People with Type 2 diabetes Managed by Group Care. *Diabetes Care* 2004; **27**: 670–675.

28. Kinnersley P, Edwards AGK, Hood K, Cadbury N, Ryan R, Prout H, et al. Interventions before consultations for helping patients address their information needs. *Cochrane Database Syst Rev* 2007; (3): CD004565.

29. Conner M, Norman P. (eds) Predicting Health Behaviour: Research and Practice with Social Cognition Models, Buckingham: Open University Press, 1995.

30. Funnell MM. Peer-based behavioural strategies to improve chronic disease self-management and clinical outcomes: evidence, logistics, evaluation considerations and needs for future research. *Family Pract* 2010; **27**: i17–i22.

31. Baker MK, Simpson K, Lloyd B, Bauman AE, Fiatarone Singh MA. Behavioral strategies in diabetes prevention programs: A systematic review of randomized controlled trials. *Diabetes Res Clin Pract* 2011; **91**: 1–12.

32. Funnell MM, Anderson RM. Empowerment and self-management of eta diabetes. *Clin Diabetes* 2004; **22**(3): 123–127.

33. Department of Health & Diabetes UK. Year of Care: Report of findings from the pilot programme. London: Department of Health, 2011.

34. Dyson PA, Beatty S, Matthews DR. An assessment of lifestyle video education for people newly diagnosed with type 2 diabetes. *J Hum Nutr Diet* 2010; **23**(4): 353–359.

35. Verhoeven F, Tanja-Dijkstra K, Nijland N, Eysenbach G, van Gemert-Pijnen L. Asynchronous and synchronous teleconsultation for diabetes care: a systematic literature review. *J Diabetes Sci Technol* 2010; **4**(3); 666–684.

36. Currell R, Urquhart C, Wainwright P, Lewis R. Telemedicine versus face to face patient care: effects on professional practice and health care outcomes. *Cochrane Database Syst Rev* 2000; (2): CD002098.

37. Gambling T, Long AF. The realisation of patient-centred care during a 3-year proactive telephone counselling self-care intervention for diabetes. *Patient Educ Couns* 2010; **80**(2): 219–226.

38. Diabetes UK. Improving supported self-management for people with diabetes. London: Diabetes UK, 2009.

39. Lawson VL, Bundy C, Harvey JN. The development of personal models of diabetes in the first 2 years after diagnosis: a prospective longitudinal study. *Diabet Med* 2008; **25**(4): 482–490.

40. WHO Working Group. Therapeutic Patient Education: continuing education programmes for healthcare providers in the field of prevention of chronic diseases. Copenhagen: World Health Organisation, 1998.

41. Anderson RM, Funnell MM. Patient empowerment: myths and misconceptions. *Patient Educ Couns* 2010; **79**(3): 277–282.

42. Glasgow RE, Peeples M, Skovlund SE. Where is the patient in diabetes performance measures? The case for including patient-centered and self-management measures. *Diabetes Care* 2008; **31**(5): 1046–1050.

43. Rubak S, Sandbaek A, Lauritzen T, Borch-Johnsen K, Christensen B. General practitioners trained in motivational interviewing can positively affect the attitude to behaviour change in people with type 2 diabetes: One year follow-up of an RCT, ADDITION Denmark. *Scand J Prim Health Care* 2009; **27**: 172–179.

44. Anderson RM, Funnell MM. Patient empowerment: reflections on the challenge of fostering the adoption of a new paradigm. *Patient Educ Couns* 2005; **57**: 153–157.

45. Simmons D, Deakin T, Walsh N, Turner B, Lawrence S, Priest L, et al. Diabetes UK Position Statement. Competency frameworks in Diabetes. *Diabet Med* 2015; DOI: 10.1111/dme.12702.

46. Bosch-Capblanch X, Abba K, Prictor M, Garner P. Contracts between patients and healthcare practitioners for improving patients' adherence to treatment, prevention and health promotion activities (Review). *Cochrane Database Syst Rev* 2007; (2): CD004808.

47. Beach MC, Price EG, Gary TL, Robinson KA, Gozu A, Palacio A, et al. Cultural competence: a systematic review of health care provider educational interventions. *Med Care* 2005; **43**(4); 356–373.

48. Lewin S, Skea Z, Entwistle VA, Zwarenstein M, Dick J. Interventions for providers to promote a patient-centred approach in clinical consultations (Review). Cochrane Consumers and Communication Group. *Cochrane Database Syst Rev* 2001; (4): CD003267.

49. Khunti K, Gray LJ, Skinner T, Carey ME, Realf K, Dallosso H, et al. Effectiveness of a diabetes education and self management programme (DESMOND) for people with newly diagnosed type 2 diabetes mellitus: three year follow-up of a cluster randomised controlled trial in primary care. *BMJ* 2012; **344**: e2333.

50. The Look AHEAD Research Group. Reduction in Weight and Cardiovascular Disease Risk Factors in Individuals with Type 2 Diabetes. One-year results of the Look AHEAD trial. *Diabetes Care* 2007; **30**: 1374–1383.

Chapter 4.6

Lifestyle issues and type 2 diabetes – physical activity and alcohol

Elaine Hibbert-Jones
Royal Gwent Hospital, Newport, UK

4.6.1 Introduction

Self-management advice for people with type 2 diabetes emphasises lifestyle change, including diet and physical activity. Chapters 4.3 and 4.5 discuss diet in relation to glycaemic control, cardiovascular risk and obesity and this chapter discusses the evidence relating to physical activity for the prevention and management of type 2 diabetes. In addition, another factor that may affect diabetes management and overall health, namely alcohol, is discussed.

4.6.2 Physical activity

Physical activity is a key component in the prevention and management of type 2 diabetes. It is now well established that regular participation in physical activity can improve blood glucose control, insulin sensitivity, lipid concentrations, blood pressure and quality of life and reduce cardiovascular events and mortality [1,2]. In addition, regular physical activity is recommended for the prevention of weight gain, the management of weight loss and the prevention of weight regain following weight loss [3].

The role of exercise in the prevention of type 2 diabetes

A number of large, multicentre trials have shown that regular participation in exercise can prevent or delay the onset of type 2 diabetes [4–6]. The Da Qing Study demonstrated that 20 minutes of mild or moderate exercise, or 10 minutes of strenuous exercise or 5 minutes of very strenuous exercise daily, reduced the risk of developing diabetes by 46% [6]. In the Finnish Diabetes Prevention Study, 30 minutes per day (150 minutes per week) of moderate intensity resistance exercise or aerobic exercise (walking, swimming) plus diet, reduced the risk of developing diabetes by 58% [5]. In the United States (US) Diabetes Prevention Program, 150 minutes of weekly aerobic activity plus diet also reduced the risk of developing type 2 diabetes by 58% [4]. At least 2.5 hours/week of moderate to vigorous physical activity should be undertaken to prevent type 2 diabetes in high risk individuals [2]. This level of exercise has also been recommended to reduce the risk of developing gestational diabetes.

Epidemiological studies show that higher levels of physical activity reduce the risk of diabetes whereas sedentary behaviours increase

Advanced Nutrition and Dietetics in Diabetes, First Edition. Edited by Louise Goff and Pamela Dyson.
© 2016 John Wiley & Sons, Ltd. Published 2016 by John Wiley & Sons, Ltd.

Table 4.6.1 Examples of aerobic and resistance training

Aerobic		Resistance
Sport/leisure	Everyday tasks	Resistance
Swimming	Brisk walking	Resistance
Jogging	Cycling	machines
Running	Vigorous	Weights e.g.
Rowing	housework	dumbbells
Racquet	Digging the	Chest presses
sports	garden	Plyometrics
Aerobics	Dancing	Hatha yoga
Football		Sit ups
Treadmill		Bench presses
Wii Fit		Shoulder
		presses

the risk [7]. It has been reported that each 2-hour increment in time spent watching television increases the risk of diabetes by 14% while each 1 hour increment of brisk walking decreases the risk by 34% [7].

Exercise and type 2 diabetes

Most of the benefits of exercise on diabetes management are achieved through acute and longer lasting improvements in insulin action, and are shown with both aerobic and resistance (anaerobic) training. Table 4.6.1 shows examples of aerobic and resistance exercise.

Energy production, substrate use and exercise type have been described in Chapter 3.5.

There are two pathways that stimulate glucose uptake by muscles. At rest and postprandially, glucose uptake into muscle is insulin-dependent. This mechanism is impaired in type 2 diabetes. During exercise, muscular contractions stimulate blood glucose uptake into working muscles via the translocation of glucose transporter proteins (Glut 4). This pathway is not impaired by insulin resistance or in type 2 diabetes [2].

Aerobic exercise

In people without diabetes, the increase in hepatic glucose production matches the glucose uptake into active muscles so that the blood glucose concentration remains stable. In people

with type 2 diabetes doing moderate intensity exercise, glucose uptake by the muscles generally exceeds hepatic glucose production and the blood glucose levels fall [8]. However, insulin levels also fall, minimising the risk of hypoglycaemia in those not taking insulin or insulin secretagogues.

Effect of aerobic exercise intensity

Aerobic exercise of moderate intensity (40–60% VO_2 max) or greater is recommended for people with type 2 diabetes [2]. A meta-analysis showed a reduction in HbA1c of 7mmol/mol (0.66%) in the exercise groups compared to the non-exercising groups. However, more intense exercise can produce greater improvements in blood glucose control, with a reduction in HbA1c of 16mmol/mol (1.5%) compared to the control group [9]. This contrasts with the findings of Hansen et al. [10] where, in a study of 50 obese males with type 2 diabetes, the groups participated in a 6 month programme of either 55 minutes at low to moderate intensity (50% VO_2 max) or 40 minutes at moderate to high intensity (75% VO_2 max) 3 times per week. Although HbA1c improved in both groups, no difference was seen between the groups, with reductions of HbA1c from 55 to 52 mmol/mol (7.2% to 6.9% $\pm$ 0.2%) in both groups.

Similar to the effect seen in type 1 diabetes, blood glucose concentration can increase following brief periods of intense aerobic activity due to an increase in plasma catecholamines that increase glucose production. This hyperglycaemia can last for 1–2 hours after the exercise session.

Metabolic effects of aerobic exercise in type 2 diabetes

- *Improvement in plasma glucose concentration and insulin resistance* Exercising muscles use 7–20 times more glucose than nonexercising muscles [1]. The effect of a single bout of exercise on insulin sensitivity and glucose tolerance lasts between 2 and 72 hours [2]. The long-term benefits are due to a cumulative effect of repeated bouts of exercise.

- *Improvement in blood pressure* Hypertension affects more than 60% of patients with type 2 diabetes [2]. Although observational studies have shown that both aerobic and anaerobic exercise can lower blood pressure in people with type 2 diabetes, the American Diabetes Association (ADA) and the American College of Sports Medicine (ACSM.) concluded that reductions in diastolic blood pressure are less common [2]. A meta-analysis of 25 studies looking at the effect of exercise on blood pressure found an average reduction of 11 and 8 mmHg respectively in systolic and diastolic blood pressures [11]. In the Look AHEAD trial, participants were given home-based exercise programmes, progressing to 175 minutes/week of moderate intensity exercise, primarily walking, as part of an intensive lifestyle intervention. Compared to those patients receiving standard diabetes support and education, this group had significantly greater reductions in diastolic and systolic blood pressure and had a significantly greater decrease in medication to treat blood pressure However, it is unlikely that these improvements are solely due to exercise. The intervention group also received specific weight reducing dietary advice. They achieved significant weight loss that was maintained over 4 years, with the intervention group showing a mean weight loss of 4.7% versus 1.1% in the control group. Weight losses of 4–7% are associated with improvements in health, including blood pressure [12,13]. Other randomised controlled trials, however, have not shown any changes in blood pressure, despite substantial increases in exercise [2,14].

- *Improvement in glycaemic control even without weight loss* A meta-analysis of controlled clinical trials found that exercise reduced HbA1c by 7 mmol/mol (0.66%), and the differences were not mediated by differences in weight loss, volume of exercise or exercise intensity [15]. One explanation given for this is the mechanisms by which insulin sensitivity is increased by exercise are not those that would necessarily be associated with body weight changes, see Box 4.6.1. The meta-analysis also found that combining diet in the

---

> **Box 4.6.1** Mechanisms by which insulin sensitivity is increased by exercise
>
> - Increased post-receptor insulin signalling
> - Increased glucose transporter protein and messenger RNA
> - Increased activity of glycogen synthase and hexokinase
> - Decreased release and increased clearance of free fatty acids
> - Increased muscle glucose delivery due to increased muscle capillary density
> - Changes in muscle composition favouring increased glucose disposal

---

exercise programme improved HbA1c more than exercise alone.

On the other hand, a randomised controlled trial, the Early ACTID study, showed no benefit in HbA1c improvements in those with newly diagnosed type 2 when exercise was combined with diet compared to diet alone [14]. In this study, subjects were assigned to usual care, diet alone or diet plus activity. The activity advice consisted of a recommendation of 30 minutes of brisk walking at least 5 days a week in addition to current activity. HbA1c was reduced in both the diet and diet plus activity groups after 6 months (–3 and –4 mmol/mol, –0.28 and –0.33%) and was maintained at 12 months. Weight loss was similar in both groups. The authors concluded that the addition of physical activity added no benefit to the use of an intensive diet intervention alone with a possible reason being that people 'reward' themselves for additional exercise with additional food, or that the form of exercise (unsupervised) was not ideal.

- *Improvement in lipid concentrations* There are mixed results of the effects of exercise on lipid concentrations, with the consensus that exercise may reduce low density lipoprotein (LDL) cholesterol but only have a small effect on high density lipoprotein (HDL) cholesterol and triglycerides [2]. In the Look AHEAD trial, the intensive lifestyle group had greater improvements in HDL and triglycerides over 4 years than the control group, but it is not possible to attribute this solely to the exercise component of the trial [13].

- *Weight management* Moderate intensity physical activity of 150–250 minutes/week with an energy equivalent of 1200–2000 kcal/week can prevent weight gain greater than 3% in most adults and may result in modest weight loss [3]. The level of exercise needed to improve blood glucose control and reduce cardiovascular risk, especially when not combined with dietary restriction, is usually insufficient for major weight loss [16]. Greater weight loss is achieved with 250–300 minutes/week or up to 60 minutes/day of exercise [2,3].

  Exercise, when combined with energy restriction provides a greater degree of weight loss compared to diet alone but this additive effect is diminished as the diet restriction is increased [3]. This may be due to the metabolic adaptations that diminish any additive effect of the energy expenditure on weight loss.

  The Look AHEAD trial combined dietary changes with activity. The intensive lifestyle group (ILI) followed diets of between 1200 and 1800 kcal/day together with 175 minutes/week of moderate intensity exercise. Compared to those patients receiving standard diabetes support and education, this group lost more weight (8.6 ± 6.9% body weight), than the control group (0.7 ± 4.8%) over 1 year and their average fitness increased by 20.9 ± 29.1% compared to 5.8 ± 22.0% in the controls [12]. The ILI group maintained a greater mean weight loss at 4 years 4.7% versus 1.1% in controls and a higher level of fitness [13]. However, it is not possible to identify which part of this multicomponent study had the greatest effect.

- *Prevention of weight regain following weight loss* There is no evidence from well-designed randomised controlled trials to judge the effectiveness of exercise for the prevention of weight regain following weight loss. Studies looking at how much exercise was associated with the least weight regain vary and include >200 minutes/week of moderate intensity exercise, 275 minutes/week of exercise above baseline levels and walking the equivalent of 16 miles/week [17].

- *Reduction or discontinuation of pharmacological treatment* Patients who undertake regular exercise use less medication than those given 'usual care' [13]. Increased exercise may enable some patients to reduce or even discontinue their medication [1].

Training effect

Aerobic training increases an individual's use of fat as an energy source, sparing glycogen and blood glucose, resulting in a lower decrease in blood glucose. The benefits of improvements in insulin action due to exercise are transient. Hence the recommendation to have no more than 2 days without aerobic exercise [2].

Recommendations for aerobic exercise

- Aerobic exercise should be performed at least 3 times a week with no more than 2 consecutive days between bouts of activity, at an intensity of 40–60% of VO_2 max (maximal aerobic capacity) for a minimum of 150 minutes/week. The activity can be performed in 10 minute bouts. Any form of aerobic exercise that uses large muscle groups and causes sustained increases in heart rate can be undertaken, see Box 4.6.2.
- The ACSM recommend 60 minutes of moderate intensity walking per day to prevent weight fluctuations <3% [3], see Table 4.6.2.

Resistance exercise

The acute effects of a single bout of resistance exercise have not been reported in type 2 diabetes but in patients with impaired fasting glucose,

---

Box 4.6.2 Exercise guidelines for adults [15]

- Moderate intensity aerobic exercise for at least 30 mins on 5 days each week. This can be in bouts of 10 or more mins *or*
- Vigorous intensity aerobic exercise for at least 20 mins on 3 days each week *or*
- A combination of the above *plus*
- Exercise to maintain or increase muscular strength and endurance (resistance exercise) at least 2 days each week

Table 4.6.2 Levels of exercise recommended for weight loss and prevention of weight regain for adults [3]

	Energy expenditure	Evidence category
To prevent weight regain	150–250 min-wk-1 (1200–2000 kcal/week)	A
For weight loss	<150 min-wk-1 – minimal weight loss	B
	>150 min-wk-1 – moderate weight loss of 2–3kg/wk	
	>225–420 min-wk-1 – weight loss of 5–7.5 kg. Dose response	
For weight maintenance after weight loss	200–300 min-wk-1 but no good evidence to recommend the amount needed to prevent weight regain after weight loss	B
Lifestyle physical activity	Useful to counter the energy imbalance in sedentary individuals that can lead to obesity	B
Physical activity and diet restriction	Physical activity increases weight loss if diet restriction is modest but not severe (<500–700 kcal/d)	A

resistance exercise reduced fasting blood glucose concentrations 24 hours after exercise [2].

Resistance training, 2–3 times a week, improves insulin action, blood glucose control and fat oxidation [2]. In an RCT, a group of older men, newly diagnosed with type 2 diabetes, participated in a twice weekly progressive resistance training programme of 45–60 mins per session, for 16 weeks, without a concomitant weight loss diet [18]. The subjects showed a 46.3% increase in insulin action, a 7% reduction in fasting blood glucose concentration and a significant loss of abdominal fat, despite a 15% increase in energy intake. These changes are thought to be due to an increase in fat free mass and muscle mass. A study of women undertaking a 12 week programme of resistance training found that although they had no change in insulin sensitivity, they had enhanced strength and muscle mass [2].

Combined aerobic and anaerobic activity

A randomised controlled trial of patients with type 2 diabetes showed a significant reduction in HbA1c of 4 mmol/mol (0.34%) over 9 months when they undertook a training programme that combined both aerobic and resistance exercises [19]. In the resistance training or aerobic training only groups, the mean changes seen in HbA1c were not significant (–2 and –3 mmol/mol,

–0.16 and –0.24% respectively). It has been suggested that patients would benefit from being given simple resistance exercises that can be done at home in addition to aerobic activity guidance.

Exercise guidelines for people with type 2 diabetes.

The most recent guidelines issued by the ACSM and ADA are summarised in Boxes 4.6.2 and 4.6.3 [15,20]. Guidance is given on the frequency, intensity and duration of both aerobic and resistance exercise to be undertaken. Examples of different types of exercise are also given.

Promotion of exercise

The Association of British Clinical Diabetologists (ABCD) recommend the best time to promote exercise in people with type 2 diabetes is around the time of diagnosis when patients are at their

---

Box 4.6.3 Physical activity guidelines for people with diabetes [2,30]

- At least 150 mins/week of moderate to vigorous intensity aerobic exercise over least 3 days with no more than 2 consecutive days between bouts of activity
- Resistance training 3 times/week
- 2.5 hours/week to prevent type 2 diabetes in high risk individuals

most motivated to make changes [1]. Although the conclusions of the early ACTID study recommend a focus on improving dietary behaviours in this group as the addition of an activity intervention conferred no additional benefits [14], further studies support physical activity at a higher intensity and volume in people with type 2 diabetes [21].

Risks of exercise

Safe exercise participation can be complicated by diabetes-related complications, such as cardiovascular disease, hypertension, microvascular changes, neuropathy and nephropathy. Worsening of pre-existing cardiovascular disease or unmasking of previously asymptomatic coronary heart disease is a major concern. Health professionals are advised to use their clinical judgement regarding recommending pre-exercise testing for low intensity exercise such as walking. No evidence suggests pre-exercise testing is routinely necessary.

For exercise more vigorous than brisk walking or exceeding the demands of everyday living, sedentary and older patients with diabetes may benefit from being assessed by a physician, for conditions associated with CVD. This may include an exercise stress test for those with an increased risk of underlying cardiovascular

disease [2], see Box 4.6.4. The ABCD recommends that every patient who wishes to start strenuous physical activity should have a thorough medical examination [1].

Exercising with long-term complications of diabetes

The presence of particular complications of diabetes may require some modification of the recommendations for exercise. More advice on this can be found in the guidelines produced by the ABCDE, ACSM and ADA [1,2] .

Many exercise programmes exclude patients with diabetic complications because of an increased risk of adverse events and, because of this, evidence for guidelines with respect to safely and exercise is lacking. Otterman et al. [22] investigated the feasibility and preliminary effectiveness of an exercise programme for 22 patients from a diabetic foot outpatient clinic completing a 12 week exercise programme. They demonstrated a 4 mmol/mol (0.4%) reduction in HbA1c and an improvement in muscle strength and perceived limitations in functioning with no training related adverse events. Further research is needed in this area to assess the effectiveness of exercise in patients with diabetic complications.

Exercise and hypoglycaemia

Although this is less of a problem for most people with type 2 diabetes compared to those with type 1 diabetes, hypoglycaemia can still occur with medications such as insulin secretagogues and insulin. For those on these medications, taking additional carbohydrate as food or fluid may be necessary to prevent low blood glucose. If the blood glucose concentration is high before exercise, hypoglycaemia is less likely to occur and additional carbohydrate is not normally necessary.

Alternatively, people treated with insulin or insulin secretagogues may need to reduce their medication to prevent exercise-induced hypoglycaemia [1,2,12]. This is the preferred strategy for those who are overweight and are exercising to lose weight, rather than increasing food intake.

Box 4.6.4 Patients at greater risk of underlying cardiovascular disease

Age >40 years with or without cardiovascular disease risk factors other than diabetes

Age >30 years and

- Type 1 or type 2 diabetes of > 10 years duration
- Hypertension
- Smoker
- Dyslipidaemia
- Proliferative or preproliferative retinopathy
- Nephropathy including microalbuminuria

Any of the following, regardless of age

- Known or suspected coronary artery disease, cerebrovascular disease and/or peripheral artery disease
- Autonomic neuropathy
- Advanced neuropathy with renal failure

Diet and exercise

Dietary advice depends on whether the person with diabetes is doing exercise for recreation, health or for competition. Physical activity, athletic performance and recovery from exercise are enhanced by optimal nutrition [23]. The key points to consider are:

- The consumption of adequate energy to support health and maximise training effects
- Sufficient carbohydrate for the maintenance of blood glucose concentration during exercise and for the restoration of glycogen stores following exercise
- Sufficient, but not excessive, fat and protein
- Prevention of dehydration that will decrease exercise performance
- The consumption of a varied diet in order to provide at least the recommended dietary allowance (RDA) for vitamins and minerals.

4.6.3 Alcohol

Risk of developing diabetes

Moderate alcohol intakes have been reported to be associated with lower prevalence of diabetes in a number of epidemiological studies. A systematic review of 32 studies in the United States [24] found:

- Moderate consumption of 1–3 drinks/day (12.6–37.8 g ethanol, 2–4 UK units) was associated with a 33–56% reduction in the incidence of type 2 diabetes and 34–55% lower incidence of diabetes-related coronary heart disease compared to non-drinkers.
- Heavy consumption (>3 drinks/day) was associated with 43% increased incidence of type 2 diabetes.

A systematic review and meta-analysis by Baliunas [25] also found a U-shaped relationship between alcohol consumption and the incidence of type 2 diabetes with a more protective effect of a moderate consumption found for women:

- In women, 24 g alcohol/day (2.4 UK units) was associated with a risk reduction of 40% compared to lifetime abstainers.

- In men, 22 g alcohol/day (2.2 UK units) was associated with 13% risk reduction.
- At higher levels of consumption (>50 g/day [>5 UK units] for women and >60 g/day [>6 UK units] for men) the risk of diabetes was increased.

The relative effects of consuming similar amounts of alcohol over a week by drinking moderate amounts daily, compared to binge drinking are unknown.

A recent study examined the relationship between high mean alcohol consumption and the metabolic syndrome and diabetes [26]. The results showed a U-shaped relationship with the metabolic syndrome, diabetes and insulin resistance. The prevalence of diabetes was 6% in non-drinkers, 3.6% in low risk (1–13 drinks/week), 3.8% in medium-high risk (14–34 drinks/week) and 6.7% in very high risk drinkers (>35 drinks/week). A meta-analysis with 12 years follow up [27] showed a U-shaped relationship with a 30–40% reduced risk of developing diabetes in those people who were consuming 1–2 drinks per day compared to heavy drinkers or abstainers.

Alcohol and glycaemic control

Although there is little evidence for the acute effect of alcohol on glycaemic control, recent studies have reported that moderate intake of alcohol is associated with improved glycaemic control in people with type 2 diabetes [28,29] although heavy drinking has a negative impact on self-care behaviours and can result in increased HbA1c levels [30].

Alcohol and blood pressure

Higher intakes of alcohol are associated with hypertension and reduction in alcohol intake in hypertensive individuals has been shown to be effective in lowering blood pressure [29].

Alcohol and medication

There is an increased risk of hypoglycaemia in those people treated with insulin or an insulin secretagogue [29], although there is no evidence for the most effective prevention and treatment of alcohol-induced hypoglycaemia. The consumption of 2–3 drinks while taking a sulfonylurea or thiazolidione does not result in adverse affects but excessive alcohol intake with metformin should be avoided because of the risk of lactic acidosis [24].

Guidelines for alcohol intake in people with type 2 diabetes

- Recommendations for most people with type 2 diabetes do not differ from national guidelines for those without diabetes
- Alcohol increases the risk of hypoglycaemia in those treated with insulin or insulin secretagogues
- There are some medical conditions where alcohol is contraindicated including hypertension, hypertryglyceridaemia, some neuropathies, retinopathy and alcohol should be avoided during pregnancy
- Alcohol should not be recommended for those people who currently do not drink.

Key points

- Regular physical activity can prevent type 2 diabetes, and improve glycaemic control and support weight maintenance in those with type 2 diabetes.
- A combination of resistance and aerobic exercise is recommended.
- Hypoglycaemia may occur in those treated with insulin or insulin secretagogues.
- Alcohol can be consumed in moderation by people with type 2 diabetes; guidelines do not differ from those for the general public.

References

1. Nagi D, Gallen I. ABCD position statement on physical activity and exercise in diabetes. *Pract Diabetes Int* 2010; **27**(4): 158–163.
2. American College of Sports Medicine and the American Diabetes Association. Joint position statement. Exercise and Type 2 diabetes. *Diabetes Care* 2010; **33**(12): e147–e167.
3. American College of Sports Medicine. Position stand. Appropriate physical activity Intervention strategies for weight loss and prevention of weight regain for adults. *Med Sci Sports Exercise* 2009; **41**(2): 459–471.
4. Diabetes Prevention Program Research Group. Reduction in the incidence of Type 2 diabetes with lifestyle intervention or Metformin. *N Engl J Med* 2002; **346**(6): 393–403.
5. Laaksonen DE, Lindstrom J, Lakka TA, Eriksson JG, Niskanen L, Wikstrom, et al. Physical activity in the prevention of type 2 diabetes. The Finnish Diabetes Prevention Study. *Diabetes* 2005; **54**(1): 158–165.
6. Pan XR, Li GW, Hu YH, Wang WY, An ZX, Hu ZX, et al. Effects of diet and exercise in preventing NIDDM in people with impaired glucose tolerance. The Da Qing IGT and Diabetes Study. *Diabetes Care* 1997; **20**(4): 537–544.
7. Hu FB. Globalization of diabetes: the role of diet, lifestyle and genes. *Diabetes Care* 2011; **34**: 1249–1257.
8. Minuk HL, Vranic M, Hanna AK, Albisser AM, Zinman B. Glucoregulatory and metabolic response to exercise in obese, non-insulin dependent diabetes. *Am J Physiol* 1981; **240**: E458–E464.
9. Boulé NG, Kenny GP, Haddad E, Wells GA, Sigal RJ. Meta-analysis of the effect of structured exercise training on cardiorespiratory fitness in type 2 diabetes mellitus. *Diabetologia* 2003; **46**: 1071–1081.
10. Hansen D, Dendale P, Jonkers RAM, Beelen M, Manders RJF, Corluy L, et al. Continuous low -to moderate- intensity exercise training is as effective as moderate- to high-intensity training at lowering HbA1c in obese type 2 diabetes patients. *Diabetologia* 2009; **52**: 1789–1797.
11. Nagi D. Benefits of regular physical activity in type 2 diabetes in: Nagi D (ed.) Exercise and Sport in Diabetes, 2nd edn. London: John Wiley & Sons Ltd., 2005.
12. Look AHEAD Research Group. Reduction in weight and cardiovascular disease risk factors in individuals with type 2 diabetes. One-year results of the Look AHEAD trial. *Diabetes Care* 2007; **30**(6): 1374–1383.
13. Look AHEAD Research Group. Long-term effects of a lifestyle intervention on weight, cardiovascular risk factors in individuals with type 2 diabetes mellitus. *Arch Intern Med* 2010; **170**(17): 1566–1575.
14. Andrews RC, Cooper AR, Montgomery AA, Norcross AJ, Peters TJ, Sharp DJ, et al. Diet or diet plus physical activity versus usual care in patients with newly diagnosed type 2 diabetes: the Early ACTID randomised controlled trial. *Lancet* 2011; **378**(9786): 129–139.
15. American College of Sports Medicine and the American Heart Association. Physical activity and public health: updated recommendation. *Med. Sci. Sports Exercise* 2007; **39**(8): 1423–1434.

16. Boulé NG, Haddad E, Kenny GP, Glen P, Wells GA, Sigal RJ. Effects of exercise on glycaemic control and body mass in type 2 diabetes mellitus: a meta-analysis of controlled clinical trials. *JAMA* 2001; **286**(10): 1218–1227.

17. Ewbank PP, Darga LL, Lucas CP. Physical activity as a predictor of weight maintenance in previously obese subjects. *Obes Res* 1995; **3**(3): 257–263.

18. Ibanez I, Izquierdo M, Arguelles I, Forga L, Larrion JL, Garcia-Unciti M, et al. Twice-weekly progressive resistance training decreases abdominal fat and improves insulin sensitivity in older men with Type 2 diabetes. *Diabetes Care* 2005; **28**(3): 662–667.

19. Church TS, Blair SN, Cocreham S, Johannsen N, Johnson W, Kramer K, et al. Effects of aerobic exercise and resistance training on haemoglobin A1c levels in patients with type 2 diabetes; a randomised controlled trial. *JAMA* 2010; **304**(20): 2253–2262.

20. American Diabetes Association. Standards of medical care in diabetes. *Diabetes Care* 2011; **34**(Suppl.): S11–S61.

21. Balducci S, Zanuso S, Pugliese G, Church T, Sigal RJ. Diet or diet or plus physical activity in patients with early type 2 diabetes. *Lancet* 2011; **378**: 2066.

22. Otterman NM, van Schie CHM, van der Schaaf M, van Bon, Busch-Westbroek TE, Nollet F. An exercise programme for patients with diabetic complications: a study on feasibility and preliminary effectiveness. *Diabet Med* 2011; **28**: 212–217.

23. American Dietetic Association , Dietitians of Canada. Nutrition and athletic performance: joint position statement. *Med Sci Sports Exercise* 2009; **41**(3): 709–731.

24. Howard AA, Arnsten J, Gourevitch MN. Effect of alcohol consumption on diabetes mellitus: a systematic review. *Ann Intern Med* 2004; **140**: 211–219.

25. Baliunas DO, Taylor BJ, Irving H, Roerecke M, Patra J, Mohapatra S, et al. Alcohol as a risk factor for type 2 diabetes: a systematic review and meta-analysis. *Diabetes Care* 2009; **32**(11): 2123–2132.

26. Clerc O, Nanchen D, Cornuz J, Marques-Vidal P, Gmels G, Daeppen J-B, et al. Alcohol drinking, the metabolic syndrome and diabetes in a population with high mean alcohol consumption. *Diabet Med* 2010; **27**: 1241–1249.

27. Koppes LL, Dekker JM, Hendriks HF, Bouter LM, Heine RJ. Moderate alcohol consumption lowers the risk of type 2 diabetes: a meta-analysis of prospective observational studies. *Diabetes Care* 2005; **28**(3): 719–725.

28. Ahmed AT, Karter AJ, Warton EM, Doan JU, Weisner CM. The relationship between alcohol consumption and glycemic control among patients with diabetes: the Kaiser Permanente Northern California Diabetes Registry. *J Gen Intern Med* 2008; **23**(3): 275–282.

29. Pietraszek A, Gregersen S, Hermansen K. Alcohol and type 2 diabetes. A review. *Nutr Metab Cardiovasc Dis* 2010; **20**(5): 366–375.

30. Engler PA, Ramsey SE, Smith RJ. Alcohol use of diabetes patients: the need for assessment and intervention. *Acta Diabetol* 2013, **50**(2): 93–99.

Chapter 4.7

Public health and the prevention of type 2 diabetes

Karen Walker

Monash University, Melbourne, Australia

4.7.1 Risk factors for type 2 diabetes

Non-modifiable risk factors

The risk of type 2 diabetes slowly increases with age and is also influenced by family history [1]. Diabetes risk doubles where both parents have the disease and again increases if the parents, particularly the mother, have been diagnosed with diabetes early in life. Women who experience an early menopause are also at higher risk [2]. Examination of the effects of inheritance suggest that generally multiple small genetic effects predominate so that the pattern of predisposing genes found in one individual may differ from those seen in another [3].

Metabolic abnormalities

Pre-diabetic conditions and diseases affecting glucose metabolism increase diabetes risk. Thus women who develop polycystic ovary syndrome or gestational diabetes are at increased risk, as are individuals with abnormalities associated with the metabolic syndrome. This is a pre-diabetic state defined by the presence of an elevated waist circumference (abdominal obesity) and raised plasma triglycerides as well as, more variably: hyperglycaemia, low plasma high density lipoproteins (HDLs) and raised blood pressure [4]. All five components of the metabolic syndrome contribute to diabetes risk, although obesity is by far the predominant factor [5].

Positive energy balance and weight gain

In modern industrialised countries energy-dense foods are very varied, plentiful and affordable while modern technologies encourage prolonged periods of sitting still. Such an environment encourages over-eating and low energy expenditure, leading many individuals to achieve a positive energy balance that when prolonged leads to steady weight gain. As a consequence, obesity now appears to be responsible for at least 80% of the population attributable risk for diabetes [5]. One meta-analysis has indicated that obesity (i.e. body mass index (BMI) >30 kg/m^2) increased diabetes risk seven-fold compared to those of normal weight, while becoming overweight (i.e. BMI >25 and ≤30 kg/m^2) increased risk almost three times [6]. Weight loss is therefore one of the most powerful means to reduce the incidence of diabetes in high-risk individuals and prevention of weight gain is the pre-eminent strategy for diabetes prevention [7]. Evidence from the effects of bariatric surgery in patients with severe obesity (mean BMI >45 kg/m^2) indicates that up to 75% of these patients can undergo complete remission of their diabetes once excess body weight is lost [8]. As discussed below, dietary interventions to induce weight loss are required for those less massively obese and can have highly beneficial outcomes. Regular physical activity is also of great importance. Modern sedentary activities, such as television viewing,

Advanced Nutrition and Dietetics in Diabetes, First Edition. Edited by Louise Goff and Pamela Dyson.
© 2016 John Wiley & Sons, Ltd. Published 2016 by John Wiley & Sons, Ltd.

have been clearly shown to increase diabetes risk [9] whereas undertaking high levels of regular physical activity can reduce diabetes risk by 20–30% [10].

Although obesity is a strong risk factor for diabetes, not all obese individuals will develop the disease.

Risk is in part determined by where adipose tissue accumulates in the body and whether or not this adipose tissue remains metabolically healthy. It is clear that the deposition of abdominal fat, as evidenced by an increased waist circumference, is particularly detrimental [11].

Adverse exposures in early life

When a growing foetus becomes subjected to conditions of malnutrition a number of adaptive changes occur that can affect later disease risk. Foetal under-nutrition can promote more efficient energy metabolism, reduction of functional elements in some developing tissues (e.g. islets or nephrons) and insulin resistance to ensure continued supply of glucose to the brain. After birth, if the child encounters an affluent post-industrial environment, these adaptations can lead to high risk of weight gain, ectopic fat deposition and diabetes in later life [12]. A trajectory of this type may to some part explain the high prevalence of diabetes in some ethnic groups such as South Asians [13].

Diet quality

Although diabetes risk is largely governed by excessive energy intake, the quality of the overall diet can modulate susceptibility. Epidemiological evidence indicates many foods impact on diabetes risk (Table 4.7.1). Foods contributing to increased diabetes risk include processed meats and red meat [14] and sugar-sweetened beverages [15] plus carbohydrate foods with high glycaemic index (GI) [16], including white rice [17] and probably (although further evidence is still needed) white potatoes [18]. Significant risk also attaches to diets with high total glycaemic load (GL) [16]. By one estimate, a 100 g/d increment in GL was associated with a 55% increase in diabetes risk [19].

Mechanisms whereby these foods exert detrimental effects remain to be fully clarified. A meal with a high GL can increase plasma glucose and non-esterified fatty acids, increase insulin demand and, if this type of meal is eaten frequently over the longer term, may lead to increased insulin resistance and contribute to weight gain [16]. Sugar-sweetened beverages lack the satiating effects of food and thus easily promote obesity and, moreover, the metabolism of their fructose component promotes the accumulation of metabolically harmful ectopic fat [20]. Processed meats contain nitrate and other preservatives as well as high amounts of sodium, these promote endothelial dysfunction and raise blood pressure [21]. Red meat in itself may contribute to lipid abnormalities by increasing saturated fat and cholesterol intake, while excessive iron intake can promote damaging oxidative stress [21].

Protective foods in relation to diabetes risk (Table 4.6.1) include wholegrain cereals [22], low fat dairy foods including yoghurt [23] and green leafy vegetables [24]. A high total fruit and vegetable intake is also protective although neither total vegetable intake nor fruit alone provides a clear effect [24]. Green leafy vegetables are rich in magnesium that is known to improve glucose metabolism and they are also a source of polyphenols that can have anti-hypertensive effects [25]. Wholegrains include the kernels and/or flour from many different cereals: wheat, oats, maize, unpolished brown rice, rye, barley, bulgur, buckwheat, amaranth and psyllium. Their protective effect is for some part associated with their insoluble dietary fibre content. High cereal fibre intake but not high vegetable fibre intake reduces diabetes risk [26]. Apart from dietary fibre, wholegrains also provide many micronutrients and phytochemicals that may mitigate oxidative stress and inflammation [27].

The protection offered by dairy foods appears attributable to nutrients in their non-fat component. Bioactive peptides in whey can stimulate the gut hormones regulating food intake [28]. Vitamin D (where dairy foods are fortified) has clear protective effects against the development of diabetes via beneficial effects on the immune system [29]. The presence of calcium in dairy

Table 4.7.1   Meta-analyses examining food intake relating to risk of Type 2 diabetes

Reference	Included studies	Number of participants	Incident cases type 2 diabetes	Length of follow-up (years)	Summary risk[a] (95% CI)
Foods increasing risk:					
Processed meat					
[14]	9	389 606	9999	4–23	1.41 [95% CI: 1.25–1.60]
White rice					
[17]	4	228 869	10 872	2–22	Western[b]: 1.12 [95% CI: 0.94–1.33]
	3	123 479	2711	5	Asian[c]: 1.55 [95% CI: 1.20–2.01]
Sugar-sweetened beverages					
[15]	8	310 819	15 819	4–20	1.26 [95% CI: 1.12–1.41]
Foods with high GI					
[16]	12	455 363	10 195	4–14	1.16 [95%CI: 1.06,1.26]
Red unprocessed meat					
[14]	10	433 070	12 226	4–23	1.12 [95%CI: 1.07, 1.38]
Foods decreasing risk:					
Decaffeinated Coffee					
[31]	6	225 516	8795	8.4–18	0.64[d] [95%CI: 0.54, 0.77]
Coffee					
[31]	18	457 922	19 319	2.6–18	0.76[d] [95%CI: 0.69–0.82]
Tea					
[31]	7	286 701	8341	8.4–18	0.82[d] [95%CI: 0.91–0.95]
Whole grains					
[22]	6	286 125	10 944	6–16	Dose[e]: 0.79 [95%CI: 0.72–0.87]
Yoghurt					
[23]	3	104 314	3480	5–12	0.83 [95%CI: 0.74–0.93]
Low fat dairy foods					
[17]	3	119 623	4810	8–12	0.82 [95%CI: 0.74, 0.90]
Green leafy vegetables					
[24]	5	192 659	18 659	4.6–18	0.84 [95%CI: 0.74,0.94]
Fruit and Vegetables					
[24]	5	179 959	19 123	6–18	0.93 [95%CI: 0.87,1.00]

[a] Highest intake *versus* lowest intake unless otherwise stated.

[b] European populations with a relatively low daily intake: <9.7 g/d vs >99 g/d.

[c] Populations from China and Japan with a relatively high daily intake: <364 g/d *versus* > 582 g/d.

[d] 3–4 cups/d *versus* 2 cups/d or less or none.

[e] For each two serve/d increment.

foods is also important although its effects may also be influenced by magnesium [30]. Consumption of coffee and tea also reduces risk [31]. The benefit of these beverages does not appear to be related to their caffeine content, but rather relates to the presence of chlorogenic acids, lignans and magnesium that can affect glucose metabolism and insulin sensitivity [31] and may also have beneficial effects on the gut microbiome [32].

While high meat intake increases diabetes risk, fish consumption can, in some circumstances, be protective. One meta-analysis indicated that high fish intake was protective in Asian populations (summary relative risk (RR) 0.89 (95% confidence interval (CI):0.81,0.98)) although this was not evident across similar studies carried out on Europeans [33]. The difference illustrates one difficulty. Protective effects of foods may depend on dietary context: other foods eaten and the way these foods are prepared. In Western populations, fish is often fried which may reduce its health benefit, whereas in Asia, fish is more frequently steamed or simmered. Understanding these complexities requires further research. In addition, meta-analyses and more primary studies are still needed to determine how other potentially protective foods such as nuts and legumes affect long-term diabetes risk.

Few studies have yet examined the effect of whole dietary patterns on diabetes risk. High adherence to a Mediterranean dietary pattern modestly reduced diabetes risk [34]. This relationship partly depended on the use of olive oil for cooking, low meat consumption and moderate alcohol intake. More studies are needed to examine the effects of this and other dietary patterns on diabetes risk.

Other risk factors

Active smoking will promote abdominal obesity and may damage the pancreas [35]. Smoking thus increases diabetes risk. One analysis found that the risk of developing diabetes was 60% higher in smokers of 20 or more cigarettes per day [35]. While moderate alcohol consumption (one to three drinks per day) appears protective and can

be part of a Mediterranean dietary pattern, heavy alcohol consumption (>3 drinks per day) is known to promote obesity and/or induce liver or pancreatic damage and will increase diabetes risk [36]. Work-related psychosocial stress does not appear to contribute to diabetes risk [37].

4.7.2 Screening for type 2 diabetes

Screening by questionnaires and risk scores

Type 2 diabetes can have a long insidious onset during which many people remain undiagnosed and unaware that they are developing the disease. The first step for public health measures is thus to identify high risk populations and to screen them regularly for the presence of diabetes. Many risk scores and screening questionnaires have now been developed for this purpose (Table 4.7.2) including one designed for global use [38]. Some are also available in electronic form. These screening tools are cost-effective in avoiding the need for an initial blood test. Identification of obesity alone is insufficient as a screening measure as some people of normal weight may exhibit insulin resistance and compromised β-cell function, while many obese people retain insulin sensitivity, particularly if they remain physically active [5].

Screening using venous plasma samples

Diabetes screening can also be carried out with blood tests using venous plasma samples. The American Diabetes Association recommends that all asymptomatic people aged 45 years or over should be screened in a healthcare setting, either by fasting plasma glucose (FPG) or by a 2 h oral glucose tolerance test (OGTT) [39]. The International Diabetes Federation suggests FPG alone can be used for screening [40]. Diabetes is present with FPG ≥7.0 mmol/L (126 mg/dL) or 2-h plasma glucose in a 75-g OGTT ≥11.1 mmol/L (200 mg/dL). More recently the use of glycated haemoglobin

Table 4.7.2 Selected screening and predictive tools for detecting undiagnosed type 2 diabetes

Test (reference)	Country of Origin	Number of variables	Items	On-line version
Screening Tools				
Cambridge DRS[a]	UK	7	age, sex, BMI, use of steroid or anti-hypertension medications, family history of diabetes, smoking habit	No
MDPPQ	UK[b]	6	age, BMI, history of diabetes or hypertension, history of GDM, ethnicity	No
Danish DRS	Denmark	6	age, sex, BMI, history of diabetes, known hypertension, physical activity	No
DRS calculator	USA	9	age, waist circumference, history of GDM, family history of diabetes, ethnicity, weight, height, hypertension, exercise	No
Patient self-assessment score	USA	6	age, sex, history of diabetes or hypertension, obesity, physical activity	No
Risk Scoring Model	China	8	age, BMI, waist:hip ratio, systolic and diastolic blood pressure, heart rate, family history of diabetes, history of hyperglycaemia	No
TOPICS diabetes screening score	Japan	6	age, sex, family history of diabetes, current smoking habit, BMI, hypertension	No
Indian DRS	India	4	age, abdominal obesity, family history of diabetes, physical activity	No
DETECT	8 countries	6	age, height, body mass index, waist circumference and systolic and diastolic blood pressure	No
Risk assessment tools				
FINDRISC	Finland	8	age, BMI, waist circumference, history of: antihypertensive treatment, hyper-glycaemia or diabetes; physical activity, daily consumption of fruits, berries and vegetables	Yes
DIFE	Germany	10	age, height, waist, hypertension, meat and fibre consumption, coffee, alcohol, physical activity, smoking	Yes
AUSDRISK	Australia	10	age, sex, waist circumference, history of diabetes or GDM, hypertensive medications, physical activity, fruit and vegetable consumption, smoking, ethnicity	Yes
Thai DRS	Thailand	5	age, BMI, waist circumference, hypertension, history of diabetes	No
Omani DRS	Oman	5	age, BMI, waist circumference, history of diabetes or hypertension	No

[a]Abbreviations: BMI: body mass index; DRS: diabetes risk score; GDM: gestational diabetes.
[b]Developed for South Asians living in the UK.

(HbA1c) has been recommended as an alternative to FPG or OGTT as it provides a measure of chronic glycaemia rather than transient blood glucose and can be determined at greater convenience for the patient, with a random non-fasting blood sample. Diabetes is present with HbA1c ≥6.5% (≥48 mmol/mol) [39,40]. Most diabetes screening is carried out in middle-aged adults, but as the obesity epidemic continues screening is now often recommended in younger individuals (including children over the age of 10 years) if they are overweight or obese and have at least one additional diabetes risk factor [39].

4.7.3 Diabetes prevention

Randomised control trials of lifestyle interventions for diabetes prevention

Overweight sedentary individuals who are developing the metabolic abnormalities associated with pre-diabetes are very good candidates for lifestyle changes to prevent the onset of type 2 diabetes. Major studies in different populations have now shown that lifestyle interventions can be very effective and cost-effective in preventing diabetes and/or slowing its progression (Table 4.7.3). For example, in the Finnish Diabetes Prevention Study (DPS) participants with impaired glucose tolerance (IGT) were randomly assigned to intensive lifestyle intervention or to a control group who received only general dietary advice. Those in the intervention group received individualised dietary counselling for a low fat healthy diet during the first year of the study, and were also encouraged to increase their physical activity and achieve modest weight loss (≥5%). After 3.2 years, diabetes incidence in the intervention group was reduced by 58% [41]. Similar interventions have also been successful either using a low fat diet [41–43], a Mediterranean diet rich in either olive oil or nuts [44], or other healthy diets low in refined carbohydrate and saturated fat [45–48]. These dietary measures were combined in most studies with support for

increased physical activity. Lifestyle interventions compare well in both cost and effectiveness with results achieved in interventions based on pharmacological agents such as metformin, alpha-glucosidase inhibitors, thiazolidinediones or Orlistat [49]. Moreover, follow-up studies to lifestyle interventions indicate that, although the interventions have only a limited duration, they can have sustained effects and bring long-lasting benefit. Thus, for example, 20 years after the Da Qing Study commenced there was a 43% lower incidence of type 2 diabetes among those who had participated in the diet plus exercise intervention than in the control group [50].

Further analyses of these lifestyle interventions provide an indication of factors that contribute to their success. An examination of the Diabetes Prevention Programme (DPP) indicated that participants were more likely to experience successful weight loss, and thus lower their diabetes risk, if they were older and more sedentary when they entered the programme and if they were older when their obesity had commenced [51]. They were also likely to be more successful if they had made few previous attempts at weight loss and had little emotionally-related eating. Development of skills in dietary restraint was found to be important to long-term success by, for example: learning to eat smaller portions of high fat foods, or to select high-fat foods less often or how to substitute a low-fat alternative for a high-fat food [51].

Long-term effects of diabetes prevention programmes

In contrast to the success of reversing progression towards diabetes in high risk individuals, once diagnosed diabetes has been evident for some time, it is more difficult but still possible to obtain a reversal through intensive lifestyle intervention. In the Look AHEAD Study, 9.2% of participants went into diabetes remission after two years of intensive lifestyle intervention, although only 3.5% remained free of diabetes after four years [52]. This illustrates the importance of screening to detect high risk individuals

Table 4.7.3 Diabetes prevention studies with lifestyle change in diverse populations

Study	Population (% female)	Follow-up (years)	Intervention	Reduction in diabetes incidence[a] (%)
Da Qing Diabetes Prevention Study [42]	577 Chinese with IGT (44%)	6	Low fat diet	56
			exercise	59
			Low fat diet *plus* exercise	51
Diabetes Prevention Study (DPS) [41]	522 Finns with IGT (67%)	3.2	Low fat diet *plus* exercise	58
Diabetes Prevention Program (DPP) [43]	3234 Americans with IGT (68%)	2.8	Low fat diet *plus* exercise	58
Indian Diabetes Prevention Program (IDPP-1) [46]	531 Indians with IGT (21%)	2.5	Low refined carbohydrate and low fat diet *plus* exercise	28.5
Taranomon Hospital Trial [45]	458 Japanese with IGT (0%)	4.0	Intensive diet plus exercise	68
The Tehran Lipid and Glucose Study (TLGS) [48]	8212 Iranians with NGT (60%)	3.6	Lifestyle intervention	39
PREDIMED-Reus [44]	7232 Spaniards with NGT (58%)	4.0	MedD (olive oil)	51
			MedD (nuts)	52
IDPP-2[b] [47]	99 Indians with IGT + IGF (21%)	3.0	Low refined carbohydrate and low fat diet *plus* exercise	20

[a]All interventions showed a significant difference from a control or standard treatment group.
[b]Non-pharmacological arms only.
IFG: impaired fasting glucose; IGT: impaired glucose tolerance; MedD: Mediterranean diet;
NGT: normal glucose tolerance.

and initiating lifestyle change at an early stage in the disease process.

Translating research into practical public health interventions

As seen in Table 4.7.3, the results accumulated from randomised control trials (RCTs) have demonstrated that lifestyle interventions to arrest progression to type 2 diabetes are both feasible and effective. The pressing concern now is how to expand the lessons learned in the controlled setting of a clinical trial to much more varied settings, translating intervention strategies into large public health programmes. Preliminary programmes are already indicating both the potential and the difficulties inherent in the translation process. Lifestyle interventions have been rolled out successfully for many different communities including: churches, community health centres, primary care settings (delivered by nurse practitioners) or provided at peoples' homes or at the workplace. New methods of programme delivery are also being trialled, such as remote coaching by telephone. The Greater Green Triangle Diabetes Prevention Project [53] provides one example of a primary-care-based intervention. Participants were patients presenting at local medical clinics in several small towns in southern Australia. They received a structured group programme comprising six 90 minute education sessions delivered by trained nurses over an 8-month period. After one year participants had successfully lost weight (−2.52 kg (95%CI: 1.85,3.19)) and waist circumference (−4.17 cm (95%CI: 3.48,4.87)) and had experienced metabolic improvement [53]. All changes that reduce diabetes risk.

Nation-wide programmes for diabetes prevention in high risk individuals are now slowly being developed in many countries. Finland commenced with the National Type 2 Diabetes Prevention Program (FIN-D2). Results from a one year follow-up of nearly 4000 participants has indicated that 19% lost at least 5% body weight and over 30% experienced improvement in glucose tolerance [54]. Other large scale programmes such as the European *Prevention using Lifestyle, Physical Activity and Nutritional Intervention* (DE-PLAN) have also been initiated [55]. A start has therefore now been made but considerable effort is still required to develop effective, culturally appropriate programs for the diverse populations worldwide who are at high risk of diabetes.

Key points

- The risk factors for type 2 diabetes include both non-modifiable (age, gender, family history, ethnicity) and modifiable (diet, physical activity, body weight).
- Certain foods, including coffee, wholegrains and green leafy vegetables appear to decrease risk and others, including red and processed meat, white rice and sugar-sweetened beverages increase the risk.
- Screening for diabetes can be achieved by direct blood sampling or by use of composite risk scores.
- There is strong evidence for diabetes prevention from randomised controlled trials in high-risk subjects, although little evidence of translation of this at the population level.

References

1. Wilson PW, Meigs JB, Sullivan L, Fox CS, Nathan DM, D'Agostino RB Sr. Prediction of incident diabetes mellitus in middle-aged adults: the Framingham Offspring Study. *Arch Intern Med* 2007; **167**: 1068–1074.
2. Brand JS, van der Schouw YT, Onland-Moret NC, Sharp SJ, Ong KK, Khaw KT, et al. Age at menopause,
   reproductive life span, and type 2 diabetes risk: results from the EPIC-InterAct study. *Diabetes Care* 2013; **36**: 1012–1019.
3. Phillips CM. Nutrigenetics and metabolic disease: current status and implications for personalised nutrition. *Nutrients* 2013; **5**: 32–57.
4. Alberti KG, Eckel RH, Grundy SM, Zimmet PZ, Cleeman JI, Donato KA, et al. Harmonizing the metabolic syndrome: a joint interim statement of the International Diabetes Federation Task Force on Epidemiology and Prevention;National Heart, Lung, and Blood Institute; American Heart Association; World Heart Federation; International Atherosclerosis Society; and International Association for the Study of Obesity. *Circulation* 2009; **120**: 1640–1645.
5. Laaksonen MA, Knekt P, Rissanen H, Härkänen T, Virtala E, Marniemi J, et al. The relative importance of modifiable potential risk factors of type 2 diabetes: a meta-analysis of two cohorts. *Eur J Epidemiol* 2010; **25**: 115–124.
6. Abdullah A, Peeters A, de Courten M, Stoelwinder J. The magnitude of association between overweight and obesity and the risk of diabetes: a meta-analysis of prospective cohort studies. *Diabetes Res Clin Pract* 2010; **89**: 309–319.
7. Liberopoulos EN, Tsouli S, Mikhailidis DP, Elisaf MS. Preventing type 2 diabetes in high risk patients: an overview of lifestyle and pharmacological measures. *Curr Drug Targets* 2006; **7**: 211–228.
8. Buchwald H, Estok R, Fahrbach K, Banel D, Jensen MD, Pories WJ, et al. Weight and type 2 diabetes after bariatric surgery: systematic review and meta-analysis. *Am J Med* 2009; **122**: 248–256.
9. Grøntved A, Hu FB. Television viewing and risk of type 2 diabetes, cardiovascular disease, and all-cause mortality: a meta-analysis. *JAMA* 2011; **305**: 2448–2455.
10. Gill JM, Cooper AR. Physical activity and prevention of type 2 diabetes mellitus. *Sports Med* 2008; **38**: 807–824.
11. Lee MJ, Wu Y, Fried SK. Adipose tissue heterogeneity: implication of depot differences in adipose tissue for obesity complications. *Mol Aspects Med* 2013; **34**: 1–11.
12. Brenseke B, Prater MR, Bahamonde J, Gutierrez JC. Current thoughts on maternal nutrition and fetal programming of the metabolic syndrome. *J Pregnancy* 2013; **2013**: 368461. doi: 10.1155/2013/368461. Epub 2013 Feb 14.
13. Bhopal RS. A four-stage model explaining the higher risk of Type 2 diabetes mellitus in South Asians compared with European populations. *Diabet Med* 2013; **30**: 35–42.
14. Aune D, Ursin G, Veierød MB. Meat consumption and the risk of type 2 diabetes: a systematic review and meta-analysis of cohort studies. *Diabetologia* 2009; **52**: 2277–2287.

15. Malik VS, Popkin BM, Bray GA, Després JP, Willett WC, Hu FB. Sugar-sweetened beverages and risk of metabolic syndrome and type 2 diabetes: a meta-analysis. *Diabetes Care* 2010; **33**: 2477–2483.

16. Dong JY, Zhang L, Zhang YH, Qin LQ. Dietary glycaemic index and glycaemic load in relation to the risk of type 2 diabetes: a meta-analysis of prospective cohort studies. *Br J Nutr* 2011; **106**: 1649–1654.

17. Hu EA, Pan A, Malik V, Sun Q. White rice consumption and risk of type 2 diabetes: meta-analysis and systematic review. *BMJ* 2012; **344**: e1454.

18. Halton TL, Willett WC, Liu S, Manson JE, Stampfer MJ, Hu FB. Potato and french fry consumption and risk of type 2 diabetes in women. *Am J Clin Nutr* 2006; **83**: 284–290.

19. Livesey G, Taylor R, Livesey H, Liu S. Is there a dose-response relation of dietary glycemic load to risk of type 2 diabetes? Meta-analysis of prospective cohort studies. *Am J Clin Nutr* 2013; **97**: 584–596.

20. Stanhope KL, Schwarz JM, Havel PJ. Adverse metabolic effects of dietary fructose: results from the recent epidemiological, clinical, and mechanistic studies. *Curr Opin Lipidol* 2013; **24**: 198–206.

21. Micha R, Michas G, Mozaffarian D. Unprocessed red and processed meats and risk of coronary artery disease and type 2 diabetes–an updated review of the evidence. *Curr Atheroscler Rep* 2012; **14**: 515–524.

22. de Munter JS, Hu FB, Spiegelman D, Franz M, van Dam RM. Whole grain, bran, and germ intake and risk of type 2 diabetes: a prospective cohort study and systematic review. *PLoS Med* 2007; **4**: e261.

23. Tong X, Dong JY, Wu ZW, Li W, Qin LQ. Dairy consumption and risk of type 2 diabetes mellitus: a meta-analysis of cohort studies. *Eur J Clin Nutr* 2011; **65**: 1027–1031.

24. Cooper AJ, Forouhi NG, Ye Z, Buijsse B, Arriola L, Balkau B, et al. Fruit and vegetable intake and type 2 diabetes: EPIC-InterAct prospective study and meta-analysis. *Eur J Clin Nutr* 2012; **66**: 1082–1092.

25. Rodrigo R, Gil D, Miranda-Merchak A, Kalantzidis G. Antihypertensive role of polyphenols. *Adv Clin Chem* 2013; **58**: 225–254.

26. Schulze MB, Schulz M, Heidemann C, Schienkiewitz A, Hoffmann K, Boeing H. Fiber and magnesium intake and incidence of type 2 diabetes: a prospective study and meta-analysis. *Arch Intern Med* 2007; **167**: 956–965.

27. Belobrajdic DP, Bird AR. The potential role of phytochemicals in wholegrain cereals for the prevention of type-2 diabetes. *Nutr J* 2013; **12**: 62.

28. Jakubowicz D, Froy O. Biochemical and metabolic mechanisms by which dietary whey protein may combat obesity and Type 2 diabetes. *J Nutr Biochem* 2013; **24**: 1–5.

29. Forouhi NG, Ye Z, Rickard AP, Khaw KT, Luben R, Langenberg C, et al. Circulating 25-hydroxyvitamin D concentration and the risk of type 2 diabetes: results from the European Prospective Investigation into Cancer (EPIC)-Norfolk cohort and updated meta-analysis of prospective studies. *Diabetologia* 2012; **55**: 2173–2182.

30. Dong JY, Qin LQ. Dietary calcium intake and risk of type 2 diabetes: possible confounding by magnesium. *Eur J Clin Nutr* 2012; **66**: 408–410.

31. Huxley R, Lee CM, Barzi F, Timmermeister L, Czernichow S, Perkovic V, et al. Coffee, decaffeinated coffee, and tea consumption in relation to incident type 2 diabetes mellitus: a systematic review with meta-analysis. *Arch Intern Med* 2009; **169**: 2053–2063.

32. Moco S, Martin FP, Rezzi S: Metabolomics view on gut microbiome modulation by polyphenol-rich foods. *J Proteome Res* 2012; **11**: 4781–4790.

33. Zheng JS, Huang T, Yang J, Fu YQ, Li D. Marine N-3 polyunsaturated fatty acids are inversely associated with risk of type 2 diabetes in Asians: a systematic review and meta-analysis. *PLoS ONE* 2012; **7**: e44525.

34. InterAct Consortium, Romaguera D, Guevara M, Norat T, Langenberg C, Forouhi NG, et al. Mediterranean diet and type 2 diabetes risk in the European Prospective Investigation into Cancer and Nutrition (EPIC) study: the InterAct project. *Diabetes Care* 2011; **34**: 1913–1918.

35. Willi C, Bodenmann P, Ghali WA, Faris PD, Cornuz J. Active smoking and the risk of type 2 diabetes: a systematic review and meta-analysis. *JAMA* 2007; **298**: 2654–2664.

36. Howard AA, Arnsten JH, Gourevitch MN. Effect of alcohol consumption on diabetes mellitus: a systematic review. *Ann Intern Med* 2004; **140**: 211–219.

37. Cosgrove MP, Sargeant LA, Caleyachetty R, Griffin SJ. Work-related stress and Type 2 diabetes: systematic review and meta-analysis. *Occup Med (Lond)* 2012; **62**: 167–173.

38. Vistisen D, Lee CM, Colagiuri S, Borch-Johnsen K, Glümer C. A globally applicable screening model for detecting individuals with undiagnosed diabetes. *Diabetes Res Clin Pract* 2012; **95**: 432–438.

39. American Diabetes Association. Executive summary: standards of medical care in diabetes – 2012. *Diabetes Care* 2012; **35**(Suppl. 1): 4–10.

40. IDF Task Force. Global Guideline for Type 2 Diabetes. Brussels: IDF, 2005, pp. 1–11.

41. Tuomilehto J, Lindström J, Eriksson JG, Valle TT, Hämäläinen H, Ilanne-Parikka P, et al. Prevention of type 2 diabetes mellitus by changes in lifestyle among subjects with impaired glucose tolerance. *N Engl J Med* 2001; **344**: 1343–1350.

42. Pan XR, Li GW, Hu YH, Wang JX, Yang WY, An ZX, et al. Effects of diet and exercise in preventing NIDDM in people with impaired glucose tolerance. The Da Qing IGT and Diabetes Study. *Diabetes Care* 1997; **20**: 537–544.

43. Knowler WC, Barrett-Connor E, Fowler SE, Hamman RF, Lachin JM, Walker EA, et al. Diabetes Prevention Program Research Group: Reduction in the incidence of type 2 diabetes with lifestyle intervention or metformin. *N Engl J Med* 2002; **346**: 393–403.

44. Salas-Salvadó J, Bulló M, Babio N, Martínez-González MÁ, Ibarrola-Jurado N, Basora J, et al. Reduction in the incidence of type 2 diabetes with the Mediterranean diet: results of the PREDIMED-Reus nutrition intervention randomized trial. *Diabetes Care* 2011; **34**: 14–19.

45. Kosaka K, Noda M, Kuzuya T. Prevention of type 2 diabetes by lifestyle intervention: a Japanese trial in IGT males. *Diabetes Res Clin Pract* 2005; **67**: 152–162.

46. Ramachandran A, Snehalatha C, Mary S, Mukesh B, Bhaskar AD, Vijay V, et al. The Indian Diabetes Prevention Programme shows that lifestyle modification and metformin prevent type 2 diabetes in Asian Indian subjects with impaired glucose tolerance (IDPP-1). *Diabetologia* 2006; **49**: 289–297.

47. Ramachandran A, Arun N, Shetty AS, Snehalatha C. Efficacy of primary prevention interventions when fasting and postglucose dysglycemia coexist: analysis of the Indian Diabetes Prevention Programmes (IDPP-1 and IDPP-2). *Diabetes Care* 2010; **33**: 2164–2168.

48. Harati H, Hadaegh F, Momenan AA, Ghanei L, Bozorgmanesh MR, Ghanbarian A, et al. Reduction in incidence of type 2 diabetes by lifestyle intervention in a middle eastern community. *Am J Prev Med* 2010; **38**: 628–636.

49. Shin JA, Lee JH, Kim HS, Choi YH, Cho JH, Yoon KH. Prevention of diabetes: a strategic approach for individual patients. *Diabetes Metab Res Rev* 2012; **28**(Suppl. 2): 79–84.

50. Li G, Zhang P, Wang J, Gregg EW, Yang W, Gong Q, et al. The long-term effect of lifestyle interventions to prevent diabetes in the China Da Qing Diabetes Prevention Study: a 20-year follow-up study. *Lancet* 2008; **371**: 1783–1789.

51. Delahanty LM, Peyrot M, Shrader PJ, Williamson DA, Meigs JB, Nathan DM, et al. Pretreatment, psychological, and behavioral predictors of weight outcomes among lifestyle intervention participants in the Diabetes Prevention Program (DPP). *Diabetes Care* 2013; **36**: 34–40.

52. Gregg EW, Chen H, Wagenknecht LE, Clark JM, Delahanty LM, Bantle J, et al. Association of an intensive lifestyle intervention with remission of type 2 diabetes. *JAMA* 2012; **308**: 2489–2496.

53. Laatikainen T, Dunbar JA, Chapman A, Kilkkinen A, Vartiainen E, Heistaro S, et al. Prevention of type 2 diabetes by lifestyle intervention in an Australian primary health care setting: Greater Green Triangle (GGT) Diabetes Prevention Project. *BMC Public Health* 2007; **7**: 249.

54. Rautio N, Jokelainen J, Saaristo T, Oksa H, Keinänen-Kiukaanniemi S; FIN-D2D Writing Group. Predictors of success of a lifestyle intervention in relation to weight loss and improvement in glucose tolerance among individuals at high risk for type 2 diabetes: The FIN-D2D Project. *J Prim Care Community Health* 2013; **4**: 59–66.

55. Schwarz PE, Lindström J, Kissimova-Scarbeck K, Szybinski Z, Barengo NC, Peltonen M, et al. The European perspective of type 2 diabetes prevention: diabetes in Europe–prevention using lifestyle, physical activity and nutritional intervention (DE-PLAN) project. *Exp Clin Endocrinol Diabetes* 2008; **116**: 167–172.

SECTION 5

Pregnancy and diabetes

Chapter 5.1

Epidemiology, aetiology and pathogenesis of diabetes in pregnancy

Anne Dornhorst and Shivani Misra

Imperial College Healthcare NHS Foundation Trust, London, UK

5.1.1 Introduction

Understanding the different types of diabetes encountered in pregnancy is important for the pregnant woman, the management of the pregnancy and the long-term implications for both mother and child. This chapter addresses the epidemiology, aetiology and pathogenesis of diabetes in pregnancy and reviews the influence of subtypes of diabetes and degree of maternal hyperglycaemia on pregnancy outcome.

5.1.2 Epidemiology

The incidence of pregnancies complicated by diabetes is increasing and will continue to increase over the foreseeable future.

Pre-gestational diabetes

An audit of 3808 pregnancies in England, Wales and Northern Ireland between 2002 and 2003 identified that 1 in 250 pregnancies occurred in women with established (pre-gestational) diabetes, with 27.6% classified as having type 2 diabetes [1]. Five years later, from 2007 to 2008, an audit of 1381 pregnancies from the Northern, North West and East Anglia regions of England found that type 2 diabetes accounted for 40.3% of women with pre-gestational diabetes [2]. Currently most antenatal clinics serving urban industrialised areas in the United

Kingdom (UK), like other parts of the world, are encountering more pregnant women with type 2 rather than type 1 diabetes [3–5].

The rise in pregnant women with type 2 diabetes is not surprising. In the UK the prevalence of type 2 diabetes has increased on average by 4.9% per year over the last two decades, reflecting the dramatic rise in obesity [6]. Meanwhile, the age of onset of type 2 diabetes has declined, with the most notable decrease occurring among younger women, and in ethnic minorities. The proportion of new diagnoses of diabetes in the UK among the age group 30 to 44 years increased from 7.5 to 15.8% between 1996 and 2006 [7].

Antenatal clinics in the UK, like many other urbanised areas of the world are frequently encountering pregnancies with diabetes due to the combination of increasing obesity, delayed age at first pregnancy and greater ethnic diversity. More women from ethnic backgrounds that carry an increased risk of type 2 diabetes are giving birth.

The prevalence of obesity in pregnant women has more than doubled in the UK in recent years, with a rise from 7.6 to 15.6% occurring between 1987 and 2007 [8]. Maternal obesity, independently of diabetes, is associated with poor pregnancy outcomes, including an increased risk of congenital malformations and stillbirth [4,9]. This effect of obesity may partially explain why outcomes in pregnant women with type 2 and type 1 diabetes are similar despite the duration

Advanced Nutrition and Dietetics in Diabetes, First Edition. Edited by Louise Goff and Pamela Dyson.
© 2016 John Wiley & Sons, Ltd. Published 2016 by John Wiley & Sons, Ltd.

of diabetes being considerably less in women with type 2 diabetes [1,10,11].

A two- to three-fold increase in congenital malformations occurs in pregnancies of women with either type 1 or type 2 diabetes. This risk is highly dependent on the level of maternal hyperglycaemia at conception, therefore ensuring good glycaemic control peri-conception is extremely important [1,12,13].

Furthermore, women of reproductive age with type 2 diabetes are more likely to experience greater social deprivation than those with type 1 diabetes and are less likely to either access pre-conception counselling or plan their pregnancies [1]. In addition, women with type 2 are more likely to be managed in primary rather than secondary care, where access to tailored pre-conception counselling and advice may be less available [14].

Whilst the background prevalence of type 1 diabetes is slowly rising [15], this increase is comparatively lower than that for type 2 diabetes. Therefore the proportion of women with pre-gestational type 2 diabetes will continue to rise. However, since the age of onset of type 1 diabetes is falling across Europe [16] the cumulative duration of type 1 diabetes among pregnant women is increasing. The duration of type 1 diabetes is important when considering pregnancy outcomes, as the risk of pregnancy-induced hypertension, pre-eclampsia, deterioration of retinopathy and severe maternal hypoglycaemia all increase with increasing duration of diabetes [17–19]. In addition, women with type 1 diabetes are, like the background population, becoming more obese and this similarly can compromise pregnancy outcomes, particularly the risk of foetal macrosomia [20,21].

Gestational diabetes

Gestational diabetes (GDM) is defined as any degree of glucose intolerance first recognised in pregnancy [22]. The majority of women develop glucose intolerance in the late second or early third trimester of pregnancy. This glucose intolerance arises as a consequence of the inability to secrete sufficient insulin to overcome the pregnancy-related increase in insulin resistance [23].

Estimates of the prevalence of GDM are highly dependent on the diagnostic criteria used to diagnose the condition; its prevalence also reflects the background rates of type 2 diabetes within that population, which may be present pre-gestationally but not detected until screening during the pregnancy. Thus the prevalence of GDM ranges between 2 and 20% depending on these factors [24,25].

Gestational diabetes is a heterogeneous condition [22]. The current definition of GDM encompasses women with undiagnosed pre-existing diabetes or glucose intolerance. This will therefore include women with previously undiagnosed type 2 diabetes; pre-clinical type 1 diabetes [26] and those with the rarer monogenic forms of diabetes, commonly known as MODY (maturity onset diabetes of the young) [27] or mitochondrial diabetes [28].

Those with previously undiagnosed type 2 diabetes are an important subset of women to recognise and the proportions in this category are rapidly increasing as the prevalence of type 2 diabetes increases in women of reproductive age [29]. This is a particularly concerning group, as in comparison to GDM developing later in pregnancy these women will be hyperglycaemic at the time of conception and organogenesis and thus carry excess risk of congenital malformation [30]. Early testing for type 2 diabetes in pregnancy is thus recommended [24].

Another smaller group of women who will initially be referred to as having GDM are those who are in the subclinical phases of type 1 diabetes [31,32]. There is an almost four-fold increase in the incidence of diabetes during the third trimester of pregnancy, in comparison to age-matched non-pregnant women [26]. Women in the preclinical phases of type 1 diabetes, already have compromised β-cell function but may still maintain normal glycaemia if not pregnant. However, during pregnancy they will not be able to meet the additional insulin demands required in late pregnancy due to increased insulin resistance and will present with diabetes at this time.

Women with asymptomatic, previously undetected monogenic forms of diabetes are also likely to be detected during pregnancy, due to a combination of screening programmes and the metabolic changes occurring in pregnancy. Women with monogenic forms of diabetes will also be over-represented in this age group [33,34]. Although these cases will be initially classified as GDM, post-partum the underlying metabolic process will continue and their type of diabetes will need to be reclassified.

Accurately separating the type of diabetes in young pregnant women is difficult, and sophisticated laboratory testing is often required, with close follow-up in the post-partum period [29].

5.1.3 Aetiology

Pre-gestational type 1 diabetes

Type 1 diabetes can occur at any age, although typically has its onset in the first three decades of life. It is caused by an autoimmune destruction of the pancreatic β-cells that produce insulin [35]. The current evidence points to an initial environmental trigger, possibly from a virus such as an enterovirus, in an individual with a background genetic susceptibility profile that responds to that trigger. The immune response involves both T- and B-lymphocytes and this finally results in the autoimmune destruction of functioning β-cells [36]. This inherent genetic susceptibility to type 1 diabetes also confers a susceptibility to other autoimmune diseases, for example autoimmune thyroid disease that occurs in 15–30% of type 1 diabetes cases and coeliac disease in 4–9% [35]. Pregnant women with type 1 diabetes should therefore routinely have their thyroid function tested at the start of their pregnancy.

Pre-gestational type 2 diabetes

Type 2 diabetes is characterised by hyperglycaemia due to a relatively impaired and insufficient insulin response to the affected individual's level of insulin resistance [37]. Type 2 diabetes is a polygenic condition that requires an underlying genetic susceptibility, as well as the presence of adverse environmental and lifestyle factors, to be fully expressed [38]. This is reflected in migration studies that demonstrate that populations with similar gene pools only develop high levels of type 2 diabetes when they migrate from rural environments with active lifestyles to a more sedentary setting, characteristically associated with an urbanised lifestyle, including increased exposure to energy-dense foods and decreased levels of physical activity [39].

Type 2 diabetes used to be a condition of late middle age but over the last three decades has occurred increasingly in younger age groups [29,40,41]. This earlier onset of type 2 diabetes is now occurring among most industrialised populations due to increased levels of obesity and physical inactivity.

An interesting and recognised contributor to early onset type 2 diabetes is exposure to a hyperglycaemic intrauterine environment [42]. This represents an example of foetal programming; a process through which *in utero* nutritional and metabolic exposure can influence long-term foetal outcomes [43]. Epigenetic changes are thought to be the molecular process mediating foetal programming [44]. Epigenetic changes influence gene expression by modifying DNA structure through methylation or acetylation of histone proteins, that form part of the complex protein packaging material supporting DNA.

In the Pima Indian population, which has one of the highest prevalence rates for early onset type 2 diabetes, the strongest single risk factor for type 2 diabetes in children aged between 5 and 19 years, is the exposure to diabetes *in utero* [45].

Gestational diabetes

Glucose intolerance occurring *de novo* in pregnancy arises when maternal insulin secretion cannot respond sufficiently to maintain euglycaemia. Maternal insulin secretion should increase two- to three-fold during the latter half of pregnancy to compensate for the changes in maternal insulin sensitivity [46]. These changes include increasing levels of placental hormones, for example human placental growth hormone and cytokines such as TNF-α and leptin [4]. These hormones increase in the maternal circulation throughout pregnancy from 8 weeks gestation, reaching maximum levels at week 35 of gestation, and have a direct inhibitory effect on insulin signalling [47] as well as raising maternal free fatty acid levels. The resulting pregnancy-related increase in maternal insulin resistance is advantageous for the developing foetus, as it facilitates the maternal-foetal transfer of glucose, especially in the post-prandial period, effectively preferentially diverting glucose away from maternal tissues to the foetus.

Glucose is the main foetal substrate stimulating foetal insulin production, which acts as the major foetal growth factor. In GDM the increased maternal glucose levels are sufficient to cause foetal hyperinsulineamia and thus accelerated foetal growth, manifesting as a large for gestational-age infant with increased adiposity and foetal macrosomia [48].

Following parturition, maternal insulin resistance rapidly returns to normal with evidence of enhanced skeletal muscle insulin signalling during this period [49]. In the post-partum phase, if the glucose intolerance of GDM resulted purely from the metabolic changes of pregnancy, normal glucose tolerance is restored. However, it is important to note that these women are still metabolically susceptible to future diabetes, if and when their insulin sensitivity decreases, either due to a further pregnancy or as a consequence of lifestyle factors such as weight gain or physical inactivity. Importantly, pregnant women with evolving late-onset type 1 diabetes, may also show restoration of euglycaemia post-partum, but will gradually become insulinopenic in the ensuing months.

Women with a previous history of GDM are therefore at risk of future type 2 diabetes [50]. The progression to type 2 diabetes can be delayed with lifestyle intervention and by oral hypoglycaemic agents such as metformin [51,52]. However, over the last 20 years the progression to type 2 diabetes has been faster in all populations studied due to rising levels of obesity [53,54]. It is also faster in those ethnic groups with a higher background prevalence of type 2 diabetes [55]. Women who develop impaired glucose tolerance post-GDM have a more accelerated progression to overt type 2 diabetes than women who have no history of prior GDM [52].

The degree of maternal hyperglycaemia that predicts future glucose intolerance in offspring appears to occur at relatively low levels. There is increasing evidence that the degree of hyperglycaemia that occurs in women with GDM may be considered relatively mild, when compared with women who have overt pre-gestational diabetes. However this is still high enough to affect foetal programming [56]. This phenomenon is important, as if the epidemic of type 2 diabetes is to be halted, ensuring good maternal glycaemic control in pregnancy will be a necessary part of any prevention programme.

5.1.4 Risk factors

Pre-gestational diabetes

Deciding who has type 1 or type 2 diabetes based on classical risk factors, for example ethnicity, body habitus and age of onset is no longer reliable. The clinical phenotypes of women diagnosed with type 1 and type 2 diabetes during childbearing ages have become increasingly blurred. This is due to the emergence of young-onset type 2 diabetes within these groups [29,41], increasing obesity occurring amongst women with type 1 diabetes reflecting the background prevalence of obesity [20], and the onset of type 2 diabetes in lean individuals from certain ethnic groups.

At least 40% of type 1 diabetes presents after the age of 18 years. The presentation can be more insidious than childhood-onset, and can involve a relatively mild period of hyperglycaemia that is non-insulin requiring [57]. The classical acute type 1 diabetes presentation is thus not a hallmark of type 1 diabetes in adulthood. In addition, ethnicity is not a reliable discriminator, as although early onset type 2 diabetes is more common among certain ethnic groups, these groups will also adopt the background risk of type 1 diabetes of their country of residence, as shown by South Asian children within the UK [58].

When managing a woman with pre-gestational diabetes it is always important to consider whether the subtype diagnosis is in fact correct, as treatment and advice will be influenced by the type of diabetes a woman has, and hence misclassification may lead to erroneous treatment. It may well be the first time since the initial diagnosis that the classification of subtype is being addressed. This is especially important for women with rare monogenic forms of diabetes who are over-represented in this age group, as their management may be different from those with type 1 or type 2 diabetes [59]. It is therefore always worth considering whether the following risk factors are present:

- A family history of diabetes
- A family history or a personal history of auto-immune diseases other than type 1 diabetes
- A history suggestive of increased insulin resistance, such as polycystic ovarian syndrome, acanthosis nigricans
- A history of previous gestational diabetes.

A young woman with type 2 diabetes would be expected to have a family history of type 2 diabetes and also a history of GDM in any previous pregnancy. If she has no family history and the diagnosis was made within the previous 2 years the possibility of her having type 1 diabetes should be seriously considered, regardless of her body weight and ethnic origin. Measuring autoantibodies associated with type 1 diabetes may be undertaken and, if positive, latent onset diabetes of adulthood (LADA), sometimes called pre-clinical type 1 diabetes, should be considered [60]. Making such a diagnosis would change the educational advice given during the pregnancy as key advice on the avoidance of ketoacidosis would need to be given, along with education on how and when to test blood or urine ketones.

Serum C-peptide can aid discrimination of type 1 from type 2 diabetes outside pregnancy [61], however, its interpretation during pregnancy, when maternal insulin secretion increases, will be problematic unless undetectable, though complete insulin deficiency would usually manifest clinically.

The glycaemic targets and management goals for all diabetes in pregnancy are similar regardless of the type of pre-gestational diabetes a women has. Treatment is also similar with multiple daily insulin injections alongside self-glucose monitoring 6 to 8 times throughout the day. In addition women with type 2 diabetes in the UK are also prescribed metformin while those with type 1 are not [62]. Post partum, women diagnosed with LADA in pregnancy require close follow-up for assessment of on-going insulin requirements.

In contrast, a woman previously diagnosed as having type 1 diabetes on the basis of age, for example a diagnosis during her 20s or earlier, may well carry the wrong diagnosis. If she has a strong family history of type 2 diabetes and gestational diabetes among the female members of the family, the likelihood is she will have type 2 rather than type 1 diabetes. This diagnosis would be further strengthened if the women in question had a history of polycystic ovarian disease [63] or clinical evidence of acanthosis nigricans [64]. Laboratory investigations confirming she has negative autoimmune antibodies for type 1 diabetes and a high circulating plasma C-peptide value (though these may not be routinely available) make the diagnosis of type 2 diabetes likely and the woman may therefore benefit from the addition of metformin both during and following the pregnancy. In addition, the lifestyle advice given to her family would be different. Children of mothers with type 2 diabetes are at high risk of developing type 2 diabetes and intensive lifestyle changes around diet and increased physical activity can have a very positive effect in lessening the risk of diabetes in at risk groups [65].

Although uncommon, one should always consider a diagnosis of the monogenic forms of diabetes when a pregnant woman has a very strong family history of early onset diabetes that appears to be inherited as an autosomal dominant trait. The two most common forms of MODY in Europe are mutations in the hepatocyte nuclear factor 1 alpha gene (MODY 3) and glucokinase gene (MODY 2) [66]. Although the prevalence of MODY in pregnant women is unknown it could represent up to 1.8% of all cases of diabetes in pregnancy, reflecting the proportionally lower prevalence of type 2 diabetes in this age group than reported in non-pregnant diabetic population studies [27]. Making the diagnosis of MODY can affect clinical management both during and after the pregnancy [67].

Gestational diabetes

The presence of risk factors for gestational diabetes still forms the basis for undertaking selective screening for GDM in the UK. The 2008 UK NICE (National Institute of Clinical Excellence) guidelines for diabetes in pregnancy currently do not include age as a risk factor [62], despite its inclusion in guidelines from other countries. In a tertiary obstetric hospital in Australia increasing age alongside BMI >35 kg/m^2 and previous GDM were the most significant risk factors for gestational diabetes, with age > 40 years having an ODDs Ratio of 7.0 (95% CI 2.9–17.2) [68]. Currently, UK-based advice is to offer screening for GDM in pregnancy at 28 weeks gestation using a 75 g oral glucose tolerance test (OGTT) only to women with any of the following risk factors:

- BMI more than 30 kg/m^2
- Previous macrosomic baby weighing 4.5 kg or more
- Previous GDM
- Family history of diabetes (first-degree relative with diabetes)
- Family origin with a high prevalence of diabetes (South Asian, Black Caribbean, Middle Eastern).

Prior to the 2010 International Association of Diabetes and Pregnancy Study Groups (IADPSG) recommendations for universal screening using the newly defined 75 g OGTT diagnostic criteria [24], both the American Diabetes Association (ADA) and the Australasian Diabetes in Pregnancy Society guidelines, like the NICE guidelines, advocated selective screening based on risk factors. With all guidelines having a high sensitivity (>92%) but low specificity (4–32%) for the diagnosis of GDM.

The new IADPSG guidelines advocate universal screening using a 75g OGTT, with the diagnosis of GDM based on any plasma glucose value above 5.1 mmol/L in the fasting state, 10.0 mmol/L at 1 hour or 8.5 mmol/L at 2 hours post-OGTT. These are expected to result in many more women being diagnosed with GDM in comparison to established selective screening and the WHO criteria for impaired glucose tolerance [25]. However, the level of maternal glycaemia proposed in the IADPSG guidelines was found to be associated with increased rates of macrosomia, neonatal hypoglycaemia, high cord C-peptide values and increased Caesarean section rates, in a large observational study of unselected pregnant women universally screened at 28 weeks gestation [48]. Another risk factor for GDM is maternal weight gain during the first 24 weeks of pregnancy in overweight and obese women, but not in women who are either underweight or have a normal BMI before pregnancy [69]. As maternal obesity as well as GDM are both independently associated with adverse pregnancy outcomes and have an additive effect on risk, this highlights the need to give all overweight or obese women appropriate weight gain targets early in pregnancy [70].

Gestational diabetes will present an enormous resource challenge to maternity services in coming years if up to a fifth of all pregnant women are identified as having GDM (by IADPSG criteria). However, identifying women with GDM may have the potential to limit the risk of premature obesity and type 2 diabetes in subsequent generations. If this holds true, the currently unstoppable 'juggernaut' of the obesity and diabetes epidemic may be amenable to preventative lifestyle interventions in women of childbearing age both before and during pregnancy.

Key points

- There are two types of diabetes during pregnancy; pre-gestational (established type 1 or type 2 diabetes before pregnancy) and gestational (diabetes occurring during pregnancy).
- Diabetes during pregnancy increases the risk of macrosomia, congenital malformations, stillbirth and neonatal deaths.
- Rates of both pre-gestational and gestational pregnancy are increasing.
- It is recommended that diabetes during pregnancy is diagnosed by a standard 75 g oral glucose tolerance test.

References

1. Health, C.E.i.M.a.C., *Pregnancy in women with type 1 and type 2 diabetes in 2002–03, England, Wales and Northern Ireland.* London: CEMACH, 2005.

2. Holman N, Lewis-Barned N, Bell R, Stephens H, Modder J, Gardosi J, et al. Development and evaluation of a standardized registry for diabetes in pregnancy using data from the Northern, North West and East Anglia regional audits. *Diabet Med* 2011; **28**(7): 797–804.

3. Lawrence JM, Contreras R, Chen W, Sacks DA. Trends in the prevalence of preexisting diabetes and gestational diabetes mellitus among a racially/ethnically diverse population of pregnant women, 1999–2005. *Diabetes Care* 2008; **31**(5): 899–904.

4. McIntyre HD, Thomae MK, Wong SF, Idris N, Callaway LK. Pregnancy in type 2 diabetes mellitus–problems & promises. *Curr Diabetes Rev* 2009; **5**(3): 190–200.

5. Albrecht SS, Kuklina EV, Bansil P, Jamieson DJ, Whiteman MK, Kourtis AP, et al. Diabetes trends among delivery hospitalizations in the U.S., 1994–2004. *Diabetes Care* 2010; **33**(4): 768–773.

6. Gonzalez EL, Johansson S, Wallander MA, Rodríguez LA. Trends in the prevalence and incidence of diabetes in the UK: 1996–2005. *J Epidemiol Community Health* 2009; **63**(4): 332–336.

7. Charlton J, Latinovic R, Gulliford MC. Explaining the decline in early mortality in men and women with type 2 diabetes: a population-based cohort study. *Diabetes Care* 2008; **31**(9): 1761–1766.

8. Heslehurst N, Rankin J, Wilkinson JR, Summerbell CD. A nationally representative study of maternal obesity in England, UK: trends in incidence and demographic inequalities in 619 323 births, *1989–2007. Int J Obes (Lond.)* 2010; **34**(3): 420–428.

9. Heslehurst N, Simpson H, Ells LJ, Rankin J, Wilkinson J, Lang R, et al. The impact of maternal BMI status on pregnancy outcomes with immediate short-term obstetric resource implications: a meta-analysis. *Obes Rev* 2008; **9**(6): 635–683.

10. Macintosh MC, Fleming KM, Bailey JA, Doyle P, Modder J, Acolet D, et al. Perinatal mortality and congenital anomalies in babies of women with type 1 or type 2 diabetes in England, Wales, and Northern Ireland: population based study. *BMJ* 2006; **333**(7560): 177.

11. Balsells M, García-Patterson A, Gich I, Corcoy R. Maternal and fetal outcome in women with type 2 versus type 1 diabetes mellitus: a systematic review and metaanalysis. *J Clin Endocrinol Metab* 2009; **94**(11): 4284–4291.

12. The Diabetes Control Complications Trial Research Group. Pregnancy outcomes in the Diabetes Control and Complications Trial. *Am J Obstet Gynecol* 1996; **174**(4): 1343–13453.

13. Guerin A, Nisenbaum R, Ray JG. Use of maternal GHb concentration to estimate the risk of congenital anomalies in the offspring of women with prepregnancy diabetes. *Diabetes Care* 2007; **30**(7): 1920–1925.

14. Roman M. Preconception Care for Women With Preexisting Type 2 Diabetes. *Clin Diabetes* 2011; **29**: 10–16.

15. Bruno G, Maule M, Merletti F, Novelli G, Falorni A, Iannilli A, et al. Age-period-cohort analysis of 1990-2003 incidence time trends of childhood diabetes in Italy: the RIDI study. *Diabetes* 2010; **59**(9): 2281–2287.

16. Patterson CC, Dahlquist GG, Gyürüs E, Green A, Soltész G; EURODIAB Study Group. Incidence trends for childhood type 1 diabetes in Europe during 1989-2003 and predicted new cases 2005-20: a multicentre prospective registration study. *Lancet* 2009; **373**(9680): 2027–2033.

17. Hanson U, Persson B. Epidemiology of pregnancy-induced hypertension and preeclampsia in type 1 (insulin-dependent) diabetic pregnancies in Sweden. *Acta Obstet Gynecol Scand* 1998; **77**(6): 620–624.

18. Temple RC, Aldridge VA, Sampson MJ, Greenwood RH, Heyburn PJ, Glenn A. Impact of pregnancy on the progression of diabetic retinopathy in Type 1 diabetes. *Diabet Med* 2001; **18**(7): 573–577.

19. Evers IM, ter Braak EW, de Valk HW, van Der Schoot B, Janssen N, Visser GH. Risk indicators predictive for severe hypoglycemia during the first trimester of type 1 diabetic pregnancy. *Diabetes Care* 2002; **25**(3): 554–559.

20. Persson M, Norman M, Hanson U. Obstetric and perinatal outcomes in type 1 diabetic pregnancies: A large, population-based study. *Diabetes Care* 2009; **32**(11): 2005–2009.

21. Persson M, Pasupathy D, Hanson U, Norman M. Birth size distribution in 3,705 infants born to mothers with type 1 diabetes: a population-based study. *Diabetes Care* 2011; **34**(5): 1145–1149.

22. American Diabetes Association Diagnosis and classification of diabetes mellitus. *Diabetes Care* 2004; **27**(Suppl. 1): S5–S10.

23. Homko C, Sivan E, Chen X, Reece EA, Boden G. Insulin secretion during and after pregnancy in patients with gestational diabetes mellitus. *J Clin Endocrinol Metab* 2001; **86**(2): 568–573.

24. IADPS. International association of diabetes and pregnancy study groups recommendations on the diagnosis and classification of hyperglycemia in pregnancy. *Diabetes Care* 2010; **33**(3): 676–682.

25. Ryan EA. Diagnosing gestational diabetes. *Diabetologia* 2011; **54**(3): 480–486.

26. Buschard K., Buch I, Mølsted-Pedersen L, Hougaard P, Kühl C. Increased incidence of true type I diabetes acquired during pregnancy. *BMJ (Clin Res Ed)* 1987; **294**(6567): 275–279.

27. Shields BM, Hicks S, Shepherd MH, Colclough K, Hattersley AT, Ellard S. Maturity-onset diabetes of the young (MODY): how many cases are we missing? *Diabetologia* 2010; **53**(12): 2504–2508.

28. Chen Y, Liao WX, Roy AC, Loganath A, Ng SC. Mitochondrial gene mutations in gestational diabetes mellitus. *Diabetes Res Clin Pract* 2000; **48**(1): 29–35.

29. Alberti G, Zimmet P, Shaw J, Bloomgarden Z, Kaufman F, Silink M, et al. Type 2 diabetes in the young: the evolving epidemic: the international diabetes federation consensus workshop. *Diabetes Care* 2004; **27**(7): 1798–1811.

30. Cundy T, Gamble G, Townend K, Henley PG, MacPherson P, Roberts AB. Perinatal mortality in Type 2 diabetes mellitus. *Diabet Med* 2000; **17**(1): 33–39.

31. Damm P, Kühl C, Buschard K, Jakobsen BK, Svejgaard A, Sodoyez-Goffaux F, et al. Prevalence and predictive value of islet cell antibodies and insulin autoantibodies in women with gestational diabetes. *Diabet Med* 1994; **11**(6): 558–563.

32. Jarvela IY, Juutinen J, Koskela P, Hartikainen AL, Kulmala P, Knip M, et al. Gestational diabetes identifies women at risk for permanent type 1 and type 2 diabetes in fertile age: predictive role of autoantibodies. *Diabetes Care* 2006; **29**(3): 607–612.

33. Weng J, Ekelund M, Lehto M, Li H, Ekberg G, Frid A, et al. Screening for MODY mutations, GAD antibodies, and type 1 diabetes–associated HLA genotypes in women with gestational diabetes mellitus. *Diabetes Care* 2002; **25**(1): 68–71.

34. Colom C, Corcoy R. Maturity onset diabetes of the young and pregnancy. *Best Pract Res Clin Endocrinol Metab* 2010; **24**(4): 605–615.

35. Barker JM. Clinical review: Type 1 diabetes-associated autoimmunity: natural history, genetic associations, and screening. *J Clin Endocrinol Metab* 2006; **91**(4): 1210–1217.

36. van Belle TL, Coppieters KT, von Herrath MG. Type 1 diabetes: etiology, immunology, and therapeutic strategies. *Physiol Rev* 2011; **91**(1): 79–118.

37. Kahn SE. The importance of the beta-cell in the pathogenesis of type 2 diabetes mellitus. *Am J Med* 2000; **108**(Suppl. 6a): 2S–8S.

38. Scott LJ, Mohlke KL, Bonnycastle LL, Willer CJ, Li Y, Duren WL, et al. A genome-wide association study of type 2 diabetes in Finns detects multiple susceptibility variants. *Science* 2007; **316**(5829): 1341–1345.

39. van Dam RM. The epidemiology of lifestyle and risk for type 2 diabetes. *Eur J Epidemiol* 2003; **18**(12): 1115–1125.

40. Bloomgarden Z. Type 2 Diabetes in the Young: The Evolving Epidemic. *Diabetes Care* 2004; **27**(4): 1798–1811.

41. Pinhas-Hamiel O, Zeitler P. The global spread of type 2 diabetes mellitus in children and adolescents. *J Pediatr* 2005; **146**(5): 693–700.

42. Dabelea D, Hanson RL, Lindsay RS, Pettitt DJ, Imperatore G, Gabir MM, et al. Intrauterine exposure to diabetes conveys risks for type 2 diabetes and obesity: a study of discordant sibships. *Diabetes* 2000; **49**(12): 2208–2211.

43. Yajnik CS. Fetal programming of diabetes: still so much to learn! *Diabetes Care* 2010; **33**(5): 1146–1148.

44. Ling C, Groop L. Epigenetics: a molecular link between environmental factors and type 2 diabetes. *Diabetes* 2009; **58**(12): 2718–2725.

45. Dabelea D, Hanson RL, Bennett PH, Roumain J, Knowler WC, Pettitt DJ. Increasing prevalence of Type II diabetes in American Indian children. *Diabetologia* 1998; **41**(8): 904–910.

46. Barbour LA, McCurdy CE, Hernandez TL, Kirwan JP, Catalano PM, Friedman JE. Cellular mechanisms for insulin resistance in normal pregnancy and gestational diabetes. *Diabetes Care* 2007; **30**(Suppl. 2): S112–S119.

47. Barbour LA, Shao J, Qiao L, Leitner W, Anderson M, Friedman JE, et al. Human placental growth hormone increases expression of the p85 regulatory unit of phosphatidylinositol 3-kinase and triggers severe insulin resistance in skeletal muscle. *Endocrinology* 2004; **145**(3): 1144–1150.

48. HSCR Group, Metzger BE, Lowe LP, Dyer AR, Trimble ER, Chaovarindr U, et al. Hyperglycemia and adverse pregnancy outcomes. *N Engl J Med* 2008; **358**(19): 1991–2002.

49. Kirwan JP, Varastehpour A, Jing M, Presley L, Shao J, Friedman JE, et al. Reversal of insulin resistance postpartum is linked to enhanced skeletal muscle insulin signaling. *J Clin Endocrinol Metab* 2004; **89**(9): 4678–4684.

50. Bellamy L, Casas JP, Hingorani AD, Williams D. Type 2 diabetes mellitus after gestational diabetes: a systematic review and meta-analysis. *Lancet* 2009; **373**(9677): 1773–1779.

51. Ratner RE. Prevention of type 2 diabetes in women with previous gestational diabetes. *Diabetes Care* 2007; **30**(Suppl. 2): S242–S245.

52. Ratner RE, Christophi CA, Metzger BE, Dabelea D, Bennett PH, Pi-Sunyer X, et al. Prevention of diabetes in women with a history of gestational diabetes: effects of metformin and lifestyle interventions. *J Clin Endocrinol Metab* 2008; **93**(12): 4774–4779.

53. Lauenborg J, Hansen T, Jensen DM, Vestergaard H, Mølsted-Pedersen L, Hornnes P, et al. Increasing incidence of diabetes after gestational diabetes: a long-term follow-up in a Danish population. *Diabetes Care* 2004; **27**(5): 1194–1199.

54. Dabelea D, ll-Bergeon JK, Hartsfield CL, Bischoff KJ, Hamman RF, McDuffie RS; Kaiser Permanente

of Colorado GDM Screening Program. Increasing prevalence of gestational diabetes mellitus (GDM) over time and by birth cohort: Kaiser Permanente of Colorado GDM Screening Program. *Diabetes Care* 2005; **28**(3): 579–584.

55. Kim C, Newton KM, Knopp RH. Gestational diabetes and the incidence of type 2 diabetes: a systematic review. *Diabetes Care* 2002; **25**(10): 1862–1868.

56. Tam WH, Ma RC, Yang X, Li AM, Ko GT, Kong AP, et al. Glucose intolerance and cardiometabolic risk in adolescents exposed to maternal gestational diabetes: a 15-year follow-up study. *Diabetes Care* 2010; **33**(6): 1382–1384.

57. Daneman D. Type 1 diabetes. *Lancet* 2006; **367**(9513): 847–858.

58. Raymond NT, Jones JR, Swift PG, Davies MJ, Lawrence G, McNally PG, et al. Comparative incidence of Type I diabetes in children aged under 15 years from South Asian and White or other ethnic backgrounds in Leicestershire, UK, 1989 to 1998. *Diabetologia* 2001; **44**(Suppl. 3): B32–B36.

59. Misra S, Dornhorst A. Gestational diabetes mellitus: primum non nocere. *Diabetes Care* 2012; **35**(9): 1811–1813.

60. Stenstrom G, Gottsäter A, Bakhtadze E, Berger B, Sundkvist G. Latent autoimmune diabetes in adults: definition, prevalence, beta-cell function, and treatment. *Diabetes* 2005; **54**(Suppl. 2): S68–S72.

61. Thunander M, Törn C, Petersson C, Ossiansson B, Fornander J, Landin-Olsson M. Levels of C-peptide, body mass index and age, and their usefulness in classification of diabetes in relation to autoimmunity, in adults with newly diagnosed diabetes in Kronoberg, Sweden. *Eur J Endocrinol* 2012; **166**(6): 1021–1029.

62. Guideline Development Group. Management of diabetes from preconception to the postnatal period: summary of NICE guidance. *BMJ* 2008; **336**(7646): 714–717.

63. Lo JC, Feigenbaum SL, Escobar GJ, Yang J, Crites YM, Ferrara A. Increased prevalence of gestational diabetes mellitus among women with diagnosed polycystic ovary syndrome: a population-based study. *Diabetes Care* 2006; **29**(8): 1915–1917.

64. Hermanns-Le T, Scheen A, Pierard GE. Acanthosis nigricans associated with insulin resistance: pathophysiology and management. *Am J Clin Dermatol* 2004; **5**(3): 199–203.

65. Ratner RE; Diabetes Prevention Program Research. An update on the Diabetes Prevention Program. *Endocr Pract* 2006; **12**(Suppl. 1): 20–24.

66. Estalella I, Rica I, Perez de Nanclares G, Bilbao JR, Vazquez JA, San Pedro JI, et al. Mutations in GCK and HNF-1alpha explain the majority of cases with clinical diagnosis of MODY in Spain. *Clin Endocrinol* 2007; **67**(4): 538–546.

67. Chakera AJ, Carleton VL, Ellard S, Wong J, Yue DK, Pinner J, et al. Antenatal diagnosis of fetal genotype determines if maternal hyperglycemia due to a glucokinase mutation requires treatment. *Diabetes Care* 2012; **35**(9): 1832–1834.

68. Teh WT, Teede HJ, Paul E, Harrison CL, Wallace EM, Allan C. Risk factors for gestational diabetes mellitus: implications for the application of screening guidelines. *Aust N Z J Obstet Gynaecol* 2011; **51**(1): 26–30.

69. Gibson KS, Waters TP, Catalano PM. Maternal weight gain in women who develop gestational diabetes mellitus. *Obstet Gynecol* 2012; **119**(3): 560–565.

70. Kuehn BM. Guideline for pregnancy weight gain offers targets for obese women. *JAMA* 2009; **302**(3): 241–242.

Clinical management of diabetes in pregnancy

Katie Wynne

Hunter New England Health and University of Newcastle, Newcastle, Australia

5.2.1 Introduction

The number of pregnancies complicated by maternal diabetes is rising as a function of maternal age and obesity. Type 1 diabetes, type 2 diabetes and gestational diabetes (GDM) result in hyperglycaemia that increases the frequency of adverse obstetric and perinatal outcomes [1]. There is a greater maternal risk of miscarriage, hypertension and pre-eclampsia, preterm labour and caesarian delivery; and greater foetal risk of congenital malformations, macrosomia, birth injury and perinatal mortality. The goal is to optimise glucose control at conception and maintain euglycaemia during pregnancy.

This chapter reviews the evidence-base for the management of diabetes in pregnancy. There have been several recent well-designed clinical trials [2–6] and clinical guidelines from the American Diabetes Association (ADA) [7] and National Institute for Clinical Excellence (NICE) [8], which are discussed below.

5.2.2 Pre-conception care

Routine diabetic care for women should include consistent and constructive advice about family planning. Specialist 'pre-pregnancy' clinics should be accessible for patients once they decide to conceive [8]. Well-planned pregnancies have fewer congenital malformations, stillbirths and neonatal deaths [9–13]. The Confidential Enquiry into Maternal and Child Health (CEMACH) data showed that sub-optimal pre-conception care is associated with a five-fold increase in the risk of foetal death after 20 weeks or major congenital malformation [1]. Despite this evidence, a large proportion of women with pre-gestational diabetes do not receive specific pre-conception care [1].

Women should be counselled that improving glycaemia reduces the risk of miscarriage, congenital malformation and neonatal death. Even a small improvement in HbA1c is associated with a reduced risk of complications [14] and improved obstetric surveillance and management of hyperglycaemia results in a good outcome for most women [15].

International targets recommend an optimal pre-pregnancy HbA1c of 42 mmol/mol (6%), at which level the malformation rate is similar to the non-diabetic population (2%) [14]. In one study, the rate of congenital malformation rose rapidly above a level of 42 mmol/mol (6%): at HbA1c 52 mmol/mol (6.9%) the risk of malformation was 3% and at HbA1c 98 mmol/mol (11.1%) the risk rose to 10%. Another study confirmed a high risk (16%) of serious adverse pregnancy outcome when the preconception HbA1c exceeded 90 mmol/mol (10.4%) [16]. NICE guidelines recommend avoiding pregnancy in women with HbA1c >86 mmol/mol

(10%) [8]. Women should be advised to use a reliable form of contraception until acceptable glycaemia is achieved.

An individualised and safe HbA1c target should be set pre-conception and practical steps identified to achieve the agreed goal. A structured education programme (for example DAFNE, DESMOND or X-PERT) may help women to reach this target. Although glycaemic control is key, care should be taken to avoid hypoglycaemia. HbA1c should be measured monthly until target levels are achieved and then every two to three months until conception. Oral folate supplements (5 mg/day) should be commenced and continued for the first twelve weeks of pregnancy as neural tube defects are more common in diabetic pregnancies. There should be a review of the need for potentially teratogenic drugs (e.g. ACE inhibitors and statins) and microvascular complications should be assessed and treated as appropriate. Lifestyle advice should be given to patients who are overweight and obese, as this is an independent obstetric risk factor [7,8].

5.2.3 Antenatal care

The antenatal clinic

Women with pre-gestational diabetes should be reviewed in a multidisciplinary clinic as soon as a viable pregnancy is confirmed, ideally before 12 weeks gestation. The team should include an obstetrician, midwife with a special interest in diabetes, diabetes physician, diabetes specialist nurse and dietitian. Women should be reviewed at 2–4 week intervals and more frequently in the final trimester of pregnancy. All patients should have a documented management plan that includes the pregnancy and postnatal period up to six weeks [8].

Glycaemic control

Maintaining optimal glycaemic control is crucial for optimising the outcomes of pregnancy. The strategy used to achieve this may differ, depending on whether the woman has type 1, type 2 or GDM (Table 5.2.1). Glucose monitoring is

Table 5.2.1 Interventions to maintain glycaemia in type 1 diabetes, type 2 diabetes and gestational diabetes

Type 1 diabetes	Diet and exercise
	Multiple dose insulin
	Continuous subcutaneous insulin infusion
Type 2 diabetes	Diet and exercise
	Metformin
	Multiple dose insulin
Gestational diabetes	Diet and exercise
	Metformin/glibenclamide
	Multiple dose insulin

Table 5.2.2 Target glucose concentrations during pregnancy

	American Guidelines	UK Guidelines
Fasting glucose	3.3–5.5 mmol/l 60–100 mg/dl	3.5–5.9 mmol/L 60–105 mg/dl
1 hour post prandial glucose	5.5–7.2 mmol/L 100–130 mg/dl	<7.8 mmol/L <140 mg/dl

commenced, aiming for a target fasting glucose concentration in the region of 3.5–5.9 mmol/l (60–105 mg/dl) and one hour post-prandial concentration of below 7.8 mmol/l (140 mg/dl) [8]. The American Guidelines aim for a marginally lower glucose concentration [7] (Table 5.2.2). The glycaemia targets in GDM are similar for those women with pre-gestational diabetes.

Women on insulin should test their capillary blood glucose concentration at least five times per day. Frequent testing is indicated because of the exaggerated post-prandial glycaemic excursions and rapid changes in glucose concentration that occur during pregnancy. Tests should be performed in the fasted state, one hour after meals and at bedtime. There is evidence that using one hour post-prandial glucose concentration to guide insulin requirements results in lower rates of caesarean sections for cephalo-pelvic disproportion, macrosomia and neonatal hypoglycaemia [17,18]. HbA1c should not be used later in pregnancy as the results are unreliable and levels change too slowly to be used to adjust treatment.

Hypoglycaemia

The most common adverse effect of intensive diabetes control is hypoglycaemia (defined as <3.3 mmol/l or 60 mg/dl in pregnancy). Mortality from hypoglycaemia is rare, but remains a known cause of death in women with type 1 diabetes [19] and can result in foetal growth retardation. In type 1 diabetes, insulin requirements usually fall in the first trimester, which may lead to an increased frequency of hypoglycaemia. Women with long-standing type 1, autonomic neuropathy and a history of recurrent hypoglycaemia are at particular risk. All women should be advised about the management of hypoglycaemia and women with type 1 should be given a glucagon pen that their partner or relative is trained to use.

Hypoglycaemia and unawareness are major barriers to achieving intensive glycaemic control [1,8,20]. Hypoglycaemic unawareness is more common in pregnancy, but awareness can be restored by temporarily raising glucose targets and by carefully avoiding hypoglycaemic episodes. The use of continuous glucose monitoring may provide more information on glucose fluctuations in patients who lack awareness, but its use is currently somewhat limited by availability [21].

Complications of diabetes

The microvascular complications of diabetes, retinopathy, nephropathy and autonomic neuropathy may worsen during pregnancy due to rapid improvements in glycaemia and the physiological changes of pregnancy. However, there is no evidence of a detrimental effect on long-term microvascular outcome [22,23]. Digital retinal screening identifies severe retinal disease, which allows treatment and therefore reduces the risk of sight-threatening complications during pregnancy. The United Kingdom (UK) guidelines [8] advise that screening should be organised at the first antenatal visit if not done within the last 12 months. If retinopathy is present a further test

should take place at 16–20 weeks, or otherwise at 28 weeks if the first test was normal. Other groups advise screening at least during each trimester [7].

Renal function should be assessed at the first antenatal appointment as women with moderate to severe nephropathy may experience some deterioration during pregnancy. Serum creatinine is the preferred method, as estimated glomerular filtration rate is unreliable because of the physiological changes of pregnancy [7]. The presence of microalbuminuria (ACR 3.5–30 mg/mmol) confers an increased risk of pre-eclampsia, preterm birth, interuterine growth restriction and adverse pregnancy outcome. Pre-pregnancy proteinuria (>2 g/day) or raised serum creatinine (>120 μmol/l) signals a higher risk of renal deterioration during pregnancy, these patients may require joint management with a nephrologist.

Diabetic ketoacidosis (DKA) may occur at only moderately increased blood glucose concentrations (<14 mmol/l or 250 mg/dl) and more rapidly than in non-pregnant patients. DKA should therefore be excluded in all unwell pregnant women with type 1 diabetes. The risk of DKA in women with diabetes is <1%, but is associated with foetal loss in >20% episodes and a high maternal mortality. It should be managed in a high dependency setting with joint obstetric and diabetic care.

Treatment regimens

Diet and exercise

Pregnant women with diabetes should receive individualised dietary advice, which will be dealt with in more detail in Chapter 5.3. An appropriate diet and exercise regimen has been shown to enhance insulin sensitivity and reduce post-prandial blood glucose concentrations. Indeed, lifestyle intervention alone is sufficient to meet glycaemic targets in 80–90% of patients with GDM [3,5].

Metformin and other hypoglycaemic agents

Available evidence [8] suggests that metformin is safe in pregnancy and breastfeeding. However, its use remains controversial and although metformin (with or without glibenclamide) is recommended by UK NICE Guidelines, it is not currently recommended by the ADA [7,8]. Other oral hypoglycaemics, such as gliclazide and other sulfonylureas, should be replaced as concern exists around potential tetragenicity. Thiazolidinediones, meglitinide analogues and incretin agents have not been well studied in pregnancy, so their safety and efficacy are not confirmed and they are generally avoided.

In patients with GDM, oral hypoglycaemics should be used as an adjunct to lifestyle modifications if targets are not reached. Two recent randomised controlled trials suggest that metformin [6] and glibenclamide [4] are safe and effective treatment alternatives to insulin. The 'MiG' Trial [6] randomised 751 women with GDM to metformin (up to 2.5 g/day) or insulin from 20 to 33 weeks gestation. The women in the metformin group who did not reach adequate glycaemic targets (46%) were also given insulin. The incidence of foetal complications (neonatal hypoglycaemia, respiratory distress, need for phototherapy, birth trauma, reduced Apgar score <7 or prematurity) were equivalent in the metformin group (32%) and insulin group (32.2%). UK guidelines recommend metformin and suggest that glibenclamide may also be considered for the management of GDM if hypoglycaemic therapy is required [8].

Insulin

A regimen of multiple daily injections (MDI) with short-acting and basal insulin is recommended by the American and UK guidelines for patients with type 1, and patients with type 2 or GDM who fail to achieve targets with oral medication. There is a large inter-individual variation in the change in insulin dose needed during pregnancy. In general, peak insulin sensitivity occurs around 10–14 weeks. After 20 weeks, insulin requirements may rise two- to three-fold, reaching a plateau or occasionally declining after 35 weeks.

NICE and the ADA have endorsed the newer short-acting insulin analogues and these have been used for the last decade with no evidence of harm. The analogues have the advantage of a faster onset of action with a tendency toward less hypoglycaemia [24]. The basal insulin of choice is intermediate neutral protamine hagedorn (NPH) insulin as it has extensive safety and efficacy data. Newer long-acting insulin analogues are not currently recommended by the ADA or NICE. There are theoretical concerns around the potential mitogenicity of glargine [25,26] and the results of a clinical trial of detemir are awaited. It should be borne in mind that patients who are transitioned to NPH insulin before pregnancy or at the first perinatal visit may experience an initial deterioration in their glycaemic control. The risk of poor glycaemic control at conception should therefore be balanced against the theoretical safety concerns surrounding basal analogues.

Comparisons of MDI versus continuous subcutaneous insulin infusion (CSII) in pregnancy show equivalent glycaemic control and perinatal outcomes [27,28]. Guidelines suggest that CSII should be considered in women with significant hypoglycaemia or increased insulin requirements before waking [7]. Larger, multi-centre, randomised controlled trials are required to establish whether the use of these technologies can improve outcomes in pregnancy.

Foetal monitoring

The NICE guidance recognises that women with diabetes require additional foetal monitoring to identify pregnancies at particular risk of complications. An early viability scan at 8–10 weeks is important to establish an accurate expected date of delivery. An anomaly scan at around 20 weeks, including a four-chamber view of the foetal heart and outflow tracts, should be performed. This structural scan is important as congenital heart disease is the most common foetal developmental abnormality. Growth scans to assess foetal growth and amniotic fluid volume are performed in the final trimester. These serial investigations aim to identify incipient macrosomia using measurements of abdominal circumference. Glycaemic control should be intensified if ultrasound investigation reports an abdominal circumference above the 70th centile [8]. Growth measurements may also identify growth retardation that is more common in patients with pre-eclampsia, macro-vascular disease or retinopathy [7].

5.2.4 Perinatal care

UK guidelines suggest delivery shortly after 38 weeks gestation and not beyond the expected delivery date because of the increased incidence of still birth and shoulder dystocia [8]. The obstetricians will consider factors such as gly-caemic control during pregnancy, diabetes com-plications, past obstetric history and foetal growth scans when setting a date for the induc-tion of labour (or elective caesarean section). For women with GDM, the American guidelines advocate using estimated foetal weight to guide obstetric management [29].

Labour should take place on a dedicated obstetric ward with a neonatal unit. Maternal hyperglycaemia during delivery is associated with foetal distress, neonatal hypoglycaemia and an adverse neurological outcome for the infant. Blood glucose should therefore be maintained between 4–7 mmol/l to reduce the incidence of neonatal hypoglycaemia and foetal distress syn-drome [8]. A continuous insulin and dextrose infusion may be required during established labour and birth to maintain these targets. Women with GDM controlled with diet and oral hypo-glycaemics do not usually require an insulin infusion to achieve intra-partum euglycaemia.

5.2.5 Postnatal care

Immediately postpartum, glucose metabolism returns to the non-pregnant state. Women with type 1 and type 2 diabetes should therefore recommence their pre-pregnancy regimen. Patients on insulin may have very low require-ments for the first 24 hours, predisposing them to hypoglycaemia. Women with GDM should discontinue all hypoglycaemic therapy immedi-ately after delivery, but continue to perform cap-illary glucose monitoring for several days to identify patients with underlying diabetes.

Breast-feeding is associated with a decreased risk of future obesity [30] and type 2 diabetes

[31] in the infant. This protective effect may be particularly important for the children of dia-betic mothers, as interuterine hyperglycaemia predisposes children to obesity, pre-diabetes and type 2 diabetes [32]. For women who breastfeed whilst on hypoglycaemic treatment, there is a risk of low blood glucose around the time of feeding. Metformin and glibenclamide can be continued throughout breastfeeding, but other hypoglycaemic agents should not be used [8].

Macrosomia (birth weight >4.0–4.5 kg) and neonatal hypoglycaemia (<2.6 mmol/l) are reported in half of all diabetic pregnancies [1]. To avoid the serious sequelae of hypoglycaemia, mothers should be encouraged to breastfeed within 30 minutes of birth and then initially every two to three hours. Foetal blood glucose should be monitored three to four hours after delivery. ensuring that pre-feed blood glucose concentrations remain >2.0 mmol/l [8].

Women with GDM should have a fasting glucose or glucose tolerance test performed at the six-week postnatal check to ensure that normal glucose metabolism has been restored. Women should be advised of the need to recheck their glucose concentrations when planning a subsequent pregnancy or following conception because of the high risk of GDM in future pregnancies [33]. One systematic review of more than 600 000 women, suggested that GDM conferred a seven times relative risk of developing type 2 diabetes [34]. The impor-tance of post-delivery dietary modification and weight reduction to reduce the risk of type 2 should be reinforced. Patients should be reas-sessed at least annually with fasting glucose measurements [8,29].

5.2.6 Screening for diabetes in pregnancy

Gestational diabetes is defined as hyperglycae-mia with first recognition in pregnancy. It is esti-mated that 2–5% of pregnancies are complicated by GDM [29]. Two randomised trials, ACHIOS Trial [3] and MFMU Network Trial [5] have confirmed the importance of intensive glucose management in these women. In these studies,

Table 5.2.3 Diagnosis of gestational diabetes

	Fasting	1 hour 75 g OGTT	2 hour 75 g OGTT
WHO (1999)	>7.0 mmol/L		>7.8 mmol/L
NICE (2008) [8]	>126 mg/dl		>140 mg/dl
ADA 2004 [38]	>5.3 mmol/L	>10 mmol/L	>8.6 mmol/L
	>95 mg/dl	>180 mg/dl	>155 mg/dl
HAPO (2010) [2]	>5.1 mmol/L	>10.0 mmol/L	>8.5 mmol/L
	>92 mg/dl	>180 mg/dl	>153 mg/dl

OGTT: 75g oral glucose tolerance test.

glycaemic treatment reduced average birth weight, shoulder dystocia, pre-eclampsia and caesarean delivery.

The exact glucose threshold at which gestational diabetes should be diagnosed remains controversial (Table 5.2.3) and recent data suggests that even minor degrees of hyperglycaemia can influence clinical outcome. The Hyperglycaemia and Adverse Pregnancy Outcome (HAPO) Trial [2] showed a continuous relationship between glucose concentrations and pregnancy risk. In this study, 25 000 pregnant women without diabetes had fasting glucose concentrations measured, as well as concentrations one and two hours after a 75 g glucose load. Glucose concentrations were positively associated with neonatal hypoglycaemia, increased birth weight and delivery by caesarean section. In response it has been suggested that GDM should be defined as a fasting threshold glucose > 5.1 mmol/l (92 mg/dl), a 1 hour concentration of >10.0 mmol/l (180 mg/dl) or a 2 hour concentration of >8.5 mmol/l (153 mg/dl) [35]. Screening women using the lower fasting 'HAPO' criteria would clearly result in a diagnosis of GDM in a much larger number of women with concomitant economic implications.

Current ADA and NICE guidelines recommend selective screening of women with significant risk factors for GDM, rather than all women (Box 5.2.1). The method of screening varies from a random or fasting glucose concentration to a formal oral glucose tolerance test. Testing commonly takes place at the start of the third trimester (28–32 weeks) when hyperglycaemia is usually apparent. However, in patients with previous GDM screening it usually takes place

---

Box 5.2.1 Risk factors for gestational diabetes

- Body mass index >30 kg/m^2
- A family origin with a high prevalence of diabetes (e.g. Asian, African-Caribbean, Middle Eastern)
- A current pregnancy with:
  - glycosuria
  - polyhydramnios
  - twins or triplets
- A history of:
  - gestational diabetes
  - a large baby (>4 kg at term)
  - an unexplained stillbirth or perinatal death
  - diabetes in a first degree relative

---

earlier (16–18 weeks) and then is repeated in the third trimester if the initial results are normal.

5.2.7 Conclusion

Over 20 years ago the St Vincent Declaration pledged to improve pregnancy outcomes for women with diabetes [36]. Despite significant clinical and scientific advances, there remains a two- to five-fold increase in obstetric complications [37]. Improving glycaemic control reduces perinatal morbidity and mortality in diabetic pregnancies. Therefore quality diabetes and obstetric care, using evidence-based guidelines, is crucial for the delivery of a good pregnancy outcome. Newer technologies, including continuous glucose monitoring and insulin pumps, may be the management tools of the future.

Key points

- Pre-conception care should be provided to all women with diabetes and glycaemic targets agreed before conception.
- Antenatal care should be provided by a multidisciplinary team and aim to optimise glycaemic control and weight gain.
- Insulin, metformin and glibenclamide are used for treatment in the UK, although only insulin is used in pregnancy in the US.
- Glucose metabolism returns to pre-pregnancy levels immediately postpartum, for women with pre-existing diabetes, medication should return to usual levels and for those with gestational diabetes, all hypoglycaemic medication should be stopped.

References

1. Confidential Enquiry into Maternal and Child Health. Diabetes in pregnancy: are we providing the best care? England, Wales, Northern Ireland, London: Findings of a National Enquiry, 2007 Feb.
2. Metzger BE, Lowe LP, Dyer AR, Trimble ER, Chaovarindr U, Coustan DR, et al. Hyperglycemia and adverse pregnancy outcomes. *N Engl J Med* 2008; **358**(19): 1991–2002.
3. Crowther CA, Hiller JE, Moss JR, McPhee AJ, Jeffries WS, Robinson JS. Effect of treatment of gestational diabetes mellitus on pregnancy outcomes. *N Engl J Med* 2005; **352**(24): 2477–2486.
4. Langer O, Conway DL, Berkus MD, Xenakis EM, Gonzales O. A comparison of glyburide and insulin in women with gestational diabetes mellitus. *N Engl J Med* 2000; **343**(16): 1134–1138.
5. Landon MB, Spong CY, Thom E, Carpenter MW, Ramin SM, Casey B, et al. A multicenter, randomized trial of treatment for mild gestational diabetes. *N Engl J Med* 2009; **361**(14): 1339–1348.
6. Rowan JA, Hague WM, Gao W, Battin MR, Moore MP. Metformin versus insulin for the treatment of gestational diabetes. *N Engl J Med* 2008; **358**(19): 2003–2015.
7. Kitzmiller JL, Block JM, Brown FM, Catalano PM, Conway DL, Coustan DR, et al. Managing preexisting diabetes for pregnancy: summary of evidence and consensus recommendations for care. *Diabetes Care* 2008; **31**(5): 1060–1079.
8. Guideline Development Group. Management of diabetes from preconception to the postnatal period: summary of NICE guidance. *BMJ* 2008; **336**(7646): 714–717.

9. Evers IM, de Valk HW, Visser GH. Risk of complications of pregnancy in women with type 1 diabetes: nationwide prospective study in the Netherlands. *BMJ* 2004; **328**(7445): 915.
10. Pearson DW, Kernaghan D, Lee R, Penney GC. The relationship between pre-pregnancy care and early pregnancy loss, major congenital anomaly or perinatal death in type I diabetes mellitus. *Br J Obstet Gynaecol* 2007; **114**(1): 104–107.
11. Ray JG, O'Brien TE, Chan WS. Preconception care and the risk of congenital anomalies in the offspring of women with diabetes mellitus: a meta-analysis. *Q J Med* 2001; **94**(8): 435–444.
12. Steel JM, Johnstone FD, Hepburn DA, Smith AF. Can prepregnancy care of diabetic women reduce the risk of abnormal babies? *BMJ* 1990; **301**(6760): 1070–1074.
13. Temple RC, Aldridge VJ, Murphy HR. Prepregnancy care and pregnancy outcomes in women with type 1 diabetes. *Diabetes Care* 2006; **29**(8): 1744–1749.
14. Guerin A, Nisenbaum R, Ray JG. Use of maternal GHb concentration to estimate the risk of congenital anomalies in the offspring of women with prepregnancy diabetes. *Diabetes Care* 2007; **30**(7): 1920–1925.
15. Holing EV. Preconception care of women with diabetes: the unrevealed obstacles. *J Matern Fetal Med* 2000; **9**(1): 10–13.
16. Jensen DM, Damm P, Sorensen B, Molsted-Pedersen L, Westergaard JG, Korsholm L, et al. Proposed diagnostic thresholds for gestational diabetes mellitus according to a 75-g oral glucose tolerance test. Maternal and perinatal outcomes in 3260 Danish women. *Diabet Med* 2003; **20**(1): 51–57.
17. de Veciana M, Major CA, Morgan MA, Asrat T, Toohey JS, Lien JM, et al. Postprandial versus preprandial blood glucose monitoring in women with gestational diabetes mellitus requiring insulin therapy. *N Engl J Med* 1995; **333**(19): 1237–1241.
18. Manderson JG, Patterson CC, Hadden DR, Traub AI, Ennis C, McCance DR. Preprandial versus postprandial blood glucose monitoring in type 1 diabetic pregnancy: a randomized controlled clinical trial. *Am J Obstet Gynecol* 2003; **189**(2): 507–512.
19. Leinonen PJ, Hiilesmaa VK, Kaaja RJ, Teramo KA. Maternal mortality in type 1 diabetes. *Diabetes Care* 2001; **24**(8): 1501–1502.
20. Rosenn BM, Miodovnik M, Holcberg G, Khoury JC, Siddiqi TA. Hypoglycemia: the price of intensive insulin therapy for pregnant women with insulin-dependent diabetes mellitus. *Obstet Gynecol* 1995; **85**(3): 417–422.
21. Murphy HR, Rayman G, Lewis K, Kelly S, Johal B, Duffield K, et al. Effectiveness of continuous glucose monitoring in pregnant women with diabetes: randomised clinical trial. *BMJ* 2008; **337**: a1680.

22. The Diabetes Control and Complications Trial Research Group. Effect of pregnancy on microvascular complications in the diabetes control and complications trial. *Diabetes Care* 2000; **23**(8): 1084–1091.

23. Verier-Mine O, Chaturvedi N, Webb D, Fuller JH. Is pregnancy a risk factor for microvascular complications? The EURODIAB Prospective Complications Study. *Diabet Med* 2005; **22**(11): 1503–1509.

24. Mathiesen ER, Kinsley B, Amiel SA, Heller S, McCance D, Duran S, et al. Maternal glycemic control and hypoglycemia in type 1 diabetic pregnancy: a randomized trial of insulin aspart versus human insulin in 322 pregnant women. *Diabetes Care* 2007; **30**(4): 771–776.

25. Hirsch IB. Insulin analogues. *N Engl J Med* 2005; **352**(2): 174–183.

26. Kurtzhals P, Schaffer L, Sorensen A, Kristensen C, Jonassen I, Schmid C, et al. Correlations of receptor binding and metabolic and mitogenic potencies of insulin analogs designed for clinical use. *Diabetes* 2000; **49**(6): 999–1005.

27. Farrar D, Tuffnell DJ, West J. Continuous subcutaneous insulin infusion versus multiple daily injections of insulin for pregnant women with diabetes. *Cochrane Database Syst Rev* 2007; (3): CD005542.

28. Mukhopadhyay A, Farrell T, Fraser RB, Ola B. Continuous subcutaneous insulin infusion vs intensive conventional insulin therapy in pregnant diabetic women: a systematic review and metaanalysis of randomized, controlled trials. *Am J Obstet Gynecol* 2007; **197**(5): 447–456.

29. Metzger BE, Buchanan TA, Coustan DR, de Leiva A, Dunger DB, Hadden DR, et al. Summary and recommendations of the Fifth International Workshop-Conference on Gestational Diabetes Mellitus. *Diabetes Care* 2007; **30**(Suppl. 2): S251–S260.

30. Mayer-Davis EJ, Rifas-Shiman SL, Zhou L, Hu FB, Colditz GA, Gillman MW. Breast-feeding and risk for childhood obesity: does maternal diabetes or obesity status matter? *Diabetes Care* 2006; **29**(10): 2231–2237.

31. Mayer-Davis EJ, Dabelea D, Lamichhane AP, D'Agostino RB, Jr., Liese AD, Thomas J, et al. Breast-feeding and type 2 diabetes in the youth of three ethnic groups: the SEARCh for diabetes in youth case-control study. *Diabetes Care* 2008; **31**(3): 470–475.

32. Clausen TD, Mathiesen ER, Hansen T, Pedersen O, Jensen DM, Lauenborg J, et al. High prevalence of type 2 diabetes and pre-diabetes in adult offspring of women with gestational diabetes mellitus or type 1 diabetes: the role of intrauterine hyperglycemia. *Diabetes Care* 2008; **31**(2): 340–346.

33. Kim C, Berger DK, Chamany S. Recurrence of gestational diabetes mellitus: a systematic review. *Diabetes Care* 2007; **30**(5): 1314–1319.

34. Bellamy L, Casas JP, Hingorani AD, Williams D. Type 2 diabetes mellitus after gestational diabetes: a systematic review and meta-analysis. *Lancet* 2009; **373**(9677): 1773–1779.

35. Metzger BE, Gabbe SG, Persson B, Buchanan TA, Catalano PA, Damm P, et al. International association of diabetes and pregnancy study groups recommendations on the diagnosis and classification of hyperglycemia in pregnancy. *Diabetes Care* 2010; **33**(3): 676–682.

36. Diabetes care and research in Europe: the Saint Vincent declaration. *Diabet Med* 1990; **7**(4): 360.

37. Macintosh MC, Fleming KM, Bailey JA, Doyle P, Modder J, Acolet D, et al. Perinatal mortality and congenital anomalies in babies of women with type 1 or type 2 diabetes in England, Wales, and Northern Ireland: population based study. *BMJ* 2006; **333**(7560): 177.

38. American Diabetes Association. Diagnosis and classification of diabetes mellitus. *Diabetes Care* 2004; **27**(Suppl. 1): S5–S10.

Chapter 5.3

Lifestyle management of diabetes in pregnancy

Alyson Hill
University of Ulster, Londonderry, UK

5.3.1 Introduction

Dietary management is fundamental for the effective management of diabetes and is a key component in achieving optimal glycaemic control [1] whilst also ensuring that the nutritional demands of pregnancy are achieved. Good glycaemic control throughout pregnancy and avoidance of postprandial glucose peaks are important in reducing the risks of maternal and neonatal complications [2].

5.3.2 Pre-pregnancy

All women with diabetes (both type 1 and type 2) should receive pre-pregnancy counselling to reduce the rate of congenital malformations and improve outcomes [3]. The CEMACH report, published in 2007, outlines a range of factors associated with poorer pregnancy outcomes, including unplanned pregnancy, smoking, suboptimal glycaemic control before and during pregnancy and no folic acid supplementation consumed.

Neural tube defects are more common in diabetes pregnancies compared to the general population [4], and therefore 5 mg folic acid once daily is recommended in women with diabetes pre-conceptually until the 12th week of pregnancy [5]. Women should also be advised on lifestyle modifications as summarised in Box 5.3.1, including eating a healthy diet and achieving an acceptable body weight prior to conceiving.

5.3.3 Obesity

Obesity is common in pregnant women with diabetes, with 62% of pregnant women with type 2 diabetes and 15% of women with type 1 diabetes being obese [3]. Maternal obesity (not diabetes specific) has been shown to be associated with increased maternal and infant mortality [6], with increased risk of congenital malformations, macrosomia (birth weight >4000 g), hypertensive disorders, gestational diabetes mellitus (GDM) [7] and anaesthetic and postoperative complications [8]. This risk is further increased when obesity and diabetes coexist [9] with different contributions of obesity and hyperglycaemia to different anomalies [10].

Obese women with diabetes should therefore be encouraged to lose weight before conception. United Kingdom (UK) guidelines recommend that pregnant women with diabetes who have a pre-pregnancy BMI of greater than 27 kg/m^2 be given weight reduction advice prior to pregnancy [5].

Energy requirements

Energy intake of pregnant women with diabetes should be adequate to meet nutrient needs and gain recommended amounts of weight throughout

Advanced Nutrition and Dietetics in Diabetes, First Edition. Edited by Louise Goff and Pamela Dyson.
© 2016 John Wiley & Sons, Ltd. Published 2016 by John Wiley & Sons, Ltd.

> **Box 5.3.1** Pre-pregnancy dietary advice for women with diabetes
>
> **Advice should include**
>
> - Commence 5 mg folic acid
> - Achieve an acceptable body weight
> - Eat a balanced diet to optimise glycaemic control
> - Carbohydrate education and adjustment (if appropriate)
> - Smoking cessation
> - Alcohol abstinence
> - Hypoglycaemia management
> - Food hygiene and safety for pregnancy

pregnancy according to BMI, physical activity level, foetal growth pattern and avoidance of excessive maternal weight gain and postpartum weight retention [11].

Active weight loss in pregnant women with diabetes using hypocaloric diets is not recommended due to the risk of ketonaemia and ketonuria and may also limit essential nutrients, vitamins and minerals [2]. There is, however, controversy regarding the severity of energy restriction for obese pregnant women with type 2 diabetes or GDM. Restricting energy intake in women with GDM was believed to control weight gain, improve glycaemic control and reduce the risk of macrosomia, however, severe energy restriction intake to below 1500 kcal/day is associated with increased ketonuria and ketonaemia [12] and is therefore not recommended. The American Diabetes Association [1] recommend that obese women with GDM adhere to a moderate energy restriction (reduction by 30% of estimated energy needs), which may improve glycaemic control without ketonaemia and reduce maternal weight gain. Therefore interventions during pregnancy should be aimed at limiting weight gain throughout gestation rather than weight loss.

Weight gain throughout pregnancy

Pregnancy weight gain targets for women with type1, type 2 and GDM should be the same as for women without diabetes [11,12], therefore minimising unnecessary weight gain during pregnancy. It is recommended that pregnant women with diabetes who have a pre-pregnancy BMI of greater than 27 kg/m^2 restrict their energy intake to around 25 kcals/kg/day in the second trimester [5]. There are, however, no UK guidelines for healthy weight gain targets for pregnant women with or without diabetes. However in comparison, the American Institute of Medicine (IOM) guidelines [13] (not specific to diabetes) recommend a healthy weight gain target based on pre-pregnancy BMI rather than suggesting a specific energy restriction. These IOM guidelines were based on observational studies and suggest that those who gain weight within the guidelines are more likely to have better maternal and infant outcomes than those who gain more or less weight [13]. Recommendations for pregnant women with diabetes suggest that BMI should be assessed pre-pregnancy and gestational weight gains should be targeted at the lower range of these recommendations [11].

There is a lack of evidence as to the most effective dietary intervention to promote appropriate weight gain in pregnancy, however, overall modification of energy intake should be considered. However, those on insulin with greater dependence on frequent snacks and avoidance of hypoglycaemia may gain more weight.

5.3.4 Nutritional management of diabetes in pregnancy

The evidence for the nutritional management of type 1 and type 2 diabetes has been extensively reviewed both nationally and internationally [1,14–16]. Broad consensus suggests that the composition of the diabetic diet in pregnancy is similar to that for non-pregnant diabetic women and that dietary advice should be based on a healthy balanced diet that provides all the essential macro- and micro-nutrients in appropriate amounts for growth and development of the foetus.

Evidence suggests that the exact proportion of macronutrients (carbohydrate, protein and fat) in the diabetic diet should be consistent with the general population [17] as research does not support any ideal percentage of energy from macronutrients in people with diabetes [15]. Saturated and trans-fatty acids should be limited and those with diabetes should be encouraged to adhere to a cardioprotective diet that is high in monounsaturated fats and low in saturated fats [1].

The aims of nutritional management in pregnancy

(1) Optimising glycaemic control and avoiding fluctuations of blood glucose, especially postprandial blood glucose, whilst avoiding hypoglycaemia and ketosis in women taking insulin.

(2) Provision of sufficient energy and nutrients to allow for foetal growth whilst avoiding accelerated foetal growth patterns [5].

Dietary modifications that limit postprandial glycaemia reduce the risk of macrosomia and other diabetic-related perinatal complications when the peak postprandial response is blunted [2]. Therefore targeting postprandial hyperglycaemia is particularly important during pregnancy [5] and adjusting treatment to postprandial blood glucose levels is recommended as it is associated with better outcomes in women with type1 or GDM than responding to fasting blood glucose levels [5]. Carbohydrate is the main nutrient that affects postprandial glucose levels [18].

Carbohydrate

Carbohydrate restriction is no longer part of diabetes management and there is no evidence for a recommended ideal amount [15]. Both the quantity (amount) and the type (high or low glycaemic index) or source of carbohydrate (starch or sugar) found in foods influence postprandial glycaemia [14]. It is now believed that the total carbohydrate intake from a meal or snack is a relatively reliable predictor of postprandial blood glucose [19].

Carbohydrate should be consistently distributed throughout the day and incorporated into each meal and snack to improve glycaemic control [15] and minimise the risk of both hypoglycaemia and ketoacidosis that are associated with maternal morbidity [11]. Women with type1 should not restrict carbohydrate intake (minimum 175 g carbohydrate/day) as low carbohydrate diets may increase the risk of ketosis and such foods provide important nutrients [1,11]. Adjusting insulin to the amount of carbohydrate consumed is an important strategy in achieving glycaemic control [18]. Structured education programmes that offer education in relation to carbohydrate counting and insulin dose adjustment are recommended for those pregnant women treated by multiple daily injections or by continuous subcutaneous insulin infusion (CSII) [5] where prandial insulin doses can be estimated according to dietary intake. For those on other insulin regimens consistency in the quantity and type of carbohydrate to encourage good postprandial glucose control is recommended [11].

Type and source of carbohydrate

Glycaemic index and glycaemic load

Individuals consuming a high glycaemic index (GI) diet show a modest benefit in controlling postprandial hyperglycaemia by reducing the GI [1], and most authorities recommend low GI or glycaemic load (GL) diets for the management of diabetes. There is limited evidence for the efficacy of low GI diets in diabetic pregnancies, with one small study showing no additional benefit of a low GI diet compared to a conventional high fibre diet [20].

Dietary fibre

In pregnancy (type 1 and GDM) high intakes of fibre (50–80 g) have been found to be associated with lower insulin requirements, but not to be associated with fasting blood glucose or glycated haemoglobin concentrations [21,22]. However Kalwarf et al. [23] suggest that dietary fibre may affect the management of glycaemia as fibre intake within the low to normal range (8–20 g/day) was inversely associated with insulin requirements during the second and third trimester. Therefore increasing fibre intake may be beneficial in pregnant women with diabetes, however, all women should aim to achieve the guideline for daily amounts (GDAs) for fibre of 24 g per day.

Sugar and sweeteners

Fructose has been shown to produce a lower postprandial glucose response when it replaces sucrose or starch in the diet than other carbohydrates, however, it is thought to adversely affect plasma lipids [24,25]. Therefore the use of added fructose as a sweetening agent is not recommended [1]. There is, however, no evidence to suggest avoiding naturally occurring fructose in fruits, vegetables and other foods [1].

There is no evidence for non-nutritive sweeteners in pregnancy, but it is assumed that they are safe to consume as substitutes for sucrose within the daily intake levels [20] and approved for use for those with diabetes in the UK as part of professional guidelines [14].

5.3.5 Physical activity

Pregnant women with uncomplicated pregnancies should be encouraged to continue to engage in physical activities [26]. The benefits of exercise for pregnant women include a sense of well-being, decreased weight gain, reduction of foetal adiposity, improved glucose control and better tolerance of labour [27,28] and therefore physical activity should be an integral component of a healthy pregnancy [29]. Pregnant women with diabetes without contraindications should be encouraged to use physical activity as part of their overall diabetes management and aim for at least 30 minutes each day [11]. In pregnancy moderate intensity physical activity that does not have a high risk of falling or abdominal trauma, is recommended [26]. Adjustments to diabetes regimens are essential to decrease the risk of exercise-induced hypoglycaemia that may be exacerbated in pregnancy [11].

Regular physical activity has been shown to lower fasting and postprandial plasma glucose concentrations and may be used as an adjunct to improve maternal glycaemia [1]. Supervised exercise programmes have been shown to improve maternal glucose tolerance when used

as an adjunct to dietary treatment and have the potential to obviate the need for insulin [30]. Therefore, encouraging exercise in those with type 2 diabetes or GDM may help limit postprandial hyperglycaemia and weight gain.

5.3.6 Lactation

Breastfeeding is recommended for women with pre-existing diabetes or GDM [31] as the preferred method of infant feeding due to the many multiple and long term benefits to both mother and child [32]. However, rates of breastfeeding are lower for women with diabetes than the general population [3]. Higher rates of pregnancy and neonatal complications among diabetic women can pose significant challenges to breastfeeding [33]. However, women with diabetes should be strongly encouraged to breastfeed because of maternal and childhood benefits specific to diabetes that are above and beyond other known benefits of breastfeeding [34]. Additionally, for women with GDM evidence suggests that lactation confers benefits by improving glucose tolerance in early postpartum [35]. Breastfeeding was found to show significantly lower postpartum glucose results with a two-fold higher rate of postpartum diabetes in those who did not breastfeed [36], therefore influencing the future onset of diabetes.

Breastfeeding, however, can cause life-threatening hypoglycaemia for lactating women on insulin and requires increased frequency of glucose testing, an increased carbohydrate intake and a reduced insulin dose [31]. The requirement for carbohydrate is increased during lactation for milk production [31]. It is estimated that an additional 60 g of carbohydrate/day is required to replace the carbohydrate secreted in human milk [31] therefore diabetic women should have a meal or snack with carbohydrate before or during feeds [5].

5.3.7 Summary

All women with diabetes should receive dietary education to promote healthy food choices to optimise glycaemic control before, during and after pregnancy. Postnatal follow up should be seen as an opportunity to initiate pre-pregnancy counselling for subsequent pregnancies. Although most women with GDM revert to normal glucose tolerance postpartum, they are at increased risk of GDM in subsequent pregnancies and type 2 diabetes later in life [37,38]. Lifestyle modifications after pregnancy aimed at reducing weight and increasing physical activity are recommended.

Key points

- Pre-conception advice for obese women recommends weight loss before conception.
- There are no current guidelines for weight gain during pregnancy in women with diabetes, but limits are advised for those who are overweight or obese at conception.
- Women with diabetes should take 5 mg folic acid until the 12th week of pregnancy.
- Concensus recommends a diet similar to that recommended for non-pregnant diabetic women.
- Regular physical activity is recommended during pregnancy.
- Breastfeeding is recommended.

References

1. Bantle JP, Wylie-Rosett J, Albright AL, Apovian CM, Clark NG, Franz MJ, et al. Nutrition recommendations and interventions for diabetes: a position statement of the America Diabetes Association. *Diabetes Care* 2008; **31**: S61–S78.
2. Jovanovic L. Medical nutritional therapy in pregnant women with pregestational diabetes mellitus. *J Matern Fetal Med* 2000; **9**: 21–28.
3. CEMACH. Confidential Enquiry into Maternal and Child Health: Diabetes in pregnancy; Are we providing the best care. England, Wales and Northern Ireland. Findings of a National Enquiry. London: CEMACH, 2007.
4. Macintosh MC, Fleming KM, Bailey JA, Doyle P, Modder J, Acolet D, et al. Perinatal mortality and congenital anomalies in babies of women with type 1 or type 2 diabetes in England, Wales, and Northern Ireland: population based study. *BMJ* 2006; **333**(7560): 177.
5. National Institute for Health and Clinical Excellence. Diabetes in pregnancy: Management of diabetes and its complications from pre-conception to the postnatal period. London: NICE, 2008.
6. Lewis G. The confidential enquiry into maternal and child health (CEMACH). Saving mothers lives, reviewing maternal deaths to make motherhood safer 2003–2005. The seventh report of the Confidential Enquires into Maternal Deaths in the United Kingdom. London: CEMACH, 2007.
7. Baeten J, Bukusi E, Lambe M. Pregnancy complications and outcomes among overweight and obese nulliparous women. *Am J Pub Health* 2001; **91**: 436–440.
8. Galtier-Dereure F, Boegner C, Bringer J. Obesity and pregnancy: complications and cost. *Am J Clin Nutr* 2000; **71**(Suppl. 5): 1242S–1248S.
9. Martinez-Frais ML, Frias JP, Bermejo E, Rodriguez-Pinilla E, Prieto L, Frais JL. Pre-gestational maternal body mass index predicts an increased risk of congenital malformations in infants of mothers with gestational diabetes. *Diabet Med* 2005; **22**: 775–781.
10. Garcia-Patterson A, Erdozain L, Ginovart G, Adelantado JM, Cubero JM, Gallo G, et al. In human gestational diabetes mellitus congenital malformations are related to prepregnancy body mass index and to severity of diabetes. *Diabetologia* 2004; **47**: 509–514.
11. Kitzmiller JL, Block JM, Brown FM, Catalano PM, Conway DL, Coustan DR, et al. Managing preexisting diabetes for pregnancy: summary of evidence and consensus recommendations for care. *Diabetes Care* 2008; **31**(5): 1060–1079.
12. Reader DM. Medical nutrition therapy and lifestyle interventions. *Diabetes Care* 2007; **30**(Suppl. 2): S188–S193.
13. Institute of Medicine (IOM). *Weight Gain During Pregnancy; Re-examining the Guidelines.* Washington DC: National Academies Press, 2009.
14. Dyson PA, Kelly T, Deakin T, Duncan A, Frost G, Harrison Z, et al.; Diabetes UK Working Group. *Diabet Med* 2011; **28**: 1282–1288.
15. Franz MJ, Powers MA, Leontos C, Holzmeister LA, Kulkarni K, Monk A, et al. The evidence for medical nutrition therapy for type 1 and type 2 diabetes in adults. *J Am Diet Assoc* 2010; **110**(12): 1852–1889.
16. Mann JI, De Leeuw I, Hermansen K, Karamanos B, Karlstrom B, Katsilambros N, et al. for the Diabetes and Nutrition Study Group (DNSG) of the European Association. Evidence-based nutritional approaches to the treatment and prevention of diabetes mellitus. *Nutr Metab Cardiovasc Dis* 2004; **14**(6): 373–394.
17. COMA. Report of the Panel on DRVs of the Committee on Medical Aspects of Food Policy

(COMA) Report on Health and Social Subjects 41. Dietary Reference Values (DRVs) for Food Energy and Nutrients for the UK. London: The Stationary Office, 1991.

18. Sheard NF. Clark NG. Brand-Miller JC. Franz MJ, Pi-Sunyer FX, Mayer-Davis E, et al. Dietary carbohydrate (amount and type) in the prevention and management of diabetes: a statement by the American Diabetes Association. *Diabetes Care* 2004; **27**(9): 2266–2271.

19. Franz M, Bantle JP, Beebe CA, Brunzell JD, Chiasson JL, Garg A. Evidence based nutrition principles and recommendations for the treatment and prevention of diabetes and related complications. *Diabetes Care* 2002; **25**(1); 148–155.

20. Louie JC, Markovic TP, Perera N, Foote D, Petocz P, Ross GP, Brand-Miller JC. A randomized controlled trial investigating the effects of a low-glycemic index diet on pregnancy outcomes in gestational diabetes mellitus. *Diabetes Care* 2011; **34**(11): 2341–2346.

21. Ney D, Hollingsworth DR, Cousins L. Decreased insulin requirements and improved control of diabetes in pregnant women given a high carbohydrate, high fibre, low fat diet. *Diabetes Care* 1982; **5**: 529–533.

22. Reece EA, Hagay Z, Caseria D, Gay LJ, DeGennaro N. Do fibre-enriched diabetic diets have glucose lowering effects in pregnancy? *Am J Perinatol* 1983; **10**: 272–4.

23. Kalwarf HJ, Bell RC, Khoury JC, Gouge AL, Miodovnik M. Dietary fibre intakes and insulin requirements in pregnant women with type 1 diabetes. *J Am Diet Assoc* 2001; **101**: 305–310.

24. Bantle JP, Swanson JE, Thomas W, Laine DC. Metabolic effects of dietary fructose in diabetic subjects. *Diabetes Care* 1992; **15**: 1468–1476.

25. Livesey G. Health potential of polyols as a sugar replacement, with emphasis on low glycaemic properties. *Nutr Res Rev* 2003; **16**: 163–191.

26. Artal R, O'Toole M. Guidelines of the American College of Obstetricians and Gynecologists for exercise during pregnancy and the postpartum period. *Br J Sports Med* 2003; **37**: 6–12.

27. American College of Obstetricians and Gynaecologists. ACOG committee opinion. Exercise during pregnancy and the postpartum period no 267. *Obstet Gynecol* 2002; **99**: 171–173.

28. Castorino K, Jovanovic L. Pregnancy and diabetes management: Advances and Controversies. *Clinic Chem* 2011; **57**: 221–223.

29. Zavorsky GS, Longo LD. Exercise guidelines in pregnancy: new perspectives. *Sports Med* 2011; **41**(5): 345–360.

30. Jovanovic-Peterson L, Peterson CM. Is exercise safe or useful for gestational diabetic women? *Diabetes* 1991; **40**(Suppl. 2): 179–181.

31. Reader D, Franz MJ. Lactation, diabetes and nutrition recommendations. *Curr Diabetes Rep* 2004; **4**(5): 370–376.

32. Kramer MS, Kakuma. The optimal duration of exclusive breastfeeding: A systematic review. Geneva: WHO, 2002. Available from URL:http://www.who.int/features/qa/57/en/index.html. Accessed June 2012.

33. Merlob P, Hod M. Short term implications: The neonate. in *Textbook of Diabetes and Pregnancy* eds. Hod M, Jovanovic L, Di Renzo GC, De Leiva A, Langer O. London: Informa Healthcare, 2008.

34. Taylor JS, Kacmar JE, Nothnagle M, Lawrence RA. A systematic review of the literature associating breastfeeding with type 2 Diabetes and gestational diabetes. *J Am Coll Nutr* 2005; **24**(5): 320–326.

35. Gunderson EP. Breastfeeding after gestational diabetes pregnancy. *Diabetes Care* 2007; **30**(Suppl. 2): S161–S168.

36. Kjos SL, Henry O, Lee RM, Buchanan TA, Mishell DR. The effects of lactation on glucose and lipid metabolism in women with recent gestational diabetes. *Obstet Gynaecol* 1993; **82**: 451–455.

37. Kim C, Newton KM, Knopp RH. Gestational diabetes and the incidence of type 2 diabetes: a systematic review. *Diabetes Care* 2002; **25**(10):1862–1868.

38. Kim C. Managing women with gestational diabetes mellitus in the postnatal period. *Diabet Obes Metab* 2010; **12**(1): 20–25.

SECTION 6

Diabetes in children and adolescents

Chapter 6.1

Epidemiology, aetiology and pathogenesis of childhood diabetes

Francesca Annan
Alder Hey Children's NHS Foundation Trust, Liverpool, UK

6.1.1 Introduction

Diabetes in childhood presents predominantly as type 1 diabetes, other forms of diabetes occur less commonly. The worldwide incidence of diabetes in children is increasing with an average annual increase of 2.8%.

6.1.2 Epidemiology of childhood diabetes

Incidence of diabetes varies worldwide, although 90% of all cases of diabetes in childhood are type 1 diabetes [1]. The variation in incidence shows correlation with the frequency of human leucocyte antigen (HLA) susceptibility genes in populations of white Caucasian ancestry. The HLA complex confers about 40–50% of the inherited risk. Across Europe there is a correlation between the frequency of HLA susceptibility genes and incidence of type 1 diabetes. By comparison, China and Japan have different HLA associations compared to white Caucasians and very low incidence rates of type 1 diabetes [2].

The number of children worldwide developing diabetes is increasing, with data from the EURODIAB study suggesting that the number of under-5s with type 1 diabetes will double over the next decade and the number of older children will increase by 70% [3,4]. The increase in type 1 diabetes may be due to the lowering of the age of presentation due to increased insulin resistance. Increased insulin resistance has been postulated to overload the β-cell, this is commonly called 'the Accelerator Hypothesis', and has been proposed from epidemiological findings but is not universally accepted [5–8]. Children with type 1 have been observed to be heavier and taller at diagnosis than their peers [9]. Birth weight and early growth rates have been examined as a cause of earlier presentation of type 1 diabetes in childhood, with some studies supporting the hypothesis that increased birth weight and rate of growth in the first 6 months are significant factors [10].

A number of countries have reported increasing incidence of diabetes in childhood [3,11–13]. This is predominantly type 1 diabetes, and incidence rates appear to be similar for migrant populations [13]. The International Diabetes Federation (IDF) diabetes atlas provides data on the worldwide incidence and prevalence of diabetes in children [14]. The rigour of some of the data varies from European data based on well-established, reliable national registers through to less reliable estimates of incidence across Africa, which need to be reviewed with caution. The worldwide estimate of the number of children aged 15 years and under who develop diabetes is 76 000 per year [14]. Highest rates of diabetes are found in Scandinavia, with lower incidence in central and eastern Europe, however all regions are reporting an increase in incidence in childhood diabetes.

Advanced Nutrition and Dietetics in Diabetes, First Edition. Edited by Louise Goff and Pamela Dyson.
© 2016 John Wiley & Sons, Ltd. Published 2016 by John Wiley & Sons, Ltd.

Studies that provide reports on the incidence of diabetes use different methods of data presentation, some countries using prevalence and others annual incidence figures. The data from the IDF world diabetes atlas allow comparison between different populations.

In the United Kingdom (UK), data from the 2009 national survey undertaken by the Royal College of Paediatrics and Child Health (RCPCH) to establish the number of children with diabetes in England identified the prevalence of type 1 and type 2 diabetes as 186.3 and 2.3 per 100 000, respectively [15]. The number of children with diabetes identified in England in 2009 was 22 783; the greatest number of cases occurred in the over-10s and 51.1% of the population were male. The regional variations in prevalence were 137–279.5/100 000. These figures may underestimate the actual number of cases due to missing data, but provide useful information about diabetes prevalence in age groups and across regions. Data from the Yorkshire and Humber region provide some insight into the regional and ethnic differences in type 1 diabetes in the UK. Type 1 diabetes incidence was reported as 18.1/100 000 childhood population, with an annual percentage change of 2.8%. Within this population there was difference in the annual percentage change in incidence for South Asian (1.5%) and non-South Asian populations (3.4%). These differences were not influenced by deprivation [16].

Type 2 diabetes is reported in increasing numbers in specific populations [11,17,18]. The highest prevalence rates of type 2 diabetes occur in populations of non-white-European descent. Data from the SEARCH for Diabetes in youth study [11,19] in the USA showed variable rates of diagnosis according to ethnicity in 10–19 year olds, with 76% of the Native American cohort being diagnosed with type 2 diabetes compared to 6% for non-Hispanic whites. Presentation of type 2 diabetes varies between countries; in Europe most cases of type 2 diabetes are associated with overweight and obesity, as defined by body mass index (BMI) percentile greater than the 85th for age and sex. In contrast, in Japan around 30% of cases of children presenting with type 2 are of normal body weight [20]. The incidence of type 2 diabetes in the UK is rising but remains less common than type 1 diabetes, 95% of patients are overweight (83% obese) and it is more prevalent in the non-white populations [21].

6.1.3 Aetiology, classification and pathogenesis

The American Diabetes Association (ADA) and the World Health Organisation (WHO) published the aetiological classification of diabetes, giving three categories of disorders of glycaemia that may affect children. These categories are: type 1 diabetes, type 2 diabetes and other specific types, which include genetic defects of β-cell function formerly known as MODY (maturity-onset diabetes of the young), defects of insulin action (e.g. Rabson–Mendhall syndrome) and diseases of the exocrine pancreas (e.g. cystic fibrosis-related diabetes). This classification is summarised in Table 6.1.1.

6.1.4 Pathogenesis of diabetes in childhood

Type 1 diabetes

Type 1 diabetes occurs as a result of autoimmune destruction of the insulin-producing β-cells of the pancreas and results in a deficiency of insulin production, with most cases attributed to T-cell mediated β-cell destruction. Symptoms usually present when around 90% of the function of the pancreatic β-cells has been destroyed. Development of type 1 diabetes is precipitated by genetic and environmental factors but exact mechanisms are not well understood. Autoimmune type 1 diabetes is linked to multiple genes; Barrett et al. in 2009 [22] identified over 40 genome locations associated with type 1 diabetes. The environmental triggers to the development of diabetes remain unknown, although infection is often cited as a trigger within the paediatric population [2,23]. The seasonal variation in onset of diabetes is used to support the argument for viral triggers, with some populations showing seasonal increases in colder autumn and winter months [24].

Table 6.1.1 Aetiological classification of glycaemic disorders adapted from International Society for Pediatric and Adolescent Diabetes consensus guidelines 2009

Type 1	Beta-cell destruction leading to absolute insulin deficiency Immune-mediated Idiopathic
Type 2	
Genetic defects of B-cell function	Monogenic diabetes Mitochondrial DNA mutation Chromosome 7, KCNJ11(Kir6.2)
Genetic defects in insulin secretion	Leprechaunism Rabson–Mendenhall syndrome Lipoatrophic diabetes Others
Diseases of exocrine pancreas	Pancreatitis Cystic Fibrosis Trauma/pancreatectomy Neoplasia Others
Endocrinopathies	Acromegaly Cushings syndrome Glucagonoma Others
Drug or chemical induced	
Infections	
Uncommon forms of immune mediated diabetes	
Other genetic syndromes associated with diabetes	Downs syndrome Wolfram syndrome Klinefelter syndrome Friedreich's ataxia Lawrence–Moon–Biedl syndrome Others

Type 1 diabetes does not have a recognisable pattern of inheritance, with familial aggregation occurring in approximately 10% of cases. The risk for an identical twin is reported as 36%, for a sibling the risk rises from 4% before the age of 20 years to 9.6% by 60 years, and type 1 diabetes is reported to be 2–3 times more common in offspring of diabetic men compared to diabetic women [25].

Diagnosis of type 1 diabetes in childhood is based on blood glucose concentrations and the presence of symptoms and is usually, but not exclusively, associated with the presence of autoimmune antibodies. Type 1 diabetes in childhood usually presents with polyuria, polydipsia associated with glycosuria and ketonuria/ketonaemia [12].

Type 2 diabetes

Type 2 diabetes in childhood is usually associated with overweight and obesity and features of insulin resistance [26,27] including hypertension, hyperlipidaemia, acanthosis nigricans and polycystic ovarian syndrome [28,29]. Type 2 develops when insulin production does not meet the demand posed by insulin resistance. Presentation usually occurs after 10 years of age and is more common in those of non-white European descent. Some children, commonly those with a lower body weight, present with autoimmune type 2 diabetes [28], patients who are antibody positive will usually require insulin treatment sooner than those who are antibody negative. A United States (US) study reported positive insulin antibodies in 8.1% and anti GAD in 30.3% of a study population [30,31]. Symptoms may or may not be present and problems with classification and treatment arise when ketonuria is present at diagnosis of type 2 diabetes [11].

Monogenic forms of diabetes

Genetic defects of β-cell function form a distinct group of monogenic diabetes formerly known as MODY. These types of diabetes usually present in the post-pubertal period with the exception of neonatal diabetes and glucokinase mutations and they have variable clinical presentation. Ketosis may occur in neonatal diabetes and there is usually a parent with diabetes [32]. Genetic testing to establish the diagnosis of monogenic diabetes is available in some countries, including the UK. A diagnosis of monogenic diabetes may be suspected when diabetes is diagnosed before 6 months of age, if there is evidence of continued endogenous insulin production (with detectable c-peptide) after the so-called honeymoon period, or in the absence of pancreatic auto-antibodies, particularly at diagnosis. In those initially diagnosed with type 2 diabetes, monogenic diabetes may be suspected when there is an absence of insulin resistance, that is a normal fasting c-peptide, in a specific ethnic group with low incidence of type 2 diabetes, in the absence of marked obesity or when there are family members who have diabetes and are a normal body weight [32].

The commonest familial forms of monogenic diabetes are HNF-1α mutations (formerly known as MODY 3), HNF-4α mutations (MODY 1) and glucokinase mutations (MODY 2). HNF-1α and HNF-4α can be treated with sulfonylureas in sensitive patients, glucokinase mutations result in fasting hyperglycaemia that does not require any treatment in childhood.

Neonatal diabetes

Diabetes diagnosed in the first 6 months is now recognised as unlikely to be type 1 diabetes. It is a rare condition and may be associated with intrauterine growth retardation. There are two recognised types of neonatal diabetes: permanent and transient [32]. Molecular genetic classification is available in the UK for all diagnoses of diabetes made in the first 6 months of life. These infants may present with diabetic ketoacidosis (DKA) and initial treatment is with insulin. Imprinting anomalies are the commonest cause of neonatal diabetes. Transient neonatal diabetes (TNDM) is due to imprinting anomalies and usually resolves at around 12 weeks, these patients may present with diabetes later in childhood and eventually require management with insulin. Permanent neonatal diabetes (PNDM) and some cases of TNDM are due to mutations in the ATP-sensitive potassium channel. Kir6.2 mutations are the second commonest cause of neonatal diabetes, the majority of cases are permanent and may be associated with neurological features. Despite presenting with ketoacidosis many patients with Kir6.2 mutation will be responsive to treatment with sulfonylureas [33].

Cystic fibrosis-related diabetes

Patients with cystic fibrosis (CF) have variable glucose levels, the earliest changes seen are intermittent post-prandial hyperglycaemia, followed by impaired glucose tolerance, diabetes without fasting hyperglycaemia and diabetes with fasting hyperglycaemia. A normal oral glucose tolerance test (OGTT) does not exclude abnormal post-prandial glucose levels at other times [34,35].

There is an association between CF mutations and cystic fibrosis-related diabetes (CFRD), the primary defect is not absolute insulin deficiency. First phase insulin secretion is delayed and a blunting of peak insulin levels is observed post OGTT. Insulin resistance occurs due to infection and inflammation as well as treatment with corticosteroids. Fasting hypoglycaemia is rarely seen in those without liver disease or malnutrition [36]. For further details of CFRD, see Chapter 9.5.

6.1.5 Conclusion

Type 1 diabetes remains the commonest form of diabetes in children, accounting for over 90% of childhood diabetes worldwide. The increasing incidence of diabetes across this age group presents challenges for the provision and delivery of lifestyle, clinical and nutritional management to achieve glycaemic control that will decrease the burden of diabetes complications and provide children and young people with healthy futures. A detailed and comprehensive review of the definition, epidemiology and classification of diabetes in childhood can be found in the 2009 ISPAD clinical practice consensus guidelines [2].

Key points

- Prevalence and incidence of type 1 diabetes in children varies by country, but is increasing around the world.
- Type 2 diabetes is increasing in children and is associated with obesity and physical inactivity.
- Other types of diabetes seen in children include monogenic diabetes, neonatal diabetes and cystic fibrosis-related diabetes.

References

1. Karvonen M, Viik-Kajander M, Moltchanova E, Libman I, LaPorte R, Tuomilehto J. Incidence of childhood type 1 diabetes worldwide. Diabetes Mondiale (DiaMond) Project Group. *Diabetes Care* 2000; **23**(10): 1516–1526.

2. Craig ME, Hattersley A, Donaghue K. ISPAD Clinical Practice Consensus Guidelines 2006-2007. Definition, epidemiology and classification. *Pediatr Diabetes* 2006; **7**(6): 343–351.

3. Editorial: Increase in childhood type 1 diabetes in Europe. *Arch Dis Child* 2009; **94**(11): 875.

4. Patterson CC, Gyürüs E, Rosenbauer J, Cinek O, Neu A, Schober E, et al. Trends in childhood type 1 diabetes incidence in Europe during 1989–2008: evidence of non-uniformity over time in rates of increase. *Diabetologia* 2012; **55**(8): 2142–2147.

5. Betts P, Mulligan J, Ward P, Smith B, Wilkin T. Increasing body weight predicts the earlier onset of insulin-dependant diabetes in childhood: testing the 'accelerator hypothesis' (2). *Diabet Med* 2005; **22**(2):144–151.

6. Kordonouri O, Hartmann R. Higher body weight is associated with earlier onset of Type 1 diabetes in children: confirming the 'Accelerator Hypothesis'. *Diabet Med* 2005; **22**(12): 1783–1784.

7. Knerr I, Wolf J, Reinehr T, Stachow R, Grabert M, Schober E, et al. The 'accelerator hypothesis': relationship between weight, height, body mass index and age at diagnosis in a large cohort of 9,248 German and Austrian children with type 1 diabetes mellitus. *Diabetologia* 2005; **48**(12): 2501–2504.

8. O'Connell MA, Donath S, Cameron FJ. Major increase in Type 1 diabetes: no support for the Accelerator Hypothesis. *Diabet Med* 2007; **24**(8): 920–923.

9. Ljungkrantz M, Ludvigsson J, Samuelsson U. Type 1 diabetes: increased height and weight gains in early childhood. *Pediatr Diabetes* 2008; **9**(3): 50–56.

10. Kharagjitsingh AV, de Ridder MAJ, Roep BO, Koeleman BPC, Bruining GJ, Veeze HJ. Revisiting infant growth prior to childhood onset type 1 diabetes. *Clin Endocrinol (Oxf)* 2010; **72**(5): 620–624.

11. Liese AD, D'Agostino RB, Jr, Hamman RF, Kilgo PD, Lawrence JM, Liu LL, et al. The burden of diabetes mellitus among US youth: prevalence estimates from the SEARCH for Diabetes in Youth Study. *Pediatrics* 2006; **118**(4): 1510–1518.

12. SEARCH for Diabetes in Youth: a multicenter study of the prevalence, incidence and classification of diabetes mellitus in youth. *Control Clin Trials* 2004; **25**(5): 458–471.

13. Söderström U, Aman J, Hjern A. Being born in Sweden increases the risk for type 1 diabetes - A study of migration of children to Sweden as a natural experiment. *Acta Paediatr* 2012; **101**(1): 73–77.

14. IDF. Diabetes in the Young: a global perspective. Brussels, 2009.

15. Haines LK, Z. Growing up with diabetes: children and young people with diabetes in England. London: Royal College of Paediatrics and Child Health; 2009.

16. Harron KL, McKinney PA, Feltbower RG, Bodansky HJ, Norman PD, Campbell FM, et al. Incidence rate trends in childhood type 1 diabetes in Yorkshire, UK 1978–2007: effects of deprivation and age at diagnosis in the South Asian and non-South Asian populations. *Diabet Med* 2011; **28**(12): 1508–1513.

17. Matyka KA. Type 2 diabetes in childhood: epidemiological and clinical aspects. *Br Med Bull* 2008; **86**: 59–75.

18. Ehtisham S, Hattersley AT, Dunger DB, Barrett TG. First UK survey of paediatric type 2 diabetes and MODY. *Arch Dis Child* 2004 06; **89**(6): 526–529.

19. Dabelea D, Bell RA, D'Agostino RB, Jr, Imperatore G, Johansen JM, Linder B, et al. Incidence of diabetes in youth in the United States. *JAMA* 2007; **297**(24): 2716–2724.

20. Rosenbloom AL, Silverstein JH, Amemiya S, Zeitler P, Klingensmith GJ. ISPAD Clinical Practice Consensus Guidelines 2006–2007. Type 2 diabetes mellitus in the child and adolescent. *Pediatr Diabetes* 2008; **9**(5): 512–526.

21. Haines L, Wan KC, Lynn R, Barrett TG, Shield JPH. Rising incidence of type 2 diabetes in children in the U.K. *Diabetes Care* 2007; **30**(5): 1097–1101.

22. Barrett JC, Clayton DG, Concannon P, Akolkar B, Cooper JD, Erlich HA, et al. Genome-wide association study and meta-analysis find that over 40 loci affect risk of type 1 diabetes. *Nat Genet* 2009; **41**(6): 703–707.

23. The Environmental Determinants of Diabetes in the Young (TEDDY) study: study design. *Pediatr Diabetes* 2007; **8**(5): 286–298.

24. Lévy-Marchal C, Patterson C, Green A. Variation by age group and seasonality at diagnosis of childhood IDDM in Europe. The EURODIAB ACE Study Group. *Diabetologia* 1995; **38**(7): 823–830.

25. Familial risk of type I diabetes in European children. The Eurodiab Ace Study Group and The Eurodiab Ace Substudy 2 Study Group. *Diabetologia* 1998; **41**(10): 1151–1156.

26. Liu LL, Lawrence JM, Davis C, Liese AD, Pettitt DJ, Pihoker C, et al. Prevalence of overweight and obesity in youth with diabetes in USA: the SEARCH for Diabetes in Youth study. *Pediatr Diabetes* 2010; **11**(1): 4–11.

27. Kershnar AK, Daniels SR, Imperatore G, Palla SL, Petitti DB, Pettitt DJ, et al. Lipid abnormalities are prevalent in youth with type 1 and type 2 diabetes: the

SEARCH for Diabetes in Youth Study. *J Pediatr* 2006; **149**(3): 314–319.

28. Badaru A, Pihoker C. Type 2 diabetes in childhood: clinical characteristics and role of β-cell autoimmunity. *Curr Diab Rep* 2012; **12**(1): 75–81.

29. Pinhas-Hamiel O, Zeitler P. Clinical presentation and treatment of type 2 diabetes in children. *Pediatr Diabetes* 2007; **8**(Suppl. 9): 16–27.

30. Reinehr T, Schober E, Wiegand S, Thon A, Holl R. Beta-cell autoantibodies in children with type 2 diabetes mellitus: subgroup or misclassification? *Arch Dis Child* 2006; **91**(6): 473–477.

31. Hathout EH, Thomas W, El-Shahawy M, Nahab F, Mace JW. Diabetic autoimmune markers in children and adolescents with type 2 diabetes. *Pediatrics* 2001; **107**(6): E102.

32. Hattersley A, Bruining J, Shield J, Njolstad P, Donaghue K. ISPAD Clinical Practice Consensus Guidelines 2006-2007. The diagnosis and management of monogenic diabetes in children. *Pediatr Diabetes* 2006; **7**(6): 352–360.

33. Støy J, Greeley SAW, Paz VP, Ye H, Pastore AN, Skowron KB, et al. Diagnosis and treatment of neonatal diabetes: an United States experience. *Pediatr Diabetes* 2008; **9**(5): 450–459.

34. Moran A, Brunzell C, Cohen RC, Katz M, Marshall BC, Onady G, et al. Clinical care guidelines for cystic fibrosis-related diabetes: a position statement of the American Diabetes Association and a clinical practice guideline of the Cystic Fibrosis Foundation, endorsed by the Pediatric Endocrine Society. *Diabetes Care* 2010; **33**(12): 2697–2708.

35. O'Riordan SMP, Robinson PD, Donaghue KC, Moran A. Management of cystic fibrosis-related diabetes in children and adolescents. *Pediatr Diabetes* 2009; **10**: 43–50.

36. Moran A, Becker D, Casella SJ, Gottlieb PA, Kirkman MS, Marshall BC, et al. Epidemiology, pathophysiology, and prognostic implications of cystic fibrosis-related diabetes: a technical review. *Diabetes Care* 2010; **33**(12): 2677–2683.

Clinical management of diabetes in children and adolescents

Princy Paul
Alder Hey Children's NHS Foundation Trust, Liverpool, UK

6.2.1 Introduction

Type 1 diabetes is one of the most common chronic childhood diseases and its incidence has doubled during the last decade [1]. The goals of intensive management of type 1 diabetes were established in 1993 by the Diabetes Control and Complications Trial (DCCT), when it was shown that good glycaemic control significantly reduced the risk of developing long-term complications of diabetes in both adults [2] and adolescents [3,4], and this has now been confirmed in children [5,6]. It is important to prevent both sustained hyperglycaemia, due to its association with long-term microvascular and macrovascular complications, and recurrent episodes of hypoglycaemia, especially in young children, due to its adverse effects on cognitive function, which may impede efforts to achieve the recommended glycaemic targets [7–9]. As a result, children with type 1 diabetes and their caregivers continue to face the challenge of maintaining blood glucose levels in the near-normal range.

The aim of diabetes management is to achieve glycated haemoglobin (HbA1c) of below 58 mmol/mol (7.5%), without significant hypoglycaemia. It is recommended by both the International Society for Pediatric and Adolescent Diabetes (ISPAD) and the International Diabetes Federation (IDF) that children and adolescents with type 1 diabetes should have access to care by a multidisciplinary team, including a paediatrician with experience in diabetes and a specialist diabetes nurse and dietitian trained in childhood diabetes [10]. Education should be adapted to each individual's age, maturity, stage of diabetes, lifestyle and culture. After the initial period of diagnosis and education (when frequent contact may be required), the child should be reviewed regularly throughout the year. This should be no less than three to four times per year, including one major annual review with the multidisciplinary team paying particular attention to growth, blood pressure, puberty, investigation of thyroid problems and coeliac disease, nutrition and complications [10].

6.2.2 Insulin management

All children with type 1 diabetes require treatment with insulin therapy. If the child is generally well at diagnosis and does not have diabetic ketoacidosis (DKA), insulin therapy should be commenced immediately. The choice of insulin and the regimen depends on the age of the child, the child or caregiver's preference to number of injections per day, the cost and availability of various formulations of insulin and injection devices, and also the presence of any needle phobia.

Insulin type and regimen

There are no randomised controlled studies comparing the long-term outcomes of using older, traditional (human) insulins with newer analogue

Advanced Nutrition and Dietetics in Diabetes, First Edition. Edited by Louise Goff and Pamela Dyson.
© 2016 John Wiley & Sons, Ltd. Published 2016 by John Wiley & Sons, Ltd.

insulins, when both groups receive equal educational input. However, traditional insulin does have some clinical limitations, including the need to be injected up to 30 minutes before eating (meaning that dose adjustment of insulin to carbohydrate content of meals can be challenging), and that it tends to have a longer profile, which means it may be more likely to cause hypoglycaemia than analogue insulin [11,12]. Anecdotal evidence from most Western countries has shown a move towards the use of analogue insulin via multiple daily injections (MDI) [13] or use of insulin pumps (continuous subcutaneous insulin infusion – CSII) in an attempt to reduce hypoglycaemic episodes [14] and to strive towards improved long-term diabetes control by aiming for near-normal HbA1c concentrations. Recurrent hypoglycaemic episodes can lead to cognitive impairment and hypoglycaemia unawareness in younger children and the use of analogue insulin has been shown to reduce the incidence in hypoglycaemic episodes in adolescents and younger children [15].

Biphasic (twice daily) injections

Pre-mixed insulin (fixed ratio mixtures of pre-meal and basal insulin) injected twice daily is widely used in some countries, particularly for pre-pubertal children with type 1 diabetes.

The advantages include

- Wide variety of preparations including using NPH (neutral protamine Hagedorn) insulin and premixed insulin using analogue, human or porcine/bovine insulin
- Ease of use, especially in school-aged child who cannot self-inject
- Fewer injections for children with needle phobia (consider CSII)
- Less expensive
- Many of these formulations are widely available in most countries.

Dosage of Insulin

The starting dosage of insulin varies from 0.5 units in pre-pubertal children to 0.75 units/kg body weight in adolescents. This can be administered as MDI (40 –50% as basal using intermediate acting

insulin and the rest divided as pre-meal boluses) or as a biphasic insulin regimen (two-thirds of the total insulin as the pre-breakfast dose, and one-third as the pre-evening meal dose) or as CSII via insulin pump. Insulin doses are titrated according to pre- and post-prandial blood glucose readings obtained by capillary blood glucose testing, until the target HbA1c is achieved. Pre-pubertal children may need up to 0.7–1 unit/kg/day outside the partial remission phase, and during the natural insulin resistance of puberty the requirement can go up to 1–2 units/kg/day [16].

Injection sites and devices

The insulin injections are given subcutaneously using various devices ranging from traditional insulin syringe to pen injector devices and automatic injection devices that are particularly useful in children with needle phobia. The two-finger pinch technique is recommended for all types of injections to ensure a strict subcutaneous injection, avoiding intramuscular injection [17]. The usual injection sites are abdomen, lateral/front aspect of thigh, lateral aspect of arm and buttocks (upper and outer quadrant) in smaller children. The side-effects associated with insulin injections include local hypersensitivity reactions, lipohypertrophy, painful injection, leakage of insulin, bleeding and bruising at injection sites and lipoatrophy (uncommon).

6.2.3 Diabetes emergencies

Hypoglyacemia

Hypoglycaemia is one of the most common acute complications of the treatment of type 1 diabetes. For research and therapeutic purposes, and for maintaining consistency in reporting hypoglycaemia in children, it is defined as a blood glucose concentration of ≤3.9 mmol/l [18], and this level is the recommended lower target in children and adolescents with insulin-treated diabetes. Symptoms of hypoglycaemia are similar in both adults and children, though behavioural symptoms are more common in children [19].

Treatment of hypoglycaemia should be provided promptly and should provide immediate oral, rapidly absorbed, simple carbohydrate calculated to raise blood glucose level to 5.6 mmol/l. Glucose is the preferred treatment for hypoglycaemia as it does not require digestion or metabolism, 1g oral glucose will raise blood glucose by approximately 0.17 mmol/l [20]). All children and adolescents with diabetes are advised to carry glucose tablets or readily absorbed carbohydrate on their person and have glucagon injections available at home.

Treatment of mild to moderate hypoglycaemia (blood glucose 3.5–3.9 mmol/l):

(1) It is advisable to confirm hypoglycaemia by testing capillary blood glucose concentrations before treating, if feasible

(2) The 'rule of thumb' is to use one glucose tablet (containing 3–4 g carbohydrate) per 10 kg body weight, this amount has been shown to increase blood glucose concentrations by approximately 3–4 mmol/l [21]. Approximately 10 g of carbohydrate is needed for a 30 kg child, 15 g for a 40 kg child and 20 g for adolescents and adults, half of these amounts will raise blood glucose concentrations by 2 mmol/l. Fast-acting glucose in the form of glucose tablets or glucose drinks is usually recommended, although there is evidence that sucrose in the form of boiled or fruit sweets is as effective in children [22]. Food and drinks containing fat (e.g. chocolate, milk, biscuits or milk shakes) should be avoided for initial treatment as they delay gastric emptying and the subsequent rise in blood glucose [18].

(3) Following initial oral treatment, it is advised to wait for 10–15 minutes, and then retest blood glucose concentrations. If blood glucose values have not risen to >5.0 mmol/l, oral intake should be repeated. A further test after 20–30 minutes is recommended in order to confirm that target glucose levels have been achieved.

(4) For initially lower glucose values, as symptoms improve, the next meal or snack may be ingested to prevent recurrence of hypoglycaemia, although not all hypoglycaemic episodes will require a starchy snack following resolution [20].

Treatment of severe hypoglycaemia:

Urgent treatment is required for severe hypoglycaemia associated with deterioration of consciousness, vomiting or convulsions. It is recommended that an immediate injection of glucagon is administered at the dose of 0.5 mg for age <8 years, 1.0 mg for ages >8 years (10–30 mcg/kg body weight) and this should be given either intramuscularly or subcutaneously [19]. Once the child has regained consciousness, they will require treatment with oral glucose to replenish liver stores. If there is no response to glucagaon, it is recommended the child is taken immediately to hospital.

Hyperglycaemia and diabetic ketoacidosis

Blood glucose concentrations above target (>7 mmol/l fasting, >11 mmol/l post-prandial) are caused by a variety of factors, including a missed or inadequate insulin dose, over-consumption of carbohydrate, over-treating a hypoglycaemic episode, stress or if a child becomes ill. Many illnesses and infections are accompanied by increased production of stress hormones, especially cortisol, and this decreases insulin sensitivity and increases blood glucose concentrations by promoting gluconeogenesis in the liver [23]. This insulin resistance and increased blood glucose concentrations lead to a relative lack of insulin and ketone body production that can result in DKA.

The principles of management of intercurrent illness, with and without the presence of ketones, are often called 'sick day rules' and are designed to maintain blood glucose concentrations as near to normal as possible during illness. The following summarises sick day rules [24]:

• Insulin administration should be maintained, even if the child is not eating. Additional rapid-acting insulin may be given as a correction dose if blood glucose concentrations are above target and blood ketones concentration are low (<0.5 mmol/l). Algorithms have been designed to support this decision making [25].

• Blood glucose concentrations should be checked frequently, and at two-hourly intervals

if blood ketones are moderate (>0.6 mmol) or high (>3 mmol). Additional rapid-acting insulin will be required, and algorithms are available for guidance [25].
• Re-hydration is critical, and the child should be advised to drink plenty of water or sugar-free fluids.

Diabetic ketoacidosis

Diabetic ketoacidosis is a medical emergency. The condition can occur with absolute or relative insulin deficiency in children during initial presentation, with 30% of all newly diagnosed children presenting with DKA. DKA can also occur during illness, during the pubertal growth spurt, in those who omit insulin, those with limited access to medical care and those using CSII therapy.

Principles of management include [26]:

• Emergency clinical evaluation to confirm diagnosis, to assess the degree of dehydration and level of consciousness
• Biochemical assessment including blood gas, blood glucose and ketones, electrolytes and infection markers
• Admittance to a unit with experienced nursing staff, written DKA guidelines and easy access to the laboratory services
• Goals of therapy include correcting dehydration and acidosis; restoring fluid volume and blood glucose avoiding the complications of the therapy. Fluid resuscitation and maintenance using isotonic saline along with low dose insulin therapy (0.1 unit/kg/h) is the mainstay of treatment [27]. Delaying the insulin infusion by one hour after starting the fluids, together with electrolyte and blood ketone monitoring, seems to reduce the incidence of cerebral oedema.

6.2.4 Insulin pump therapy

Continuous subcutaneous insulin infusion (CSII) is arguably the most physiological method of intensive insulin therapy available at present, allowing continual delivery of short or rapid-acting basal insulin with additional boluses with meals. There is evidence to show that CSII can reduce severe hypoglycaemia, marginally improve HbA1c, reduce glycaemic variability, reduce acute complications and improve quality of life in children [28,29]. Increasingly CSII is used as the first-line therapy for diabetes in pre-school children [30].

However CSII is still an expensive mode of insulin delivery and patient selection is variable across the world. A 'common sense' approach is recommended, particularly because CSII eligibility in children depends not only on a patient's capabilities, but also, to a large extent, on the child's family's psychological competence [28].

Structured education

Appropriate education, delivered by an experienced specialist diabetes team, to the child, family and caregivers at school or nursery is the cornerstone for starting any young person on CSII. The health care team's initial task is to assess the young person's and parent's level of expertise in the basics of diabetes management, including carbohydrate counting skills. An education and training plan can be designed to address any gaps in knowledge and to provide information about the use of an insulin pump, adjusting basal rates and boluses, together with trouble shooting. Young age (<12 years), frequent blood glucose monitoring and lower HbA1c at pump initiation have been identified as predictors of achieving glycaemic targets with CSII [28].

Basal rates and insulin delivery

If the child has reasonable glycaemic control on MDI, a reduction in the total daily dose (TDD) for CSII is recommended for children as in adults. Reduction of 10–15% is usually recommended for toddlers and preschoolers, and 15–20% reduction is required for adolescents, due to insulin resistance associated with puberty [28]. Between 40–50% of the calculated dose is administered as a basal dose and this is delivered by changeable rate according to circadian rhythms by age.

A recent large observational study has shown less prominent dawn phenomenon with marked dusk phenomenon for preschool-age children on CSII, while adolescents show typical dual rate requirement with both marked dawn and dusk phenomenon with relative increase in basal rates early morning and late afternoon [31]. Basal rates often vary during the week with changes in activity levels, and most school-age children have separate basal rate profiles for weekdays and the weekend.

Guidelines for management of hypoglycaemia for young people using CSII are similar to those treated by MDI, and it is important to find the cause for hypoglycaemia to prevent further episodes. CSII therapy offers more flexibility for treatment of hypoglycaemia as suspension of insulin delivery is an option. For example, if the blood glucose concentrations remain <4 mmol/l after two administrations of 5–15 g carbohydrate, it is appropriate to stop the pump until blood glucose rises above 4 mmol/l.

Sick days for young people on CSII can be managed more effectively by increasing basal rates by 20–50% throughout the day, and utilising meal and correction boluses as appropriate. It is essential to monitor blood glucose and blood ketones concentrations frequently and to seek professional help as soon as possible if the child is unwell and DKA is suspected or fluid intake is compromised.

Continuous glucose monitoring and closed loop systems

Standard use of glucose meters for self-monitoring provides single blood glucose levels, without giving the 'whole picture' of glucose variability during a 24 hour period, and especially during the night when blood glucose levels are seldom measured and there may be an increased risk of hypoglycaemia. The use of a device such as real-time continuous glucose monitoring (RT-CGM) can help optimise glycaemic control. RT-CGM utilises a glucose sensor worn under the skin (independent of the pump) and communicates with the pump or a separate device to alert the wearer to trends in blood glucose concentrations. At present, users must still manually adjust the pump insulin doses via the pump and use self blood glucose monitoring for calibration, although automatic closed loop systems or the 'artificial pancreas' are in development [33]. The Star 3 study of 485 patients (156 of which were children) with type 1 diabetes showed the benefit of sensor-augmented pump therapy, with a reduction in HbA1c of 5 mmol/mol (0.5%) in the intervention group, and significantly more children in this group achieving target HbA1c levels at one year [32]. Most paediatric patients with type 1 diabetes are potential candidates for the use of RT-CGM, although issues with resources mean that this technology is unavailable to many.

6.2.5 Type 2 diabetes

Type 2 diabetes was almost unknown in children and adolescents until recently, and is strongly associated with obesity [34]. Global prevalence rates vary and range from 0 to 5.3%, with the highest prevalence reported in Pima Indians in the United States (US), and the lowest rates among white Caucasian populations [35].

Young people with type 2 diabetes have an increased risk of developing both micro and macrovascular complications [36]. The aims of clinical treatment include weight loss, increased physical activity, reducing glycaemia to normal levels and treating co-morbidities including hypertension, dyslipidaemia, retinopathy and nephropathy [37]. The emphasis for treatment is on lifestyle change, especially for treating comorbidities such as hypertension and dyslipidaemia, although pharmaceutical therapy may well be required [38]. Management of glycaemia is particularly challenging, with a recent study reporting that monotherapy with metformin was effective in only 50% of a sample of 699 young people with type 2 diabetes, and that it is likely that most young people will require combination therapy or insulin treatment within a few years after diagnosis [39].

Key points

- Children with type 1 diabetes are treated with insulin, administered by injection or by an insulin pump.
- The aim of treatment is to maintain blood glucose levels as close to the normal range as possible to minimise the risk of long-term tissue damage.
- Hypoglycaemia is common in children and adolescents.
- Diabetic ketoacidosis may occur and should be treated as a medical emergency.
- Type 2 diabetes in children is managed by lifestyle and medication.

References

1. International Diabetes Federation. Incidence of diabetes. *Diabetes Atlas*. Brussels, Belgium: IDF, 2012.
2. Diabetes Control and Complications Trial Research Group (DCCT). The effect of intensive treatment of diabetes on the development and progression of long-term complications in insulin dependent diabetes. *New Eng J Med* 1993; **329**: 977–986.
3. DCCT. Effect of intensive diabetes treatment on the development and progression of long-term complications in adolescents with insulin-dependent diabetes mellitus: Diabetes Control and Complications Trial. Diabetes Control and Complications Trial Research Group. *J Pediatr* 1994; **125**: 177–188.
4. White NH, Cleary PA, Dahms W, Goldstein D, Malone J, Tamborlane WV; Diabetes Control and Complications Trial (DCCT)/Epidemiology of Diabetes Interventions and Complications (EDIC) Research Group. Beneficial effects of intensive therapy of diabetes during adolescence: outcomes after the conclusion of the Diabetes Control and Complications Trial (DCCT). *J Pediatr* 2001; **139**: 804–812.
5. Silverstein J, Klingensmith G, Copeland K, Plotnick L, Kaufman F, Laffel L, et al.; American Diabetes Association. Care of children and adolescents with type 1 diabetes: a statement of the American Diabetes Association. *Diabetes Care* 2005; **28**: 186–212.
6. Donaghue KC, Chiarelli F, Trotta D, Allgrove J, Dahl-Jorgensen K. Microvascular and macrovascular complications associated with diabetes in children and adolescents. *Pediatr Diabetes* 2009; **10**(Suppl. 12): 195–203.
7. Ryan C. Does severe hypoglycaemia disrupt academic achievement in children with early onset diabetes? *Dev Med Child Neurol* 2012; **54**(5): 393–394.
8. Hannonen R, Tupola S, Ahonen T, Riikonen R. Neurocognitive functioning in children with type-1 diabetes with and without episodes of severe hypoglycaemia. *Dev Med Child Neurol* 2003; **45**(4): 262–268.
9. Rovet JF, Ehrlich RM. The effect of hypoglycemic seizures on cognitive function in children with diabetes: a 7-year prospective study. *J Pediatr* 1999; **134**(4): 503–506.
10. International Diabetes Federation. Global IDF/ISPAD guideline for diabetes in childhood and adolescence. Brussels, Belgium: IDF/ISPAD, 2011.
11. Bangstad HJ, Danne T, Deeb L, Jarosz-Chobot P, Urakami T, Hanas R. Insulin treatment in children and adolescents with diabetes. *Pediatr Diabetes* 2009; **10**(Suppl. 12): 82–99.
12. Ford-Adams ME, Murphy NP, Moore EJ, Edge JA, Ong KL, Watts AP, et al. Insulin lispro: a potential role in preventing nocturnal hypoglycaemia in young children with diabetes mellitus. *Diabet Med* 2003; **20**: 656–660.
13. Galli-Tsinopoulu A, Stergidou D. Insulin analogues for type 1 diabetes in children and adolescents. *Drugs Today (Barc)* 2012; **48**(12): 795–809.
14. Plotnick LP, Clark LM, Brancati FL, Erlinger T. Safety and effectiveness of insulin pump therapy in children and adolescents with type 1 diabetes. *Diabetes Care* 2003; **26**: 1142–1146.
15. Miles HL, Acerini CL. Insulin analog preparations and their use in children and adolescents with type 1 diabetes mellitus. *Paediatr Drugs* 2008; **10**(3): 163–176.
16. Bangstad HJ, Danne T, Deeb LC, Jarosz-Chobot P, Urakami T, Hanas R. Global IDF/ISPAD Guidelines for diabetes in childhood and adolescence. Insulin treatment. Brussels, Belgium: IDF/ISPAD, 2011.
17. Hofman PL, Derraik JG, Pinto TE, Tregurtha S, Faherty A, Peart JM, et al. Defining the ideal injection techniques when using 5-mm needles in children and adults. *Diabetes Care* 2010; **33**(9): 1940–1944.
18. Clarke W, Jones T, Rewers A, Dunger D, Maahs DM, Klingensmith GJ. Global IDF/ISPAD Guidelines for diabetes in childhood and adolescence. Assessment and monitoring of hypoglycaemia. Brussels, Belgium: IDF/ISPAD, 2011.
19. Clarke W, Jones T, Rewers A, Dunger D, Maahs DM, Klingensmith GJ. Assessment and management of hypoglycemia in children and adolescents with diabetes. *Pediatr Diabetes* 2009; **10**(Suppl. 12): 134–145.
20. Wiethop BV, Cryer PE. Alanine and terbutaline in treatment of hypoglycaemia in IDDM. *Diabetes Care* 1993; **16**: 1131–1136.
21. Brodows RG, Williams C, Amatruda JM. Treatment of insulin reactions in diabetics. *JAMA* 1984; **252**: 3378–3381.
22. Husband AC, Crawford S, McCoy LA, Pacaud D. The effectiveness of glucose, sucrose, and fructose in

treating hypoglycemia in children with type 1 diabetes. *Pediatr Diabetes* 2010; **11**(3): 154–158.

23. Laffel L. Sick day management in type 1 diabetes. *Endocrinol Metab Clin North Am* 2000; **29**: 707–723.

24. Brink S, Laffel L, Likitmaskul S, Liu L, Maguire AM, Olsen B, et al. Sick day management in children and adolescents with diabetes. *Pediatr Diabetes* 2009; **10**(Suppl 12): 146–153.

25. Brink S, Laffel L, Likitmaskul S, Liu L, Maguire AM, Olsen B, et al. Global IDF/ISPAD Guidelines for diabetes in childhood and adolescence. Sick day management. Brussels, Belgium: IDF/ISPAD, 2011.

26. Wolsdorf J, Craig M, Daneman D, Dunger D, Edge J, Lee W, et al. Global IDF/ISPAD Guidelines for diabetes in childhood and adolescence. Diabetic ketoacidosis. Brussels, Belgium: IDF/ISPAD, 2011.

27. Dunger DB, Sperling MA, Acerini CL, Bohn DJ, Daneman D, Danne TP, et al.; ESPE; LWPES. ESPE/LWPES consensus statement on diabetic ketoacidosis in children and adolescents. *Arch Dis Child* 2004; **89**(2): 188–194.

28. Phillip M, Battelino T, Rodriguez H, Danne T, Kaufman F; European Society for Paediatric Endocrinology; Lawson Wilkins Pediatric Endocrine Society; International Society for Pediatric and Adolescent Diabetes; American Diabetes Association; European Association for the Study of Diabetes. Use of insulin pump therapy in the pediatric age-group: consensus statement from the European Society for Paediatric Endocrinology, the Lawson Wilkins Pediatric Endocrine Society, and the International Society for Pediatric and Adolescent Diabetes, endorsed by the American Diabetes Association and the European Association for the Study of Diabetes. *Diabetes Care* 2007; **30**: 1653–1662.

29. Danne T, Battelino T, Jarosz-Chobot P, Kordonouri O, Pánkowska E, Ludvigsson J, et al.; PedPump Study Group. Establishing glycaemic control with continuous subcutaneous insulin infusion in children and adolescents with type 1 diabetes: experience of the PedPump Study in 17 countries. *Diabetologia.* 2008; **51**(9): 1594–1601.

30. Levy-Shraga Y, Lerner-Geva L, Modan-Moses D, Graph-Barel C, Mazor-Aronovitch K, Boyko V, et al. Benefits of continuous subcutaneous insulin infusion (CSII) therapy in preschool children. *Exp Clin Endocrinol Diabetes* 2013; **121**(4): 225–229.

31. Bachran R, Beyer P, Klinkert C, Heidtmann B, Rosenbauer J, Holl RW; German/Austrian DPV Initiative; German Pediatric CSII Working Group; BMBF Competence Network Diabetes. Basal rates and circadian profiles in continuous subcutaneous insulin infusion (CSII) differ for preschool children, prepubertal children, adolescents and young adults. *Pediatr Diabetes* 2012; **13**(1): 1–5.

32. Bergenstal RM, Tamborlane WV, Ahmann A, Buse JB, Dailey G, Davis SN, et al.; STAR 3 Study Group. Effectiveness of sensor-augmented insulin-pump therapy in type 1 diabetes. *N Engl J Med* 2010; **363**(4): 311–320.

33. Thabit H, Hovorka R. Closed-loop insulin delivery in type 1 diabetes. *Endocrinol Metab Clin North Am* 2012; **41**(1): 105–117.

34. Pinhas-Hamiel O, Zeitler P. The global spread of type 2 diabetes mellitus in children and adolescents. *J Pediatr* 2005; **146**: 693–700.

35. Fazeli Farsani S, van der Aa MP, van der Vorst MM, Knibbe CA, de Boer A. Global trends in the incidence and prevalence of type 2 diabetes in children and adolescents: a systematic review and evaluation of methodological approaches. *Diabetologia* 2013; **56**(7): 1471–1488.

36. Eppens MC, Craig ME, Cusumano J, Hing S, Chan AK, Howard NJ, et al. Prevalence of diabetes complications in adolescents with type 2 compared with type 1 diabetes. *Diabetes Care* 2006; **29**(6): 1300–1306.

37. Rosenbloom A, Silverstein JH, Amemiya S, Zeitler P, Maahs DM, Klingensmith GJ. Global IDF/ISPAD Guidelines for diabetes in childhood and adolescence. Type 2 diabetes. Brussels, Belgium: IDF/ISPAD, 2011.

38. Springer SC, Silverstein J, Copeland K, Moore KR, Prazar GE, Raymer T, et al. American Academy of Pediatrics. Management of type 2 diabetes in children and adolescents. *Pediatrics* 2013; **131**(2): e648–e664.

39. TODAY Study Group, Zeitler P, Hirst K, Pyle L, Linder B, Copeland K, Arslanian S, et al. A clinical trial to maintain glycemic control in youth with type 2 diabetes. *N Engl J Med* 2012; **366**(24): 2247–2256.

Chapter 6.3

Lifestyle management of childhood diabetes

Francesca Annan

Alder Hey Children's NHS Foundation Trust, Liverpool, UK

6.3.1 Introduction

National and international guidelines [1–4] on the management of childhood diabetes, nutrition and lifestyle are available to inform clinical practice. Diet and lifestyle management are integral parts of diabetes care and are concerned with ensuring normal growth and development, delivering improved glycaemic control and reducing the risk of long-term complications. The delivery of management advice will depend on the availability and choice of treatment regimen.

The 2009 International Society for Paediatric and Adolescent Diabetes (ISPAD) Clinical Practice Consensus guidelines [5] describe nutrition and exercise as key components of diabetes management, together with insulin therapy. Skinner and Cameron also acknowledge the importance of psychosocial aspects of diabetes management required to achieve good glycaemic control [6,7]. Paediatric diabetes management has a limited evidence base to support the efficacy of diet, lifestyle and education methods on outcomes. Self-management education and advice should therefore be flexible, adapted to the individual and designed to promote the best possible outcome.

6.3.2 Type 1 diabetes

The management aims for type 1 diabetes, adapted from the ISPAD guidelines [2], are summarised in Box 6.3.1. Nutrition and lifestyle

---

Box 6.3.1 Type 1 diabetes management guidelines for children

- Promote normal growth and development, avoiding overweight and obesity
- Establish healthy lifelong eating habits, preserving social, cultural and psychological wellbeing
- Prevent and treat acute complications
- Reduce the risk of long term micro- and macro-vascular complications.

Source: ISPAD Guidelines, 2009 [2]

---

advice have key roles to play in achieving health and well-being, normal growth and development and glycaemic control [8]. The delivery of education should recognise the other psychosocial and cultural factors that will influence adherence to advice. The SEARCH for diabetes in youth research group have demonstrated that a large proportion of young people with type 1 and 2 diabetes do not adhere to dietary guidelines, and factors such as diabetes self-management skills, parental education, parental support and involvement and physical activity factors all impact on dietary behaviours [9,10].

Composition of the diet and education methods

Recommendations regarding dietary composition do not differ from the non-diabetic population. Teaching strategies for achieving a healthy diet in childhood include use of tools developed

---

Advanced Nutrition and Dietetics in Diabetes, First Edition. Edited by Louise Goff and Pamela Dyson.
© 2016 John Wiley & Sons, Ltd. Published 2016 by John Wiley & Sons, Ltd.

for education of populations about healthy food choices, for example, food pyramids and food plates. The use of these tools with children and adolescents with type 1 diabetes has not been evaluated in large-scale studies but is generally recommended for providing nutrition and health education [5].

Dietary choices in children and adolescents with type 1 diabetes in developed countries have been shown to be less healthy than those of non-diabetic peers; data from reviews in Western populations suggest that children and adolescents with type 1 diabetes consume more saturated fat and less carbohydrate than their peers [11,12]. This may be a result of the focus on carbohydrate education to achieve glycaemic control.

The results from the Diabetes Complication and Control Trial (DCCT) prompted a move towards intensive therapy in the paediatric population [13]. The focus of intensive therapy often relates purely to the number of injections or insulin pump therapy and has not replicated the level of input and psychosocial support to children and adolescents. The number of injections or insulin pump therapy alone has not been shown to improve glycaemic control [14]. Much of the focus of education in the paediatric population is on carbohydrate counting and insulin adjustment skills. Studies investigating psychosocial elements of diabetes education may guide delivery of education to support families to achieve improved glycaemic control [15,16].

Carbohydrate management

Current guidelines recommend treatment strategies which focus on flexible methods of managing diabetes that allow adaptation to a child or young person's lifestyle using insulin to carbohydrate ratios and carbohydrate counting [17]. Evaluation of carbohydrate counting skills is restricted to small pilot studies [18–20], which limits the conclusions that can be drawn and findings to date are somewhat contradictory. However, there is limited evidence to support the argument that consistent and accurate estimation of the carbohydrate content of food is associated with better glycaemic control. Initial data from the pilot study looking at an adapted version of the Dose

Adjustment for Normal Eating (DAFNE) programme for adolescents did not demonstrate improvements in glycaemic control [21]. Further evaluation of carbohydrate counting and insulin adjustment skills in children and adolescents is needed. Carbohydrate counting and insulin adjustment require families and patients to calculate insulin doses based on carbohydrate, blood glucose and activity. This may be a difficult process for some and consideration should be given to use of technology to support calculations through the use of bolus advice [22,23].

Educating children and adolescents about carbohydrate intake should include advice about timing and delivery of insulin in relation to the food consumed. Ideally fast-acting insulin should be delivered prior to eating [24,25]. Patients using insulin pump therapy are able to match delivery of insulin to meal composition. A small study from Pankowska [26] suggests that protein and fat content of a meal can be used to establish both the insulin requirement and duration of bolus delivery. For those using pump therapy, some small studies have investigated the use of different bolus delivery options (square or extended bolus and dual wave bolus) to improve post-prandial glucose control [27]. These have considered the role of fat and protein on the glucose response to the meal or glycaemic index. Fat digestion produces fatty acids and triglycerides and then glycerol, whilst protein digestion produces amino acids. Gluconeogenesis, which occurs in the liver in the presence of low insulin and raised glucagon concentration, creates glucose from precursors including glycerol and amino acids. However, studies using the Pankowska formula (which calculates additional does of insulin for fat and protein intake) report increased frequency of night time hypoglycaemia. Using the concept of glycaemic index to inform bolus choice [28] has demonstrated improved post-prandial control without the later increase in hypoglycaemia, as additional insulin is not calculated [28]. This is an area that requires further investigation to establish how dietary education may need to evolve to allow adjustments in insulin dose calculation and bolus delivery according to meal composition with insulin pump therapy.

Fat and protein

Current management recommendations consider protein and fat in terms of their impact on long-term health and prevention of macrovascular complications, rather than effects on glycaemic control. Protein intake during adolescence should support pubertal growth and decline to adult recommendations once growth is complete (0.8–1 g/kg body weight). Adjustments to protein intake in the presence of microalbuminuria in the adolescent population have not been fully investigated.

Total fat intake should meet population recommendations for reducing cardiovascular risk. There are no differences in the recommendations about type of fat from those made for the general paediatric population, saturated and trans-fat should be limited to less than 10% dietary energy, saturated fats can be replaced with monounsaturated fats [5].

Evidence of dyslipidaemia in adolescents from Europe, North America and United Kingdom (UK) highlights the need to ensure dietary education is not limited to carbohydrate and insulin adjustment [29–32]. A recent trial of the Dietary Approaches to Stop Hypertension (DASH) diet in youth with diabetes has been shown to be associated with a reduction in cardiovascular risk factors. Patients with type 1 diabetes, with a higher adherence score for the DASH diet had lower LDL/HDL ratio and better glycaemic control [33]. A small Italian study also suggests that lower saturated fat intakes are associated with improved glycaemic control in children with diabetes [34].

Obesity and physical activity

Promotion of a healthy lifestyle to reduce cardiovascular risk factors, including overweight and obesity, is recommended for all children. Children with diabetes have been shown to be heavier than their non-diabetic peers [35]. Lifestyle management includes the promotion of physical activity for weight management and improvements in cardiovascular risk factors. The World Health Organisation (WHO) physical activity recommendation for all children are for 60 minutes of daily moderate to vigorous physical activity [36], varying with age from play through to formal exercise. Levels of physical activity often decline with age. Studies on patterns of physical activity in diabetes show similar declines in activity that relate to age and gender as well as increased sedentary behaviours [37–39]. Levels of television viewing in a type 1 diabetes population from Norway correlated with low physical activity and overweight and obesity [40]. Data from a study of over 23 000 patients attending 209 centres in Germany and Austria examined lipid profiles, blood pressure, glycated haemoglobin and body mass index and compared them to levels of physical activity assessed by questionnaire [41,42]. Increased frequency of physical activity was associated with a lower frequency of dyslipidaemia (41% in the inactive group, 34% in the most active group) as well as lower glycated haemoglobin in the patient group with highest physical activity levels. The positive impact of exercise on glycaemic control is not demonstrated in other studies [43]. This failure to observe improvements in glycaemic control is usually accounted for by the difficulties experienced in managing exercise and the use of inappropriate management strategies to control glucose excursions during exercise.

Physical activity and exercise management

All physical activity has the potential to disrupt glucose metabolism. The metabolic consequences of exercise vary with type, intensity and duration of exercise, blood glucose and insulin concentrations and diet [44].

Education for children and young people with type 1 diabetes needs to include strategies to achieve glycaemic control during and after exercise. The DirecNet [45] group have examined the impact of exercise on overnight glycaemia, demonstrating that despite the use of American Diabetes Association recommendations on prevention of hypoglycaemia, 11 out of 50 patients developed hypoglycaemia during exercise and mean blood glucose concentrations at night were lower on exercise nights. The spontaneous nature of play in younger children makes this type of planned management difficult to implement, and therefore

Table 6.3.1 Summary of strategies to support exercise management in children with type 1 diabetes

Activity	Management advice
Exercise within peak insulin action	Check blood glucose concentration before, during and after activity. If blood glucose below 4 mmol/L, treat hypoglycaemia and delay exercise until blood glucose concentration normalises. If blood glucose concentration > 10 mmol/L delay carbohydrate intake until 20minutes into activity. If blood glucose concentration >15 mmol/L check for ketones and manage before exercise commences. Consider decreasing pre-exercise insulin food bolus by up to 50%. If exercise is aerobic or duration greater than 45 minutes then consume carbohydrate (1 g/kg/h) at 20 minute intervals to maintain blood glucose concentration. Consume adequate fluids.
Anaerobic activities e.g. basketball, athletic field events, sprint events	Check blood glucose concentration before, during and after to assess responses to exercise. If activity lasts longer than 45 minutes consume carbohydrate during exercise. Consume meal or snack within 1 hour of finishing exercise to reduce the risk of post-exercise hypoglycaemia.
Aerobic activities	Consume additional carbohydrate and/or adjust insulin dose when exercise lasts 45 minutes or longer.
Team sports	Monitor blood glucose concentration before, during and after activity. If within peak action of insulin consider reducing insulin doses Consume snack and fluid at half time, if competition stress increases blood glucose concentration consider small corrective dose of insulin.
Post-exercise	Consume carbohydrate snack or meal with fluids after exercise. If blood glucose concentration raised post exercise treat with caution. Consume pre-bedtime snack whenever exercise duration is 60 minutes or longer.

education for parents needs to include the management of spontaneous activity as well as the prevention of post-exercise hypoglycaemia. A detailed review of the management of exercise can be found in the ISPAD consensus guidelines 2009 [46]. A summary of strategies that may be used for planned regular activity can be found in Table 6.3.1.

6.3.3 Type 2 diabetes

Type 2 diabetes presenting in childhood has increased in prevalence over the last 10 years. The numbers of patients remain small and the majority of evidence about management in this group of patients comes from the SEARCH for diabetes in youth trial in the United States [47]. Most of the children presenting with type 2 diabetes are overweight or obese and therefore weight management and prevention of comorbidities are the main aims of nutritional advice [5,48] as two key risk factors are dyslipidaemia and hypertension [33,49]. A systematic review by Johnston et al. in 2010 found no high quality evidence to support lifestyle modification in children and adolescents improving either short- or long-term glycaemic control. In a study of 320 youths with type 2 diabetes, adherence to the DASH dietary intervention was associated with lower BMI and LDL concentration but not improved glycaemic control. Examples of modifications needed include increased physical activity levels, decrease in sedentary activities, for example TV watching and reduction in consumption of sugar-sweetened beverages [50]. The Treatment Options for Type 2 Diabetes in Adolescents and Youth (TODAY) study has reported improvements in glycaemic control with metformin monotherapy, although lifestyle intervention plus metformin was not significantly better than metformin alone [51]. Education and support to engage families in lifestyle changes and parental involvement in management has been shown to predict better outcomes [52].

Eating disorders and disordered eating

Type 1 diabetes management provides opportunities for manipulation of treatment to control body weight [53]. There is some controversy about the prevalence of eating disorders, with some studies reporting that they do not occur more commonly in adolescents with diabetes [54–56], and others suggesting anorexia nervosa and bulimia are 2.4 times more common in teenage girls with type 1 diabetes [57] Insulin omission is common, in one study, 30–40% of a young female population with type 1 diabetes reported deliberately omitting their insulin [58]. The most frequently cited reason for deliberate insulin omission in this group is body image and weight control [55]. Disturbed eating behaviours significantly affect the physical and emotional health of the individuals concerned and are associated with impaired metabolic control, diabetic ketoacidosis and a high risk of diabetic complications [59].

Management of diabetes needs to include assessment of insulin regimen, insulin omission, food manipulation, body dissatisfaction and family functioning to identify those at risk [60–62].

6.3.4 Summary

Nutritional management of diabetes in children and adolescents is delivered as part of a package of care that must be set within the context of the family and social support systems. Good nutrition

and lifestyle behaviours are important for normal growth and development as well as improved glycaemic control. Further research is needed to guide how best to deliver nutritional care. Studies currently taking place will help us to understand how to deliver effective nutritional management to children and carers throughout their diabetes journey.

Key points

- Dietary advice aims to promote normal growth and development and avoid overweight and obesity.
- There is no evidence for the ideal macronutrient composition of the diet, but carbohydrate management is key to glycaemic control.
- Physical activity is recommended, but children with type 1 need strategies to reduce the risk of hypoglycaemia.
- Weight management is key for those with type 2 diabetes who are overweight or obese.
- Disordered eating and insulin omission is common in young people with type 1 diabetes.

References

1. Craig ME, Twigg SM, Donaghue KC, Cheung NW, Cameron FW, Conn J, et al for the Australian Type 1 Diabetes Guidlines Expert Advisory Group. National evidence-based clinical care guidelines for type 1 diabetes in children, adolescents and adults. Canberra: Australian Government Department of Health and Ageing, 2011.
2. Hanas R, Donaghue KC, Klingensmith G, Swift PGF. (Eds). ISPAD clinical consensus practice guidelines. *Pediatr Diabetes* 2009; **10**(Suppl. 12): 1–2.
3. NICE. Type 1 Diabetes:Diagnosis and management of type 1 diabetes in children, young people and adults. London: National Institute of Clinical Excellence, 2004.
4. American Diabetes Association position statement: evidence-based nutrition principles and recommendations for the treatment and prevention of diabetes and related complications. *J Am Diet Assoc* 2002; **102**(1): 109–118.
5. Smart C, Aslander-van Vliet E, Waldron S. Nutritional management in children and adolescents with diabetes. *Pediatr Diabetes* 2009; **10**(Suppl. 12): 100–117.
6. Skinner TC, Cameron FJ. Improving glycaemic control in children and adolescents: which aspects of therapy really matter? *Diabet Med* 2010; **27**(4): 369–375.

7. Cameron FJ, Skinner TC, de Beaufort CE, Hoey H, Swift PGF, Aanstoot H, et al. Are family factors universally related to metabolic outcomes in adolescents with Type 1 diabetes? *Diabet Med* 2008; **25**(4): 463–468.

8. Mehta SN, Volkening LK, Anderson BJ, Nansel T, Weissberg-Benchell J, Wysocki T, et al. Dietary behaviors predict glycemic control in youth with type 1 diabetes. *Diabetes Care* 2008; **31**(7): 1318–1320.

9. Bortsov A, Liese AD, Bell RA, Dabelea D, D'Agostino RB, Jr, Hamman RF, et al. Correlates of dietary intake in youth with diabetes: results from the SEARCH for diabetes in youth study. *J Nutr Educ Behav* 2011; **43**(2): 123–129.

10. Patton SR, Dolan LM, Powers SW. Dietary adherence and associated glycemic control in families of young children with type 1 diabetes. *J Am Diet Assoc* 2007; **107**(1): 46–52.

11. Mehta SN, Haynie DL, Higgins LA, Bucey NN, Rovner AJ, Volkening LK, et al. Emphasis on carbohydrates may negatively influence dietary patterns in youth with type 1 diabetes. *Diabetes Care* 2009; **32**(12): 2174–2176.

12. Rovner AJ, Nansel TR. Are children with type 1 diabetes consuming a healthful diet? A review of the current evidence and strategies for dietary change. *Diabetes Educ* 2009; **35**(1): 97–107.

13. DCCT. Effect of intensive diabetes treatment on the development and progression of long-term complications in adolescents with insulin-dependent diabetes mellitus: Diabetes Control and Complications Trial. Diabetes Control and Complications Trial Research Group. *J Pediatr* 1994; **125**(2): 177–188.

14. de Beaufort CE, Swift PGF, Skinner CT, Aanstoot HJ, Aman J, Cameron F, et al. Continuing stability of center differences in pediatric diabetes care: do advances in diabetes treatment improve outcome? The Hvidoere Study Group on Childhood Diabetes. *Diabetes Care* 2007; **30**(9): 2245–2250.

15. Murphy HR, Wadham C, Rayman G, Skinner TC. Approaches to integrating paediatric diabetes care and structured education: experiences from the Families, Adolescents, and Children's Teamwork Study (FACTS). *Diabet Med* 2007; **24**(11): 1261–1268.

16. Christie D, Strange V, Allen E, Oliver S, Wong ICK, Smith F, et al. Maximising engagement, motivation and long term change in a Structured Intensive Education Programme in Diabetes for children, young people and their families: Child and Adolescent Structured Competencies Approach to Diabetes Education (CASCADE). *BMC Pediatr* 2009; **9**: 57.

17. Kawamura T. The importance of carbohydrate counting in the treatment of children with diabetes. *Pediatr Diabetes* 2007; **8**(Suppl. 6): 57–62.

18. Smart CE, Ross K, Edge JA, Collins CE, Colyvas K, King BR. Children and adolescents on intensive insulin therapy maintain postprandial glycaemic control without precise carbohydrate counting. *Diabet Med* 2009; **26**(3): 279–285.

19. Mehta SN, Quinn N, Volkening LK, Laffel LMB. Impact of carbohydrate counting on glycemic control in children with type 1 diabetes. *Diabetes Care* 2009; **32**(6): 1014–1016.

20. Smart CE, Ross K, Edge JA, King BR, McElduff P, Collins CE. Can children with Type 1 diabetes and their caregivers estimate the carbohydrate content of meals and snacks? *Diabet Med* 2010; **27**(3): 348–353.

21. Waller H, Eiser C, Knowles J, Rogers N, Wharmby S, Heller S, et al. Pilot study of a novel educational programme for 11–16 year olds with type 1 diabetes mellitus: the KICk-OFF course. *Arch Dis Child* 2008; **93**(11): 927–931.

22. Anderson DG. Multiple daily injections in young patients using the ezy-BICC bolus insulin calculation card, compared to mixed insulin and CSII. *Pediatr Diabetes* 2009; **10**(5): 304–309.

23. Hassan K, Heptulla RA. Glycemic control in pediatric type 1 diabetes: role of caregiver literacy. *Pediatrics* 2010; **125**(5): e1104–e1108.

24. Scaramuzza AE, Iafusco D, Santoro L, Bosetti A, De Palma A, Spiri D, et al. Timing of bolus in children with type 1 diabetes using continuous subcutaneous insulin infusion (TiBoDi Study). *Diabetes Technol Ther* 2010; **12**(2): 149–152.

25. Luijf YM, van Bon A,C., Hoekstra JB, Devries JH. Premeal injection of rapid-acting insulin reduces postprandial glycemic excursions in type 1 diabetes. *Diabetes Care* 2010; **33**(10): 2152–2155.

26. Pańkowska E, Szypowska A, Lipka M, Szpotańska M, Błazik M, Groele L. Application of novel dual wave meal bolus and its impact on glycated hemoglobin A1c level in children with type 1 diabetes. *Pediatr Diabetes* 2009; **10**(5): 298–303.

27. O'Connell MA, Gilbertson HR, Donath SM, Cameron FJ. Optimizing Postprandial Glycemia in Pediatric Patients With Type 1 Diabetes Using Insulin Pump Therapy. *Diabetes Care* 2008; **31**(8): 1491–1495.

28. Ryan RL, King BR, Anderson DG, Attia JR, Collins CE, Smart CE. Influence of and optimal insulin therapy for a low-glycemic index meal in children with type 1 diabetes receiving intensive insulin therapy. *Diabetes Care* 2008; **31**(8):1485–1490.

29. Kershnar AK, Daniels SR, Imperatore G, Palla SL, Petitti DB, Pettitt DJ, et al. Lipid abnormalities are prevalent in youth with type 1 and type 2 diabetes: the SEARCH for Diabetes in Youth Study. *J Pediatr* 2006; **149**(3): 314–319.

30. Edge JA, James T, Shine B. Longitudinal screening of serum lipids in children and adolescents with Type 1 diabetes in a UK clinic population. *Diabet Med* 2008; **25**(8): 942–948.

31. Guy J, Ogden L, Wadwa RP, Hamman RF, Mayer-Davis E, Liese AD, et al. Lipid and lipoprotein profiles in youth with and without type 1 diabetes: the SEARCH for Diabetes in Youth case-control study. *Diabetes Care* 2009; **32**(3): 416–420.

32. Petitti DB, Imperatore G, Palla SL, Daniels SR, Dolan LM, Kershnar AK, et al. Serum lipids and glucose control: the SEARCH for Diabetes in Youth study. *Arch Pediatr Adolesc Med* 2007; **161**(2):159–165.

33. Liese AD, Bortsov A, Günther AL, Dabelea D, Reynolds K, Standiford DA, et al. Association of DASH diet with cardiovascular risk factors in youth with diabetes mellitus: the SEARCH for Diabetes in Youth study. *Circulation* 2011; **123**(13): 1410–1417.

34. Maffeis C, Morandi A, Ventura E, Sabbion A, Contreas G, Tomasselli F, et al. Diet, physical, and biochemical characteristics of children and adolescents with type 1 diabetes: relationship between dietary fat and glucose control. *Pediatr Diabetes* 2012; **13**(2): 137–146.

35. Ljungkrantz M, Ludvigsson J, Samuelsson U. Type 1 diabetes: increased height and weight gains in early childhood. *Pediatr Diabetes* 2008; **9**(3): 50–56.

36. World Health Organization. Global Recommendations on Physical Activity for Health. Geneva: WHO, 2010.

37. Schweiger B, Klingensmith G, Snell-Bergeon J. Physical activity in adolescent females with type 1 diabetes. *Int J Pediatr* 2010; **2010**: 328318.

38. Edmunds S, Roche D, Stratton G. Levels and patterns of physical activity in children and adolescents with type 1 diabetes and associated metabolic and physiologic health outcomes. *J Phys Act Health* 2010; **7**(1): 68–77.

39. Michaliszyn SF, Faulkner MS. Physical activity and sedentary behavior in adolescents with type 1 diabetes. *Res Nurs Health* 2010; **33**(5): 441–449.

40. Øverby NC, Margeirsdottir HD, Brunborg C, Anderssen SA, Andersen LF, Dahl-Jørgensen K. Physical activity and overweight in children and adolescents using intensified insulin treatment. *Pediatr Diabetes* 2009; **10**(2): 135–141.

41. Herbst A, Kordonouri O, Schwab KO, Schmidt F, Holl RW. Impact of physical activity on cardiovascular risk factors in children with type 1 diabetes: a multicenter study of 23,251 patients. *Diabetes Care* 2007; **30**(8): 2098–2100.

42. Herbst A, Bachran R, Kapellen T, Holl RW. Effects of regular physical activity on control of glycemia in pediatric patients with type 1 diabetes mellitus. *Arch Pediatr Adolesc Med* 2006; **160**(6): 573–577.

43. Åman J, Skinner TC, de Beaufort CE, Swift PG, Aanstoot HJ, Cameron F. Associations between physical activity, sedentary behavior, and glycemic control in a large cohort of adolescents with type 1 diabetes: the Hvidoere Study Group on Childhood Diabetes. *Pediatr Diabetes* 2009; **10**(4): 234–239.

44. Riddell MC, Iscoe KE. Physical activity, sport, and pediatric diabetes. *Pediatr Diabetes* 2006; **7**(1): 60–70.

45. Tsalikian E, Mauras N, Beck RW, Tamborlane WV, Janz KF, Chase HP, et al. Impact of exercise on overnight glycemic control in children with type 1 diabetes mellitus. *J Pediatr* 2005; **147**(4): 528–534.

46. Robertson K, Adolfsson P, Scheiner G, Hanas R, Riddell MC. Exercise in children and adolescents with diabetes. *Pediatr Diabetes* 2009; **10**: 154–168.

47. SEARCH for Diabetes in Youth: a multicenter study of the prevalence, incidence and classification of diabetes mellitus in youth. *Control Clin Trials* 2004; **25**(5): 458–471.

48. Rosenbloom AL, Silverstein JH, Amemiya S, Zeitler P, Klingensmith GJ. ISPAD Clinical Practice Consensus Guidelines 2006–2007. Type 2 diabetes mellitus in the child and adolescent. *Pediatr Diabetes* 2008; **9**(5): 512–526.

49. Günther ALB, Liese AD, Bell RA, Dabelea D, Lawrence JM, Rodriguez BL, et al. Association between the dietary approaches to hypertension diet and hypertension in youth with diabetes mellitus. *Hypertension* 2009; **53**(1): 6–12.

50. Lobelo F, Liese AD, Liu J, Mayer-Davis E, D'Agostino RB, Jr, Pate RR, et al. Physical activity and electronic media use in the SEARCH for diabetes in youth case-control study. *Pediatrics* 2010; **125**(6): e1364–e1371.

51. Zeitler P, Hirst K, Pyle L, Linder B, Copeland K, Arslanian S, et al. A clinical trial to maintain glycemic control in youth with type 2 diabetes. *N Engl J Med* 2012; **366**(24): 2247–2256.

52. Waitzfelder B, Pihoker C, Klingensmith G, Case D, Anderson A, Bell RA, et al. Adherence to guidelines for youths with diabetes mellitus. *Pediatrics* 2011; **128**(3): 531–538.

53. Lawrence JM, Liese AD, Liu L, Dabelea D, Anderson A, Imperatore G, et al. Weight-loss practices and weight-related issues among youth with type 1 or type 2 diabetes. *Diabetes Care* 2008; **31**(12): 2251–2257.

54. Kelly SD, Howe CJ, Hendler JP, Lipman TH. Disordered eating behaviors in youth with type 1 diabetes. *Diabetes Educ* 2005; **31**(4): 572–583.

55. Bryden KS, Neil A, Mayou RA, Peveler RC, Fairburn CG, Dunger DB. Eating habits, body weight, and insulin misuse. A longitudinal study of teenagers and young adults with type 1 diabetes. *Diabetes Care* 1999; **22**(12): 1956–1960.

56. Colton PA, Olmsted MP, Daneman D, Rydall AC, Rodin GM. Natural history and predictors of disturbed eating behaviour in girls with Type 1 diabetes. *Diabet Med* 2007; **24**(4): 424–429.

57. Jones JM, Lawson Ml, Daneman D, Olmsread MP, Rodin G. Eating disorders in adolescent females with and without type 1 diabetes: cross sectional study. *BMJ* 2000; **320**: 1563–1566.

58. Polonsky WH, Anderson BJ, Lohrer PA, Aponte JE, Jacobsen AM, Cole CF. Insulin omission in women with IDDM. *Diabetes Care* 1994; **17**(10): 1178–1185

59. Goebel-Fabbri AE, Fikkan J, Franko DL, Pearson K, Anderson BJ, Weinger K. Insulin restriction and associated morbidity and mortality in women with type 1 diabetes. *Diabetes Care* 2008; **31**(3): 415–419.

60. Ackard DM, Vik N, Neumark-Sztainer D, Schmitz KH, Hannan P, Jacobs, David R Jr. Disordered eating and body dissatisfaction in adolescents with type 1 diabetes and a population-based comparison sample: comparative prevalence and clinical implications. *Pediatr Diabetes* 2008; **9**(4): 312–319.

61. Neumark-Sztainer D, Patterson J, Mellin A, Ackard DM, Utter J, Story M, et al. Weight control practices and disordered eating behaviors among adolescent females and males with type 1 diabetes: associations with sociodemographics, weight concerns, familial factors, and metabolic outcomes. *Diabetes Care* 2002; **25**(8): 1289–1296.

62. Maharaj SI, Rodin GM, Olmsted MP, Connolly JA, Daneman D. Eating disturbances in girls with diabetes: the contribution of adolescent self-concept, maternal weight and shape concerns and mother-daughter relationships. *Psychol Med* 2003; **33**(3): 525–539.

SECTION 7

Diabetes in older people

Chapter 7.1

Epidemiology, aetiology, pathogenesis and management of diabetes in older people

Ahmed H. Abdelhafiz[1] and Alan J. Sinclair[2]
[1] Rotherham General Hospital, Rotherham, UK
[2] Bedfordshire & Hertfordshire PG Medical School, Luton, UK

7.1.1 Introduction

Diabetes is associated with increasing age, family history, ethnicity, obesity and sedentary life style. It causes premature morbidity, mortality and is a substantial health burden on individuals, health systems and society. Diabetes is the seventh leading cause of death in the United States (US) and the incidence, prevalence and mortality caused by diabetes and diabetic complications (mainly cardiovascular disease) increase with ageing [1]. Diabetes is similar to the ageing process itself; as it accelerates, ageing increases atherosclerosis and degenerative processes such as premature cataracts and is associated with geriatric syndromes, such as cognitive dysfunction, physical disability, falls and fractures. With increasing ageing of the population and changes in lifestyle worldwide, the prevalence of diabetes is likely to reach epidemic levels in most countries. Because type 2 diabetes is the most common type affecting older people, it will be the main focus of this chapter.

7.1.2 Epidemiology

Global changes in lifestyle leading to increased obesity and urbanisation, combined with an ageing population are predicted to increase diabetes prevalence, especially among individuals aged ≥75 years.

7.1.3 Incidence and prevalence

The worldwide prevalence of diabetes is rising with increasing age. In France, the prevalence has increased to 14.2% in those aged 65–74 years, peaking at 19.7% in men and 14.2% in women aged 75–79 years. More than half of those with diabetes were ≥ 65 years [2]. In the US, total diabetes prevalence is estimated to be 14% of the population and is highest in those aged ≥65 years and by the year 2050 diabetes prevalence could be as high as 33% of the whole population [3]. However, the prevalence of undiagnosed diabetes is much higher. In the National Health and Nutrition Examination Survey the prevalence of diagnosed diabetes in those ≥75 years old was 14.9%, undiagnosed diabetes based on fasting plasma glucose and 2 hours oral glucose tolerance test was 13.4%. This makes a total prevalence of diagnosed and undiagnosed diabetes of 28.3% and undiagnosed diabetes constitutes a proportion of around 47%. Pre-diabetes, defined as either impaired fasting glycaemia (IFG) or impaired glucose tolerance (IGT) was prevalent in 46.7% of those ≥75 years old. Therefore, the total prevalence of diabetes (diagnosed and

Advanced Nutrition and Dietetics in Diabetes, First Edition. Edited by Louise Goff and Pamela Dyson.
© 2016 John Wiley & Sons, Ltd. Published 2016 by John Wiley & Sons, Ltd.

undiagnosed) and pre-diabetes (IFG and IGT) reaches a peak of around 75% of older people ≥75 years of age [4].

Race and ethnicity

The burden of diabetes is likely to grow faster in the low and middle-income countries (LMIC). It is estimated that between 2010 and 2030, there will be a 69% increase in numbers of adults (aged 20–79 years) with diabetes in LMIC countries and a 20% increase in higher income countries [5]. This is likely due to growth and ageing of the population and urbanisation associated with lifestyle change. The prevalence of diabetes among older Chinese in rural Taiwan was 16.9% in 2000 (mean (SD) age 72.6 (6) years at baseline) and increased to 23.7% in 2005. The overall 5-year cumulative incidence of new onset diabetes was 6.8% [6]. In minority ethnic groups living in the developed world the incidence and prevalence of diabetes is higher than white populations. For example, the prevalence of diabetes in Mexican American older adults (≥75 years) has nearly doubled between 1993–1994 and 2004–2005 from 20.3 to 37.2%, respectively, in comparison to the increase in the general population of the same age group from 10.4 to 16.4% [7]. Prevalence of diabetes among African Americans and Hispanics has consistently been higher than whites and is projected to triple by the year 2050 while only doubling in whites. In addition, prevalence rates for Native Americans ranges from 5 to 50% in some tribes [8]. In the United Kingdom (UK), diabetes in people of South Asian descent and African or African-Caribbean descent is six and three times, respectively, more common, than in the white population.

Care homes

In the US around 24.6% of nursing home residents had diabetes in 2004. Among residents aged 65–74, 75–84, and ≥85 years, diabetes prevalence was 36.1, 29.5, and 18.3%, respectively [9]. There was a steady increase in the prevalence of diabetes in US nursing homes from 1995 to 2004 (16.9 to 26.4% in males and 16.1 to 22.2% in females). The overall increase

was from 16.3 to 23.4% with an average change of 0.8% per year. Level of comorbidity also increased. Residents aged ≥85 years and those with high functional impairment showed a significant increasing trend as well as increasing prevalence of cardiovascular disease from 59.6 to 75.4% for men and 68.1 to 78.7% for women [10]. A more recent survey showed a further increase in the prevalence of diabetes affecting 32.8% of residents of nursing homes and subjects with diabetes tended to have a greater comorbid burden, more medications, and had more hospitalisations than residents with no diabetes [11]. Ethnic disparities in diabetes prevalence are also well documented in care home settings. In US nursing homes, the odds of diabetes are about two times higher in black and Hispanic residents relative to white residents and diabetes was present in 22.5 and 35.6% of whites and non-whites, respectively [9].

7.1.4 Aetiology and pathogenesis

Aetiology and pathogenesis of diabetes in older people is complex. Increased adiposity and decreased physical activity with increasing age predispose older people to develop insulin resistance. On the other hand, normal ageing is associated with impaired insulin secretion and progressive increase in both fasting and postprandial glucose levels, see Box 7.1.1.

Box 7.1.1 Determinants of glucose intolerance in older people

Age
Reduced number of glucose transport units
Defect in post-receptor insulin signalling pathway
Increased β-cell dysfunction
Mitochondrial dysfunction
Reduced β-cell mass
Reduced muscle mass
Low concentrations of adiponectin
High concentrations of TNF-α
Reduced levels of insulin-like growth factor-I
Physical inactivity
Increased body fat
Changes in body fat distribution.

Increased insulin resistance

Ageing is associated with changes in body fat distribution with a reduction in subcutaneous fat and increased visceral fat [12] that is linked to glucose intolerance and diabetes, and a decline in skeletal muscle mass or sarcopenia [13]. As the muscle tissue is the main site of glucose consumption, the loss of muscle mass increases the risk of developing glucose intolerance and diabetes. Increasing muscle mass by resistance training in older people has been shown to improve glucose tolerance [14]. Increased truncal obesity (visceral fat accumulation) with ageing leads to altered lipid metabolism. The rate of lipolysis increases causing high levels of free fatty acids that may have a role in reducing peripheral insulin sensitivity [15]. Accumulation of lipids within the muscles is another factor leading to insulin resistance. A reduction in mitochondrial function [16] may also contribute to age-related glucose intolerance by reduced oxidative metabolism and decline in physical fitness and oxidative capacity of older people. Low concentrations of adiponectin (secreted by adipose tissue that improves insulin resistance by increasing fat oxidation), low concentration of leptin (secreted by adipose tissue that decreases appetite and its decline may contribute to the increased adiposity and body composition changes seen in the elderly), high concentrations of tumour necrosis factor alpha (which induces anorexia, weight loss and insulin resistance) and reduced levels of insulin-like growth factor-I (a peptide hormone that stimulates glucose uptake) are associated with ageing and linked to increased insulin resistance and incident diabetes [17–19].

Decreased insulin secretion

Ageing is associated with a reduction in insulin secretion of 0.7% per year due to a combination of β-cell dysfunction and reduced β-cell mass (apoptosis) and individuals with glucose intolerance demonstrate a 50% reduction in β-cell mass [20]. β-cell autoimmunity may lead to activation of acute phase response in older people with diabetes [21]. In genetically predisposed individuals long-term hypersecretion of interleukins, C reactive protein and tumour necrosis factor alpha may contribute to impaired β-cell insulin secretion and insulin resistance [21]. Disturbances in the physiology of the gut-derived incretins, gastric inhibitory polypeptide (GIP) and glucagonlike peptide-1 (GLP-1), may be another factor involved in β-cell dysfunction [22]. Both peptides enhance insulin secretion after meals and may have a role in maintaining β-cell growth, proliferation, and inhibition of apoptosis. Ageing is associated with reduced level and function of these peptides [23].

Progression to diabetes

Normal glucose homeostasis requires normal insulin secretion by β-cells of the pancreas combined with normal peripheral glucose utilisation by peripheral tissues sensitive to insulin. In older people with diabetes, abnormalities in both insulin secretion and insulin sensitivity underlie the development of diabetes with a principle defect of insulin secretion in lean individuals and insulin resistance in obese ones. It is likely that both genetic and environmental factors are involved in the pathogenesis of insulin secretory dysfunction and insulin resistance. As older people are heterogeneous the extent and rate of deterioration in glucose homeostasis is variable, leading to insignificant changes in some individuals and diabetes in others. It is possible that insulin resistance develops in the pre-diabetes state and β-cells compensate by increasing insulin secretion, causing hyperinsulinaemia and initially maintaining normal glucose tolerance. Eventually, a combination of reduced insulin secretory capacity of β-cells to compensate for insulin resistance and further diminution of peripheral tissue sensitivity to insulin, insulin secretion becomes inadequate, leading to the progression to persistent hyperglycaemia, glucose intolerance and then to diabetes, see Figure 7.1.1.

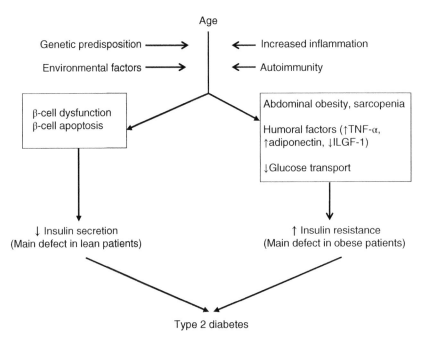

Figure 7.1.1 Pathogenesis of type 2 diabetes in older people

Box 7.1.2 Risk factors for diabetes in older people

Age
Family history (two or more close relatives)
Abdominal obesity (waist circumference
    >100 cm in men, 92 cm in women)
High body mass index (>30.0 kg/m²)
Hypertension
Dyslipdaemia
Depression
Vitamin D deficiency
Sleep disturbance
Undernutrition
Low socioeconomic status
High carbohydrate diet

7.1.5 Risk factors

Age per se is associated with changes that predispose to development of diabetes. Physiological changes, as outlined above, are important. Additionally, psychosocial factors, such as depressive illness, stress, lower social support and poor nutrition appear to contribute to incident diabetes in older people, see Box 7.1.2.

Abdominal obesity

Body mass index (BMI) may not accurately reflect percentage of body fat in the elderly due to age-associated loss of height caused by compression of vertebral bodies combined with age-related decrease in muscle mass and increase in abdominal fat [24]. This may overestimate the BMI value in older people. Risk of diabetes associated with overweight, expressed as BMI, tends to decline with age [25]. Recently BMI in the overweight range was not shown to be associated with diabetes in the elderly cohort but obesity (BMI≥ 30.0 kg/m²) was a significant risk factor for diabetes [25]. Therefore the definition of healthy weight, expressed as BMI, may need to be set at a higher value in older people, but this needs further research. On the other hand waist circumference (WC) of 100 cm in men and 92 cm in women was a predictor of incident diabetes in older people. BMI and WC yielded similar risk prediction in older men whereas WC was a superior predictor in older women. The use of BMI combined with WC does not improve identification of diabetes risk beyond single measures of BMI (in men) or WC (in women)

[26]. Rate of change in central adiposity is another determinant risk factor for diabetes. In the Cardiovascular Health Study participants with >10 cm increase in WC from baseline had a hazard ratio of diabetes of 1.7 (95% CI 1.1 to 2.8) compared with those who gained or lost 2 cm or less in a cohort of 4193 subjects ≥65 years of age [27].

Vitamin D deficiency

Vitamin D receptors are present on the pancreatic β-cells, suggesting that vitamin D deficiency may inhibit insulin secretion and vitamin D administration may improve insulin secretion, thus reducing the risk of developing diabetes. However, the relationship between low vitamin D levels and the risk of developing diabetes is not consistent. One meta-analysis found an association between low vitamin D status and increased risk of incident diabetes [28], although vitamin D supplementation in another study had no effect on glycaemia or incident diabetes [29]. Recently, lower serum vitamin D levels have not been shown to be associated with increased risk of developing diabetes in 5140 postmenopausal women (mean age 66 years) participating in the Women's Health Initiative Clinical Trials and Observational Study who were free of diabetes at baseline and followed up for 7.3 years [30]. The protective effect of vitamin D in reducing the diabetes risk in older people may need higher doses of vitamin D supplementation. Also, exposure to sun implies greater outdoor physical activity, which in itself may have beneficial effects on insulin sensitivity, unrelated to vitamin D levels.

Depression

Depressive illness is another risk factor for diabetes although the nature of the association is not clear. Several factors are common in depression that may predispose to diabetes, such as lack of physical activity and obesity. However, it has been shown that depression is a risk for diabetes independent of these factors. In a longitudinal study of 4803 community sample of adults aged 55 years incident diabetes was associated with depression, independent of sociodemographic variables, antidepressant or antipsychotic use after 5 years of follow up [31]. Depression increased the risk of diabetes by 65% and the characteristics of depression that may play a role in the development of diabetes were non-severe depression, persistent depression and untreated depression. The chronic stress state associated with depression may be an underlying factor leading to development of diabetes.

Sleep disturbance

Long day napping (≥1 h) and short night sleeping (<5 h) have been shown to be associated with high risk of diabetes in older people. This association may be partially explained by obesity and napping itself could be a marker of other health conditions that increase the risk of diabetes [32]. Insomnia is another factor associated with ageing and increasing risk of insulin resistance. Sleep disturbances may cause insulin resistance through inducing sympathetic over-activity or increasing secretion of counter regulatory hormones during sleep [33].

Low socioeconomic status

Incident diabetes was associated with lower wealth (P 0.05 for men and 0.004 for women) after adjusting for socio-economic and demographic factors among 9053 older adults selected from the English Longitudinal Study of Ageing and followed up for 4 years [34]. In Canada, prevalence of diabetes decreases steadily as income goes up. There is a graded association between income and diabetes with the lowest compared to those with the highest income [35]. This could be partly explained by differences in the distribution of obesity by socioeconomic status.

Undernutrition

Underweight may be associated with increased risk of diabetes among older adults. In a cohort of 127 213 older adults (aged 40–79 years), subjects (aged 60–79 years) with a BMI <18.5 kg/m^2 had a higher risk of incident diabetes in men and women compared with those with a BMI of 18.5–24.9 kg/m^2 while no association was found in younger subjects (40–59 years old) after a mean of follow up of 5.3 years [36]. The explanation for the association of underweight and diabetes is uncertain but it could be related to malnutrition leading to impaired insulin release.

Other factors

Metabolic syndrome is common in older people and is associated with increased risk of diabetes. In a cross-sectional study, around one-sixth (19.9% of males and 12.2% of females) of 623 non-diabetic older adults (aged 58 to 93 years) had undetected diabetes. The likelihood of having diabetes was higher for males, those with systolic blood pressure ≥130 mmHg, triglycerides ≥1.7 mmol/l and large waist circumference, all are components of the metabolic syndrome [37]. The main pathophysiology of metabolic syndrome leading to diabetes is insulin resistance. Other factors, such as sedentary lifestyle, smoking, excess alcohol and high carbohydrate diet may be associated with increasing risk of insulin resistance and development of diabetes [38].

7.1.6 Screening

Screening and identification of diabetes in high risk individuals is of clinical interest as preventive interventions are likely to be cost effective [39]. Older people with fasting plasma glucose in the range 6.1–6.9 mmol/L or 2-hour plasma glucose in the range 7.8–11.0 mmol/L are at increased risk for development of diabetes [40]. Due to the practical barriers of testing the fasting or post-prandial blood sugar, the use of HbA1c alone, in the range 5.5 to <6.5% has been shown to identify a population with risk for developing diabetes (32.4%) over 7.5 years. This suggests that HbA1c-based testing could be used in clinical settings to identify subjects who would benefit from intensive prevention programmes [41]. Persons with hypertension will also benefit

from screening as blood pressure targets for persons with diabetes are lower than for those without diabetes. Obesity, dyslipidaemia, sedentary lifestyle, family history of diabetes and ethnicity are other factors to be considered in screening that may help reduce numbers of undiagnosed diabetes.

7.1.7 Prevention

Methods of prevention are summarised in Box 7.1.3. Lifestyle modification with a focus on weight loss and physical activity may improve insulin sensitivity and reduce development of diabetes. Resistance training may have an impact on improving body composition, body fat distribution, inflammatory markers and blood glucose homeostasis reducing insulin resistance [42]. Any type of physical activity is useful in older age groups. Low-intensity physical activity at least once a week was associated with reduced risk of diabetes in older people (≥70 years) compared with no activity, while in relatively younger adults (aged 50 to 69 years) physical activity has to be at least moderate in intensity to have an impact on diabetes prevention [43]. Even short-term exercise, for only seven days, improves insulin resistance and β-cell function in older people with impaired glucose tolerance, independent of change in weight or lipid profile [44]. This emphasises the importance of exercise programmes in old age as a preventive measure for diabetes. Addressing poor nutrition and socioeconomic inequalities are other important factors, see Figure 7.1.2.

Box 7.1.3   Prevention of diabetes in older people

Weight loss
Increased physical activity
Exercise programmes

   Low intensity
   Resistance training
   Repeated short term

Good nutrition
Addressing socioeconomic inequalities.

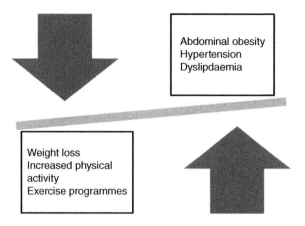

Figure 7.1.2 Main risk factors and prevention of type 2 diabetes in older people

7.1.8 Conclusion

Ageing is associated with changes in body fat distribution that predispose to increased insulin resistance and decreased insulin secretion, leading to glucose intolerance and diabetes in genetically susceptible individuals. The prevalence of diabetes in older people, therefore, is increasing as a result of the growing ageing of the population and sedentary lifestyle with increased obesity. There remain a significant number of older people with either undetected diabetes or in a pre-diabetes state. Increased physical activity and healthy diet are the main focus for diabetes prevention.

Key points

- Normal ageing is associated with changes in body fat distribution, leading to decreased insulin secretion and increased insulin resistance that progress to glucose intolerance and diabetes in genetically predisposed individuals.
- Prevalence of diabetes is increasing due to ageing of the population and increasing obesity and this remains higher in the developing world and ethnic minorities living in western countries.
- Significant numbers of older people remain undiagnosed or have a pre-diabetes state.
- Healthy lifestyle is the cornerstone of diabetes prevention.

References

1. Liu L. Changes in cardiovascular hospitalization and comorbidity of heart failure in the United States: Findings from the National Hospital Discharge Surveys 1980–2006. *Int J Cardiol* 2011; **149**: 39–45.
2. Ricci P, Blotière PO, Weill A, Simon D, Tuppin P, Ricordeau P, et al. Diabète traité en France : quelles évolutions entre 2000 et 2009? *Bull Epidemiol Hebd* 2010; **43**: 425–431.
3. Boyle JP, Thompson TJ, Gregg EW, Barker LE, Williamson DF. Projection of the year 2050 burden of diabetes in the US adult population: dynamic modeling of incidence, mortality, and prediabetes prevalence. *Popul Health Metrics* 2010; **8**(1): 29. doi:10.1186/1478-7954-8-29.
4. Cowie C, Rust KF, Ford ES, Eberhardt MS, Byrd-Holt DD, Li C, et al. Full accounting of diabetes and pre-diabetes in the U.S. population in 1988–1994 and 2005–2006. *Diabetes Care* 2009; **32**: 287–294.
5. Shaw JE, Sicree RA, Zimmet PZ. Global estimates of the prevalence of diabetes for 2010 and 2030. *Diabetes Res Clin Pract* 2010; **87**: 4–14.
6. Peng LN, Lin MH, Lai HY, Hwang SJ, Chen LK, Chiou ST. Risk factors of new onset diabetes mellitus among elderly Chinese in rural Taiwan. *Age Ageing* 2010; **39**(1): 125–128.
7. Beard HA, Al Ghatrif M, Samper-Terent R, Gerst K, Markides KS. Trends in diabetes prevalence and diabetes-related complications in older Mexican Americans from 1993–1994 to 2004–2005. *Diabetes Care* 2009; **32**: 2212–2217.
8. Deshpande AD, Harris-Hayes M, Schootman M. Epidemiology of diabetes and diabetes-related complications. *Phys Ther* 2008; **88**: 1254–1264.
9. Resnick HE, Heineman J, Stone R, Shorr RI. Diabetes in U.S. nursing homes, 2004. *Diabetes Care* 2008; **31**: 287–288.

10. Zhang X, Decker FH, Luo H, Geiss LS, Pearson WS, Saaddine JB, et al. Trends in the prevalence and co-morbidities of diabetes mellitus in nursing home residents in the United States: 1995–2004. *J Am Geriatr Soc* 2010; **58**: 724–730.

11. Dybicz SB, Thompson S, Molotsky S, Stuart B. Prevalence of diabetes and the burden of comorbid conditions among elderly nursing home residents. *Am J Geriatr Pharmacother* 2011; doi:10.1016/j.amjopharm.2011.05.001

12. Kuk JL, Saunders TJ, Davidson LE, Ross R. Age-related changes in total and regional fat distribution. *Ageing Res Rev* 2009; **8**: 339–348.

13. Evans WJ. Skeletal muscle loss: cachexia, sarcopenia, and inactivity. *Am J Clin Nutr* 2010; **91**: 1123S–1127S.

14. Balducci S, Zanuso S, Nicolucci A, Fernando F, Cavallo S, Cardelli P, et al. Anti-inflammatory effect of exercise training in subjects with type 2 diabetes and the metabolic syndrome is dependent on exercise modalities and independent of weight loss. *Nutr, Metab Cardiovasc Dis* 2010; **20**: 608–617.

15. Guilherme A, Virbasius JV, Puri V, Czech MP. Adipocyte dysfunctions linking obesity to insulin resistance and type 2 diabetes. *Nat Rev Mol Cell Biol* 2008; **9**: 367–377.

16. Kim JA, Wei Y, Sowers RJ. Role of mitochondrial dysfunction in insulin resistance. *Circulation Res* 2008; **102**: 401–414.

17. Rabe K, Lehrke M, Parhofer KG, Broedl UC. Adipokines and insulin resistance. *Mol Med* 2008; **14**: 741–751.

18. Nieto-Vazquez I, Fernandez-Veledo S, Kramer DK, Vila-Bedmar R, Garcia-Guerra L, Lorenzo M. Insulin resistance associated to obesity: the link TNF-alpha. *Arch Physiol Biochem* 2008; **114**: 183–194.

19. Benbassat CA, Maki KC, Unterman TG. Circulating levels of insulin-like growth factor (IGF) binding protein- 1 and -3 in aging men: relationships to insulin, glucose, IGF, and dehydroepiandrosterone sulfate levels and anthropometric measures. *J Clin Endocrinol Metab* 1997; **82**: 1484–1491.

20. Szoke E, Shrayyef MZ, Messing S, Woerle HJ, van Haeften TW, Meyer C, et al. Effect of aging on glucose homeostasis: accelerated deterioration of β-cell function in individuals with impaired glucose tolerance. *Diabetes Care* 2008; **31**: 539–543.

21. Dehghan A, Kardys I, de Maat MPm, Uitterlinden AG, Sijbrands EJ, Bootsma AH, et al. Genetic variation, C-reactive protein levels, and incidence of diabetes. *Diabetes* 2007; **56**: 872–878.

22. Kim W, Egan JM. The role of incretins in glucose homeostasis and diabetes treatment. *Pharm Rev* 2008; **60**: 470–512.

23. Farilla L, Bulotta A, Hirshberg B, Li Calzi S, Khoury N, Noushmehr H, et al. Glucagon-like peptide 1 inhibits cell apoptosis and improves glucose responsiveness of freshly isolated human islets. *Endocrinology* 2003; **144**: 5149–5158.

24. Villareal DT, Apovian CM, Kushner RF, Klein S; American Society for Nutrition; NAASO, The Obesity Society. Obesity in older adults: technical review and position statement of the American Society for Nutrition and NAASO, The Obesity Society. *Am J Clin Nutr* 2005; **82**: 923–934.

25. Kvamme JM, Wilsgaard T, Florholmen J, Jacobsen BK. Body mass index and disease burden in elderly men and women: The Tromsø Study. *Eur J Epidemiol* 2010; **25**: 183–193.

26. Wannamethee SG, Papacosta O, Whincup PH, Carson C, Thomas MC, Lawlor DA, et al. Assessing prediction of diabetes in older adults using different adiposity measures: a 7 year prospective study in 6,923 older men and women. *Diabetologia* 2010; **53**: 890–898.

27. Biggs ML, Mukamal KJ, Luchsinger JA, Ix JH, Carnethon MR, Newman AB, et al. Association between adiposity in midlife and older age and risk of diabetes in older adults. *JAMA* 2010; **24**: 2504–2512.

28. Pittas AG, Chung M, Trikalinos T, Mitri J, Brendel M, Patel K, et al. Systematic review: Vitamin D and car-diometabolic outcomes. *Ann Intern Med* 2010; **152**: 307–314.

29. Song Y, Manson JE. Vitamin D, insulin resistance, and type 2 diabetes. *Curr CardioRisk Rep* 2010; **4**: 40–47.

30. Robinson JG, Manson J, Larson J, Liu S, Song Y, Howard BV, et al. Lack of association between 25(OH)Dlevels and incident type 2 diabetes in older women. *Diabetes Care* 2011; **34**: 628–634.

31. Campayo A, de Jonge P, Roy JF, Saz P, de la Cámara C, Quintanilla MA, et al. Depressive disorder and incident diabetes mellitus: The effect of characteristics of depression. *Am J Psych* 2010; **167**: 580–588.

32. Xu Q, Song Y, Hollenbeck A, Blair A, Schatzkin A, Chen H. Day napping and short night sleeping are associated hith Higher risk of diabetes in older adults. *Diabetes Care* 2010; **33**: 78–83.

33. Yamamoto N, Yamanaka G, Ishizawa K, Ishikawa M, Murakami S, Yamanaka T, et al. Insomnia increases insulin resistance and insulin secretion in elderly people. *J Am Geriatr Soc* 2010; **58**: 801–804.

34. Tanaka T, Gjonça E, Gulliford MC. Income, wealth and risk of diabetes among older adults: cohort study using the English longitudinal study of ageing. *Eur J Public Health* 2011; doi: 10.1093/eurpub/ckr050.

35. Dinca-Panaitescua S, Dinca-Panaitescub M, Bryantc T, Daiski I, Pilkington B, Raphael D. Diabetes prevalence and income: Results of the Canadian Community Health Survey. *Health Policy* 2011; **99**: 116–123.

36. Sairenchi T, Iso H, Irie F, Fukasawa N, Ota H, Muto T. Underweight as a Predictor of Diabetes in Older Adults *Diabetes Care* 2008; **31**: 583–584.

37. Dankner R, Geulayov G, Olmer L, Kaplan G. Undetected type 2 diabetes in older adults. *Age Ageing* 2009; **38**: 56–62.

38. O'Sullivan TA, Bremner A, O'Neill S, Lyons-Wall P. Glycaemic load is associated with insulin resistance in older Australian women. *Eur J Clin Nutr* 2010; **64**: 80–87.

39. Li R, Zhang P, Barker LE, Chowdhury FM, Zhang X. Cost-Effectiveness of Interventions to Prevent and Control Diabetes Mellitus: A Systematic Review. *Diabetes Care* 2010; **33**: 1872–1894.

40. Gerstein HC, Santaguida P, Raina P, Morrison KM, Balion C, Hunt D, et al. Annual incidence and relative risk of diabetes in people with various categories of dysglycemia: a systematic overview and meta-analysis of prospective studies. *Diabetes Res Clin Pract* 2007; **78**: 305–312.

41. Ackermann RT, Cheng YJ, Williamson DF, Gregg EW. Identifying adults at high risk for diabetes and cardiovascular disease using haemoglobin A1c. National Health and Nutrition Examination Survey 2005–2006. *Am J Prev Med* 2011; **40**: 11–17.

42. Flack KD, Davy KP, Hulver MW, Winett RA, Frisard MI, Davy BM. Aging, resistance training, and diabetes prevention. *J Aging Res* 2011; doi:10.4061/2011/127315.

43. Demakakos P, Hamer M, Stamatakis E, Steptoe A. Low-intensity physical activity is associated with reduced risk of incident type 2 diabetes in older adults: evidence from the English Longitudinal Study of Ageing. *Diabetologia* 2010; **53**: 1877–1885.

44. Bloem CJ, Chang AM. Short-term exercise improves beta cell function and insulin resistance in older people with impaired glucose tolerance. *J Clin Endocrinol Metab* 2008; **93**: 387–392.

Chapter 7.2

Lifestyle management, including nutrition, of diabetes in older people

Trisha Dunning
Deakin University and Barwon Health, Victoria, Australia

7.2.1 Introduction

Diabetes is common in older people, affecting approximately 20% of older Caucasians [1,2] with a further 20% having diabetes risk factors but undiagnosed. Increasing age is a major risk factor for diabetes but the diagnosis is often missed or delayed because the clinical presentation differs from the 'textbook' signs and symptoms, thus recognising and managing diabetes in older people can be complex. Diabetes is a major cause of morbidity and mortality in older people [3]. Poor glycaemic control and chronic hyperglycaemia is associated with short- and long-term complications in older people, such as ketoacidosis, hyperosmolar states and myocardial infarction [4]. Diabetes is rated as the sixth leading cause of death in older people, excluding deaths attributed to cardiovascular and other diseases, many of which are associated with diabetes.

7.2.2 Brief overview of the pathogenesis of diabetes in older people

Diabetes in older people is metabolically different from that in younger people. Fasting hepatic glucose production is not increased as it is in younger people with type 2 diabetes [5,6]. Lean older people with type 2 diabetes have impaired insulin secretion but insulin action is relatively normal. In contrast, overweight older people have relatively normal insulin secretion but significant insulin resistance. It is likely that autoimmunity may be a factor in the pathogenesis of diabetes in lean older people [7], thus it is important to measure autoimmune markers, such as antiglutamic acid decarboxylase and/or islet cell antibodies to aid diagnosis and management decisions. These metabolic differences suggest management is likely to differ for lean and obese older people: lean people are likely to need insulin at, or soon after, diagnosis, whereas overweight older people might benefit initially from insulin sensitising medicines such as metformin, providing the individual does not have risk factors for lactic acidosis.

7.2.3 Clinical features of diabetes in older people

Diabetes usually presents differently in older people than in younger adults; the signs and symptoms are often non-specific. The renal threshold increases; thus glycosuria might not be present until the blood glucose is very high and thirst recognition is often impaired. The diagnosis is often made during routine health checks, during a hospital admission or when the individual presents with a diabetes complication or in a hyperosmolar state.

Advanced Nutrition and Dietetics in Diabetes, First Edition. Edited by Louise Goff and Pamela Dyson.
© 2016 John Wiley & Sons, Ltd. Published 2016 by John Wiley & Sons, Ltd.

The risk of complications increases with duration of diabetes and persistent hyperglycaemia [7]. Complications exacerbate functional decline and reduce independence, self-care capacity and quality of life [8]. Vascular dementia and Alzheimer's disease are associated with diabetes and older people with diabetes have higher rates of depression [9]. Complications put older people at significant risk of under-recognised and under-treated pain, increased risk of pressure ulcers and falling and sustaining significant injuries, such as fractures [10]. Renal disease affects medicine pharmacodynamics and pharmacokinetics that predispose the individual to anaemia and medicine-related adverse events [10].

Therefore, primary prevention programmes and screening programmes to diagnose diabetes early are essential. Fasting blood glucose is not reliable in many older people and is not recommended as a screening test [7]. The United States Centre for Disease Control and Prevention [11] recommend that people with diabetes risk factors and who are overweight and those over 45 years be screened every one to three years using fasting glucose, HbA1c or an oral glucose tolerance test. HbA1c may be a viable option providing interfering factors that affect HbA1c assays are considered [12] but more research in this area is needed.

Geriatric syndromes and delirium

Geriatric syndromes (Box 7.2.1) and delirium are also common in older people. Delirium presents as changes over hours or days in a person's mental state. Symptoms include confusion, inability to focus, hallucinations, disorientation and personality changes, such as agitation and irritability not explained by dementia [13]. Delirium is due to many interrelated factors, such as age, especially over 80 years, dementia/cognitive impairment, multiple comorbid conditions, functional impairments, sensory deficits, depression and some medicines, such as hypnotics and sedatives, narcotics and anticholinergic agents such as frusemide [14]. Serotonin syndrome can result from interactions between two or more medicines; usually one is a serotonin reuptake inhibitor or a monoamine oxidase

---

Box 7.2.1 Common geriatric syndromes

Geriatric syndromes are a group of conditions not usually present in younger people. Geriatric syndromes are subtle and often under-recognised by individuals and caregivers (family and health professionals). When present, self-care capacity is compromised. Inadequate self-care or not achieving targets should trigger an assessment of the individual to determine whether one or more geriatric syndromes are present.

- Falls
- Pain
- Urinary tract infection
- Cognitive impairment, e.g. using Mini-Mental State Examination, Mini-Cog, Clock drawing test
- Depression, e.g. Geriatric Depression Scale, Patient Health Questionnaire (PHQ2)
- Hypoglycaemia
- Delirium
- Polypharmacy.

---

inhibitor [15]. Diabetes-related predisposing factors include cardiovascular disease, renal disease, changes in electrolytes in hyperglycaemic and hyperosmolar states, infections and hypoglycaemia.

7.2.4 Overview of management strategies

There is little randomised control trial data for people over 70 years, thus, management recommendations are often extrapolated from studies involving younger people with diabetes and/or are based on consensus opinion. Generally diabetes management strategies for high functioning older people with diabetes are similar to younger age groups [16], but there are some significant differences, especially in residential aged care facilities (RACF) where older people are likely to have several comorbidities and are more vulnerable. Diabetes management is often suboptimal in older people, especially those living in RACFs [17–19]. Many older people do not achieve optimal management targets and macrovascular and/or microvascualar disease and neuropathy is often present at diagnosis.

Some countries are introducing 'aging in place programmes' to maintain older people in the community with appropriate support for as long as possible. In addition to maintaining/ supporting functional health status, such programs could adopt a proactive risk management approach to care that encompasses:

• screening for diabetes
• identifying and prioritising risks such as nutritional deficiencies, pain, falls, delirium, increasing frailty, compromised driving and hypo- and hyper-glycaemia
• regular comprehensive medicine reviews, including herbal medicine use and other complementary therapies
• regular mental status, cognitive functioning and self-care assessments
• a plan to stop driving
• advanced care planning and a plan for end of life care
• the need for medical alert and call systems to enhance safety
• support for carers.

Management aims focus on safety, maintaining independence, functional status and quality of life, managing symptoms, reducing the impact of diabetes complications and comorbidities, and pharmacovigilance. The importance of individualising management targets has been recognised [12,20] and involving the older person and their family/ other carers in management decisions is essential.

Controlling blood pressure and lipids has a significant impact on the risk of complications and quality of life [21–23]. The benefit of tight glycaemic control for older people is still debated [24], but there is some evidence that it is beneficial if it can be achieved early in the course of diabetes, especially before complications develop; however, complications are often present at diagnosis and hypoglycaemia and related risks need to be considered. Nevertheless, good glycaemic control could reduce the risk of microvascular complications in older people with longer duration of diabetes.

There is a significant risk of hypoglycaemia with some glucose-lowering medicines that puts older people at risk of serious falls and myocardial infarction. The symptoms of hypoglycaemia and myocardial infarction are often atypical and unrecognised. Regular blood glucose testing can help identify hypo- and hyper-glycaemia. Likewise, the individual, his or her carers and health professionals might need to learn to recognise cues that signify hypoglycaemia for the individual.

The European Geriatrics Society and The International Diabetes Federation guidelines for blood glucose and blood pressure and lipid targets for healthy and frail older people are given in Table 7.2.1. Table 7.2.2 outlines *some* of the multifactorial interrelated factors that influence management decisions.

Table 7.2.1 European Geriatrics Society and the International Diabetes Federation blood glucose, blood pressure and lipid targets for healthy and frail older people

	Healthy older people with diabetes	Frail older people with diabetes
Blood glucose		
Fasting	<7.0 mmol/L	<10.0 mmol/L
Two hours post-prandial	<10.0 mmol/L	<14.0 mmol/L
HbA1c	<7%	<8%
Blood pressure		<150/90 mmHg
Lipids		
Low density lipoprotein	<140/80 mmHg	–
cholesterol (LDL-C)	<3.0 mM	
Triglycerides (TG)	<2.3 mM	–

Table 7.2.2 Overview of some of the factors that affect management decisions in older people with diabetes

Issue	Consequences
Hyperglycaemia	Symptoms may be atypical and hyperglycaemia can be missed. Hyperglycaemia can lead to:
	Urinary frequency
	Incontinence
	Disturbed sleep
	Dehydration and hyperosmolar states
	Delirium
	Increased risk of falls
	Changed cognitive function and/or delirium
	Infections
	Exacerbated pain
	Weight loss and nutritional deficiencies
	Long term diabetes complications.
	Other comorbidities such as cancer and sleep apnoea
	may be caused/exacerbated by corticosteroid, antipsychotic or thiazide diuretic medicines.
Hypoglycaemia	Often difficult to recognise because symptoms can occur at lower blood glucose levels.
	Neuroglycopenic symptoms often predominate and include confusion, delirium, dizziness, weakness and falls.
	Increases falls risk and likelihood of injury such as fractures.
Polypharmacy	Risk of interactions and other adverse events.
	Increased risk of falls.
	Complicated regimens that make medicine self-management difficult and non-adherence likely.
	Increased risk of delirium.
	Serotonin syndrome especially if analgesics are used with antidepressant medicines.
	Herbal medicine and other complementary therapy use can contribute to polypharmcay and interact with conventional medicines and use should be considered and documented.
Nutrition	Age- and disease-related changes in saliva production, swallowing, appetite, smell, and digestion affect food intake and enjoyment
	May not tolerate high fibre diets.
	Nutritional deficiencies such as vitamin D are common.
	Anaemia often accompanies renal disease.
	May require supplements to correct deficiencies and to enhance wound healing.
	Nutritional deficiencies and changed eating habits can be due to some medicines, e.g. metformin affects vitamin B 12 and can cause bloating.
	Alcoholism
	In aged care facilities may be receiving enteral feeds, which influence medicine choices and hypoglycaemia management
Changed activity levels	May be due to medicines, nutritional deficiencies, functional decline, fear of falling and about safety.
	Affects mobility and balance.

(*continued*)

Table 7.2.2 *(continued)*

Issue	Consequences
Presence of diabetes complications and comorbidities	Affects self-care (vision and hearing impairments, cognitive impairment) safety, functional status, independence and motivation. Some complications such as gastric autonomic neuropathy can affect absorption of food and oral medicines. Renal disease affects medicine excretion and affects appetite. Can contribute to depression and cognitive changes. Pain Falls risk Cognitive impairment, dementia and delirium Hypoglycaemia Risk of sudden death Capacity to learn Consider geriatric syndromes Box 7.2.1.

7.2.5 Management guidelines

A range of guidelines for managing diabetes in older people is shown in Box 7.2.2.: In addition, comprehensive guidelines for managing diabetes in RACF have been published [25]. Interviews have been conducted with older people and their carers to ensure their perspectives are reflected in the management recommendations, promoting person-centred care. The information will be combined with the best available evidence to develop a guiding philosophy that underpins the guidelines.

Although there is little randomised control trial evidence to support care recommendations for older people, there is a considerable degree of consensus among the available guidelines:

- Care of older people needs to be individualised regardless of whether they live in the community or in RCAFs, and the care needs to be revised regularly including at any change in status or treatment, especially medicines.
- It is important to prevent cardiovascular disease if possible. If cardiovascular disease is present, it needs to be treated early and effectively using healthy diet and activity, lipid-lowering agents, aspirin and antihypertensive agents.
- Hyperglycaemia should be controlled to promote comfort, reduce cardiovascular risks and microvascular disease, enhance self-care capacity, reduce falls risk, manage hyperglycaemia-related symptoms and prevent dehydration and consequent risk of ketoacidosis, hyperosmolar states, delirium, cognitive impairment and depression.

Box 7.2.2 Some guidelines for managing diabetes in older people

- International Diabetes Federation. *Managing older people with type 2 diabetes: Global guidelines.* IDF, Belgium 2014. Available at: http://www.idf.org/sites/default/files/IDF-Guideline-for-older-people-T2D.pdf
- A section in The American Diabetes Association (ADA) Diabetes Management Guidelines (2004), which was based on the Californian Healthcare Foundation/American Geriatrics Society Guidelines (AGS) [26].
- Australian Diabetes Educators Association (ADEA) (2003) Guidelines for Managing Diabetes in the Elderly, ADEA, Canberra.
- British Geriatrics Society Best Practice Guide (2009) reviewed 2012. http://www.bgs.org.uk/Publishing%2DDownloads/good_practice_full/diabetes>6-4 (accessed September 2012).
- Joslin Diabetes Centre and Diabetes Clinic (2007) Guidelines for the Care of the Older Adult with Diabetes [27].
- Diabetes Australia (2012) Diabetes Management in Aged Care: a Practical Guide. Diabetes Australia, Canberra.
- Royal Australian College of General Practitioners (RACGP) (2005) Medical Care of Older Persons in Residential Aged Care Facilities http://www.racgp.org.au/silverbookonline/11-2.asp (accessed September 2012).
- Sinclair et al. Diabetes Mellitus in Older People Position statement on behalf of the International Association of Gerontology and Geriatrics (IAGG), the European Diabetes Working Party for Older People (EDWPOP) and the International Task Force of Experts in Diabetes [20].

- Regular screening for and managing geriatric syndromes is essential, including in hospital, see Box 7.2.1.
- Parmacovigilance, which can be achieved using quality use of medicines (QUM) [28]. QUM is a decision-making framework that applies to the entire medication pathway but clinically it means:
  o selecting medicines options wisely based on a comprehensive assessment
  o using non-medicine options where possible but choosing a suitable medicines/s if medicines are indicated
  o using medicines safely and effectively and monitoring the outcomes, which encompasses regular clinical assessment and medicine reviews.

Significantly, older people are not a homogeneous group; therefore, research, even when it is well designed, cannot always be generalised to individual older people, which highlights the need to provide individualised, holistic, person-centred care that takes account of the individual's social situation and support systems. The significant number of diabetes complications and comorbidities and their severity in older people highlights the importance of involving an interdisciplinary team, including general practitioners, diabetes experts, geriatricians and other experts as required.

7.2.6 General health care

It is essential that general health care is incorporated into diabetes management plans and guidelines for older people. General health care includes immunisation, health screening such as mammograms and bowel and prostate checks, oral health and hearing assessments, and assessing functional status and capabilities, such as driving and self-care.

In addition, it is important to regularly assess quality of life, for which standardised, valid tools can be used. It can be more useful to determine the individual's top three to five quality of life issues and monitor changes in them, for example using a likert scale [26]. The latter is a patient-generated quality of life tool and is likely to reflect issues relevant to the individual, such as pets. Such tools can be combined with standardised quality of life tools.

7.2.7 Blood glucose monitoring and blood glucose targets

Blood glucose monitoring

The value of blood glucose self-monitoring in type 2 diabetes is debated and there is no evidence that it reduces morbidity and mortality in older people [29]. It is argued that it is of limited value in improving glycaemic control in people with type 2 diabetes on oral glucose-lowering medicines or diet unless it is accompanied by appropriate health professional and individual education about how to use the information to titrate medicine doses[30].

However, Murata et al. [31] demonstrated intensive blood glucose monitoring improved HbA1c in veterans with type 2 diabetes (mean age of 65) on insulin. Blood glucose monitoring may depend on the treatment modality and glycaemic control and the individual's capability [27]. It is imperative in older people with type 1 diabetes, those with hypoglycaemic unawareness and older people with type 2 diabetes on insulin and sulfonylureas to detect hypo- and hyper-glycaemia and prevent short-term complications that could lead to hospital admission. In addition it is useful when the management plan is being actively modified. Blood glucose self-monitoring is important for improving glycaemia and is a useful risk assessment and management strategy.

Blood glucose targets

The UKPDS [32] showed the benefits of good blood glucose control take at least eight years to manifest, whereas the benefits of controlling blood pressure and lipids are usually evident in two to three years [33] thus, considering the expected life span is important when determining management targets. Likewise, moderate blood glucose control enhances wound healing, reduces hyperglycaemia-related symptoms such as lethargy, pain and lowered mood, and improves cognitive functioning.

There is little evidence that tight blood glucose control is beneficial in older people with functional deficits in activities of daily living [34]. However, older people with few functional deficits may benefit from optimising glycaemic control because they currently have worse morbidity than age-matched older people without diabetes [34].

The target blood glucose range should be individualised; generally 4–11 mmol/L, and regularly reviewed. Hypoglycaemia risk must be assessed and monitored, remembering hypoglycaemia, including serious hypoglycaemia, can be difficult to recognise in older people. Neuroglycopaenic symptoms, such as confusion, delirium, dizziness, weakness and falls, often predominate in older people with diabetes [27]. Consequently, hypoglycaemia is often overlooked and has serious mental and physical consequences.

7.2.8 Nutrition and activity

Although several countries have dietary guidelines for older people, there is little evidence to support most of them. While overweight older people benefit from weight loss, rigorous diets do not result in significant improvements in glycaemic control in older people living in RACFs [35]. Many older people with diabetes are deficient in essential amino acids and trace elements, thus supplements containing magnesium, zinc and vitamins C, D and E may be beneficial.

Underweight and undernutrition are key considerations in older people. Nutritional deficiencies can affect medicine transport and affect medication safety; therefore regular nutritional assessments are essential. Indicators of poor nutrition include:

• Significant change in weight: 10% of weight and/or unplanned weight loss or gain of >12 kg in six months.
• Body mass index <22 or >27, mid arm circumference <10th percentile.
• Serum prealbumin <15 mg/dl, albumin <3.5 g/dl, transferrin <200 mg /dl, cholesterol <160 mg/dl [1].

Older people often require less energy, depending on gender, body composition and activity. Carbohydrate and fat content should be individualised. Protein requirements often increase during wound healing, such as after surgery and pressure and venous ulcers and other stressors, and may need to be modified in end-stage renal disease.

Physical activity is also essential for optimal health and wellbeing, maintaining strength and mobility and managing blood glucose levels. Strength training and exercises to promote strength and balance are important and contribute to blood glucose control, improve mobility and prevent falls [36,37]. However, diet and exercise are often inadequate and glucose-lowering medicines are required. Smoking cessation is also essential.

7.2.9 Medicines: The need for pharmacovigilance

Many older people take several medicines (polypharmacy) at various dose intervals throughout the day and are at significant risk of interactions and adverse events due to medicines mismanagement, and altered renal and liver function, which affects the pharmaocodynamics and pharmacokinetics of medicines and increases the risk of medicine-related adverse events. Thus, regular medicines reviews are essential, including when doses or the dose regimen change. In addition, individualised medicines education for the person with diabetes and carers is essential. As indicated, QUM and considering the Beers Criteria recommendations [38] are helpful when making medicine decisions.

Glucose-lowering medicines

Long acting oral agents are contraindicated because of the risk of hypoglycaemia. Short acting agents that have a lower hypoglycaemia risk are preferable. Renal function should be monitored when using metformin. It should not be used in older men with serum creatinine 1.5 mg/dL, women with serum creatinine of 1.4 mg/ dL or in either gender if there is a risk of lactic acidosis. Older people on metformin should have serum creatinine measured at least annually. A timed urine collection to assess creatinine clearance should be used for people over 80 who have reduced muscle mass. Metformin and alpha glucosidase inhibitors might also be contraindicated in coexisting gastrointestinal disease.

There is concern about the risk of fluid retention, the effects on bone mineral density and cardiovascular risks with thiazolidinediones in older people [7]. Some short-term trials indicate that dipeptidyl peptidase-4 inhibitors (DPP-4) are effective in older people [39]. Although insulin is classified as a high risk medicine, and the Beers criteria suggest sliding scales should not be used in older people, rapid-acting insulins and long-acting insulin analogues can reduce polypharmacy and have a lower hypoglycaemia risk than other insulins, including premixed insulins. However, the latter can enable community-dwelling older people to safely manage their insulin, especially if insulin pens are used [40].

Lipid-lowering medicines

Where possible, and safe, dyslipidaemia should be corrected to reduce the risk of cardiovascular events, but clinical judgement is important. Controlling blood glucose helps control lipids. Diet and exercise should be first line treatment, but lipid-lowering agents may be needed [8]. Lowering LDL cholesterol and increasing HDL is generally important; but the choice of lipid-lowering agent depends on the underlying lipid abnormality, life expectancy, age and frailty level. Frailty is associated with increasing age, lower cholesterol and increased mortality. High cholesterol in the very old is associated with longevity [41]. Lipid targets are shown in Table 7.2.1. Liver function needs to be monitored within 12 weeks of prescribing niacin, statins and fibrates and when doses change [42].

Antihypertensive agents

Targets are shown in Table 7.2.1. The risk of postural hypotension and consequent falls must be considered. Diuretics, angiotensin converting enzyme inhibitors (ACE), beta blockers and calcium channel blockers are used, depending on the underlying abnormality. Older people are less tolerant of rapid changes in blood pressure, therefore, using the lowest effective dose and slowly titrating the dose is likely to be safer and enhance medicine adherence. Renal function and serum potassium and electrolytes need to be monitored when using thiazide diuretics.

Aspirin

Aspirin might be beneficial if the individual is not using any other anticoagulant therapy and does not have contraindications to aspirin. Generally the dose ranges between 81 and 325 mg [29].

Education

Education programs for groups and individuals need to be adapted to suit the cognitive capability and learning style and sometimes include family and carers. Education should be individualised where possible. For example, when older people are sick and hyperglycaemic they are likely to have cognitive changes that affect their ability to make decisions. At such times the best advice for managing sick days might be to tell them or their carer to call the doctor. Significantly, cognitive and functional capability can change rapidly in older people. Therefore, educating health professionals about managing diabetes in older people is important.

7.2.10 Surgical care

Older people require surgery for a number of reasons. Recently, the American College of Surgeons and the American Geriatrics Society released guidelines to help improve the surgical care of people over 65 [43]. The Guidelines emphasise the need for interdisciplinary team care and comprehensive pre-operative assessment to reduce surgical risks. Recommended assessments are encompassed in 13 key areas that reflect physical and mental functioning, geriatric syndromes (Box 7.2.3), nutritional status, cardiac and respiratory risk, and medicines.

Interestingly, although the guidelines suggest ascertaining whether the person is using herbal

---

Box 7.2.3 Strategies to improve the care of older people with diabetes

- Keep the regimen as simple as possible
- Individualise care based on:

  ° Individual's preferences
  ° Self-care capabilities
  ° Mental health
  ° Cognitive status
  ° Renal and liver status
  ° Functional status
  ° Life expectancy
  ° Availability of social and self-care support.

- Monitor blood glucose to detect hypo- and hyper-glycaemia early
- Treat hypertension and dyslipidaemia
- Manage hyperglycaemia: generally HbA1c < 7% but HbA1c < 8% in vulnerable and frail older people at risk of hypoglycaemia and related risks.
- Undertake comprehensive complication screening that includes functional capacity, cognitive status, oral health, self-care capacity, falls risk, hypolycaemia risk, risk of nutritional deficiencies and presence of geriatric syndromes
- Regularly review medicine regimen, especially when introducing new medicines or stopping existing medicines and when health status changes.

---

medicines, they do not provide guidance about herbal medicines that could pose a risk in surgical patients. For example, commonly used herbal medicines such as *Hypericum perforatum* (St John's wort), *Echinacea* species, *Angelica sinensis* (Dong qua) interact with warfarin and increase the risk of bleeding. Others interact with oral glucose-lowering medicines and increase the risk of hypoglycaemia, yet others interact with antihypertensive and lipid-lowering agents and sedatives [44]. In addition, some need to be stopped several days before surgery.

7.2.11 Annual health assessment

Comprehensive health assessments are essential *in addition to regular diabetes-related assessments* and may be required more frequently than annually, for example when health status changes. As well as diabetes-related assessments,

the following issues should be assessed and included in a holistic care plan:

- Functional status and the effect on independence, driving safely and pain. Pain is under assessed and under treated in older people and contributes to hyperglycaemia, depression and reduced quality of life.
- Geriatric syndromes and delirium see Box 7.2.1.
- Hearing and vision
- Advanced care planning
- Home medicine review
- Proactive risk assessment for pain, falls, hypoglycaemia and hyperglycaemia
- Health screening: mammogram, pap smear, prostate check
- There is strong evidence that many commonly prescribed medicines should not be used in older people. These include antipsychotic medicines to manage behavioural problems associated with dementia, long-acting sulfonylureas, sliding insulin scales [38]. Thus, regular comprehensive medicines reviews are needed especially when multiple prescribers are involved and can be undertaken at home. As indicated, QUM and The Beers Criteria [38] and the risks associated with high risk medicines influence medicine choices.

7.2.12 Summary

Managing diabetes in older people is complex. Hyperglycaemic and hypoglycaemic symptoms are often atypical and under-recognised. Physical and mental changes are common and affect self-care capacity and safety. Delirium and geriatric

---

Key points

- Diabetes is common in the elderly.
- The elderly are not a homogeneous group and treatment and management should be individualised.
- Weight management should address undernutrition and weight loss as well as obesity and overweight.
- There is little evidence for nutritional guidelines for the elderly with diabetes.

---

syndromes must be considered. Care should be individualised and holistic and the adoption of early detection and risk assessment and risk minimising strategies is essential.

References

1. Mooradian A, Mclaughlin S, Boyer C, Winter J. Diabetes care for older adults. *Diabetes Spectrum* 1999; **12**(2): 70–77.

2. Chiasson J, Josse R, Gomis. STOP-NIDDIM trial Research Group. Acarbose for the prevention of type 2 diabetes mellitus. The STOP-NIDDIM randomised trial. *Lancet* 2002; **359**(9323): 2072–2077.

3. Gu K, Cowie C, Harris M. Mortality differences between adults with and without diabetes in a national sample 1973–1993. *Diabetes* 1997; **46**(Suppl): 26A.

4. Zhang Y, Hu G, Yuan Z, Chen L. Glycosylated haemoglobin in relationship to cardiovascular outcomes and death in patients with type 2 diabetes; a systematic review and meta-analysis. *PloS ONE* 2012; **7**(8): e42551.

5. Amer P, Pollare T, Lithell H. Different aetiologies of type 2 (non-insulin dependent) diabetes mellitus in obese and non-obese subjects. *Diabeteologia* 1991; **34**: 483–487.

6. Meneilly G, Elliott T. Metabolic alterations in middle aged and elderly obese patients with type 2 diabetes. *Diabetes Care* 1999; **22**: 12–118.

7. Meneilly GS, Knip A, Tessier D, Canadian Diabetes Association Clinical Practice Guidelines Expert Committee. Diabetes in the elderly. *Can J Diabetes* 2013; **37**(Suppl. 1): S184–S190.

8. Kirkman MS, Briscoe VJ, Clark N, Florez H, Haas LB, Halter JB, et al. Diabetes in older adults. *Diabetes Care* 2012; **35**(12): 2650–2664.

9. Cahoon C. Depression in older adults *Am J Nurs* 2012; **112**(11): 22–30.

10. Californian Healthcare Foundation and the American Geriatrics Society Panel (AGS) on Improving Care of the Older Person with Diabetes. Guidelines for improving the care of the older person with diabetes mellitus. *J Am Geriatr Soc* 2003; **51**(Suppl. 5): s25–s27.

11. United States Department of Health and Human Services Centres for Disease Control and Prevention. National Diabetes Fact Sheet on Diabetes in the United States in 2011. Atlanta GA: Centres for Disease Control and Prevention, 2011.

12. Australian Diabetes Society (ADS). Position Statement: Individualisation of HbA1c Targets for Adults with Diabetes https://diabetessociety.com.au/downloads/positionstatements/HbA1ctargets.pdf (accessed 22 June 2015).

13. American Psychiatric Association. Diagnostic and Statistical Manual of Mental Disorders (DSM-1V-TR). Washington DC, 2000.

14. Inouye S. Delirium. in Cassel C (ed.) Geriatric Medicine, New York: Springer-Verlag, 2003.

15. Hall M. Serotonin syndrome. *Aust Prescriber* 2003; **26**: 62–63.

16. European Diabetes Working Party for Older People 2001–2004. Clinical Guidelines for Type 2 Diabetes www.euroage-diabetes.com (accessed September 2012).

17. Sinclair A, Allard I, Bayer A. Observations of diabetes care in long-term institutional settings with measures of cognitive function and dependency. *Diabetes Care* 1997; **20**(5): 778–784.

18. Brown A, Mangione C, Saliba D, Sarkison C. Californian Healthcare Foundation and the American Geriatrics Society Panel (AGS) on Improving Care of the Older Person with Diabetes. Guidelines for improving the care of the older person with diabetes mellitus. *J Am Geriatr Soc* 2003; **51**(Suppl. 5): s265–s280.

19. Haas L. Management of diabetes mellitus medications in nursing homes. *Drugs Aging* 2005; **22** (3): 309–218.

20. Sinclair A. Diabetes mellitus in older people: Position statement on behalf of the International Association of Gerontology and Geriatrics (IAGG), the European Diabetes Working Party for Older People (EDWPOP) and the International Task Force of Experts in Diabetes. *JAMA* 2012; **13**(8) 487–502.

21. Keech A, Colquhoun D, Best J. LIPID Study group Secondary prevention of cardiovascular events with long term pravastatin in patients with diabetes or impaired fasting glucose, results form the LIPID trial. *Diabetes Care* 2003; **26**: 2713–2721.

22. Collins R, Armitage J, Parish S. Health Protection Collaborative Study group. Effects of cholesterol lowering with simvastatin on stroke and other major vascular events in 20536 people with cerebrovascular disease or other high risk conditions. *Lancet* 2004; **363**: 737–767.

23. Expert Panel on Detection, Evaluation, And Treatment of High Blood Cholesterol In Adults (Adult Treatment Panel III) Executive Summary of The Third Report of The National Cholesterol Education Program (NCEP). *JAMA* 2001; **285**: 2486–2497.

24. Duckworth W, Abraira C, Moritz T, Reda D, Emanuele N, Reaven PD, et al.; VADT Investigators. Glucose control and vascular complications in veterans with type 2 diabetes. *N Engl J Med* 2009; **360**(2): 129–139.

25. Dunning T, Savage S, Duggan N. McKellar guidelines for managing older people with diabetes in residential

and other care settings. Centre for Nursing and Allied Health Research, Geelong, Australia, 2014.

26. Olson D Norris S. Diabetes in older adults: overview of AGS guidelines for treatment of diabetes mellitus in geriatric populations *Geriatrics* 2004; **59** (4): 18–25.

27. Joslin Diabetes Centre and Joslin Clinic. Guideline for the Care of the Older Adult https://www.joslin.org/docs/Guideline_For_Care_Of_Older_Adults_with_Diabetes.pdf (accessed 22 June 2015).

28. Department of Health and Ageing. National Strategy for Quality Use of Medicines http://www.health.gov.au/internet/main/publishing.nsf/Content/nmp-quality.htm (accessed 22 June 2015).

29. Jenkinson C, McGee H. Health Status Measurement. Oxford: Radcliffe Medical Press, 1998.

30. Clar C, Barnard K, Cummins E, Royle P, Waugh N. Self-monitoring of blood glucose in type 2 diabetes: systematic review *High Technol Assess* 2010, **14** (12) 1–140.

31. Murata G, Shah J, Hoffman R, Wendel C, Adam K, Solvas P, et al. Intensified blood glucose monitoring improves glycaemia control in stable, insulin-treated veterans with type 2 diabetes: the Diabetes outcomes in Veterans Study (DOVES) *Diabetes Care* 2003; **26:** 1759–1763.

32. United Kingdom Prospective Study Group (UKPDS) Intensive blood glucose control with sulphonylureas or insulin compared with conventional treatment and risk of complications in patients with type 2 diabetes. (UKPDS 33) *Lancet* 1998; **352**(9131): 837–853.

33. United Kingdom Prospective Study Group (UKPDS). Tight blood pressure control and risk of macrovascular and microvascular complications in type 2 diabetes: (UKPDS 38) *BMJ* 1998; **317**: 703–713.

34. Blaum C, Ofstedal M, Langa K, Wray L. Functional status and health outcomes in older Americans with diabetes. *J Am Geriatr Soc* 2003; **51**(6): 745–753.

35. Coulson A, Mandelbaum D, Reaven G. Dietary management in nursing home residents with non-insulin dependent diabetes mellitus. *Am J Clin Nutr* 1990; **51**: 67–71.

36. Nelson M, Rejeski W, Blaor S. Physical activity and public health in older adults: recommendations from the American College of Sports Medicine and the American Heart Association. *Med Sci Sports Exercise* 2007; **39**: 328–336.

37. Kayani R, Saudek C, Brancati F. Association of diabetes, comorbidities and A1c with functional disability in older adults: results from the National Health and Nutrition Examination Survey (NHANES 1999–2006) *Diabetes Care* 2010; **33**: 1055–1060.

38. American Geriatrics Society. American Geriatrics Society updated Beers criteria for potentially inappropriate medication use in older adults. *J Am Geriatr Soc* **60**(4): 616–631.

39. Pratley R, McCall T, Fleck P. Alogiptin use in elderly people: a pooled analysis from phase 2 and 3 studies *J Am Geriatr Soc* 2009; **57**: 2011–2019.

40. Corsi A, Torree E, Coronel G. Prefilled insulin pen in newly insulin treated diabetic patients over 60 years *Diabetes Nutr Metab* 1990; **10**: 78–81.

41. Schupf N, Costa R, Luchsinger J, Tang MX, Lee JH, Mayeux R. Relationship between plasma lipids and all-cause mortality in non-demented elderly. *J Am Geriatr Soc* 2005; **53**: 219–226.

42. Streja D, Streja E. Management of dyslipidaemia in the elderly. *EndoText*, Ch. 4, 2011. http://www.ncbi.nlm.nih.gov/books/NBK279133/ (accessed 22 June 2015).

43. Chow W, Rosenthal R, Merkow R, Ko C, Esnaola N. Clinical Perioperative Assessment of the geriatric Patient: A Best Practice Guideline form the American College of Surgeons National Quality Improvement Program and the American Geriatrics Society. *J Am Coll Surg* 2012; **216**(4): 463–496.

44. Braun L, Cohen M. Herbs and Natural Supplements: an Evidence-based Guide. Australia: Churchill Livingstone, 2010.

SECTION 8

Diabetes in ethnic groups

Chapter 8.1

Epidemiology, aetiology and pathogenesis of diabetes in ethnic groups

Louise Goff
King's College London, London, UK

8.1.1 Introduction

Ethnicity can be described as a group to which people belong or are perceived to belong, according to a variety of individual factors they share, including ancestral origins, genetic traits, social, economic, geographical, dietary and cultural traditions and languages [1,2]. The term 'ethnic minority group' is often used to describe migrant populations, that is people residing in a country different to that of their birth. However, in many regions of the world there are second and third generations of migrants for whom country of birth does not represent their ethnic origin, hence the use of terminology such as Black-British and Asian-American, which accounts for ancestry and place of birth.

In any region of the world there is considerable variability in the prevalence of diabetes amongst different ethnic groups. Furthermore, within a given ethnic group there are significant differences in the prevalence of diabetes between different environments, suggesting there are both genetic and environmental factors contributing to the development of diabetes.

Whilst in any given region of the world there are minority ethnic groups that have disproportionately high prevalence of diabetes compared to both the relevant traditional population and the host population, it is important to also consider that in some regions of the world there are indigenous or native populations, for example the Aborigines of Australia and the Native Indians of North America, who may not be defined as 'minority ethnic groups' but who are minority populations at very high risk of diabetes and therefore should be a target for prevention strategies.

8.1.2 Epidemiology

Within the United States (US), African-Americans, Hispanics and Asian Americans are the minority ethnic groups of most importance when considering diabetes prevalence. Data from the National Health Interview Survey (NHIS, 2007–2009) are listed in Table 8.1.1 and

Table 8.1.1 Diabetes prevalence, by ethnicity, in the United States

Ethnic group	Diabetes prevalence (%)
Non-Hispanic white	7.1
Asian American	8.4
Hispanic	11.8
Cubans and Central & South American	7.6
Mexican American	13.3
Puerto Rican	13.8
Non-Hispanic black	12.6

2007–2009 NHIS data for people aged 20 years or older, adjusted for population age differences.

Advanced Nutrition and Dietetics in Diabetes, First Edition. Edited by Louise Goff and Pamela Dyson.
© 2016 John Wiley & Sons, Ltd. Published 2016 by John Wiley & Sons, Ltd.

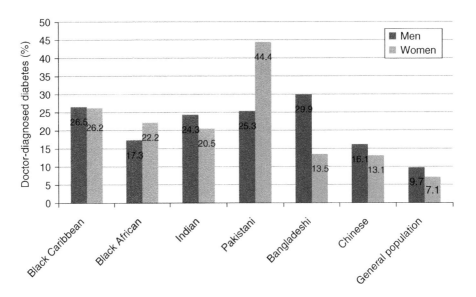

Figure 8.1.1   Prevalence of doctor-diagnosed diabetes, by sex, within minority ethnic groups aged 55 years and over

show the prevalence of diabetes (types 1 and 2 combined) amongst the main minority ethnic groups of the US, adjusted for age differences [3]. When compared to non-Hispanic white adults, the risk of diagnosed diabetes was 18% higher among Asian Americans, 66% higher among Hispanics, and 77% higher among non-Hispanic blacks, driven predominantly by the high prevalence of type 2 diabetes in these communities [3]. The Strong Heart Study assessed the prevalence of diabetes and impaired glucose tolerance amongst native American Indian tribes from three geographical locations and reported age-standardized diabetes prevalence of 44 and 54% for men and women, respectively [4].

In the United Kingdom (UK), data from the 2004 'Health Survey for England: the health of minority ethnic groups' provides information on the prevalence of diabetes amongst important minority ethnic groups of the UK [5]. In all ethnic groups, diabetes prevalence is highest in the 55 years+ age group; the prevalence rates can be seen in Figure 8.1.1. As in the US, Black African and Caribbean and South Asian communities show higher prevalence, and although the prevalence appears higher in the UK compared to the US, this is likely due to the older age of the population in the UK data.

In Australasia, minority ethnic groups with a particularly high prevalence of diabetes include those from the Pacific Islands (e.g. Tonga, Samoa, Fiji), Singapore, Pakistan, India, the Philippines and Sri Lanka [6,7], although it is acknowledged that African and Middle Eastern communities are becoming increasingly important. The prevalence of diabetes amongst the indigenous groups of Aborigines and Torres Strait Islanders has been reported as 8.9 and 45.2% for male and female Aborigines, respectively, and 34.2 and 41.8% for male and female Torres Strait Islanders, respectively [8].

Type 2 diabetes is increasingly recognized in childhood and, similarly to adult prevalence, children from ethnic minority groups experience significantly higher risks of developing type 2 diabetes than do children of White-European ancestry. Data from the UK have estimated the relative risk of type 2 diabetes in South Asian children is 14 times greater than in White-European children [9], which may be driven by higher body fat and central fat accumulation [10]. Recent data from the US SEARCH for Diabetes in Youth study has demonstrated a 30.5% increase in type 2 diabetes prevalence amongst 10–19 year olds between 2001 and

2009, driven predominantly by high rates amongst ethnic minority children: in 2009 the prevalence of type 2 diabetes was highest amongst American Indian youth (1.20 per 1000), followed by Black youth (1.06 per 1000), Hispanic youth (0.79 per 1000), with lowest rates amongst White American youth (0.17 per 1000) [11]. Native American Indian children are also recognized for disproportionately high rates of type 2 diabetes [12].

Whilst much of the literature focuses on type 2 diabetes amongst ethnic minority groups, there are other types of diabetes that are particularly prevalent amongst specific ethnic groups, for example atypical ketosis prone diabetes (AKPD). AKPD, also known as Flatbush diabetes and ketosis-prone type 2 diabetes, was originally described by Winter et al. [13] amongst African-American patients who presented with diabetic ketoacidosis but subsequently resemble the progression of type 2 diabetes (i.e. spontaneous remission requiring discontinuation of insulin therapy within a few weeks). This presentation has mainly been reported in people of African ancestry but also in Chinese [14], Japanese [15] and South Asian patients [16]. The natural course of AKPD is distinct from either type 1 diabetes or type 2 diabetes, however, its pathogenesis is poorly understood.

8.1.3 Aetiology

The identification of ethnic patterns of health and disease has led to a wealth of research exploring the genetic and environmental or lifestyle factors that may be responsible. Epidemiological evidence, recognizing different rates of disease within an ethnic group living in different countries (migration), shows that the prevalence of diabetes is influenced by environmental factors. For example, Asian-Indians living in rural areas of India have a prevalence of diabetes of about 2%. Asian-Indians living in urban India have a prevalence of diabetes of about 8%. Asian-Indians migrated to the UK or other westernized countries, such as Singapore, have about four times higher prevalence of diabetes compared to those living in India [17,18]. Similarly African-Americans

have been shown to have a prevalence of diabetes at least 12 times greater than that observed among native African blacks (12 and 1%, respectively) [19–22].

Migration studies have been important in identifying, in more detail, the impact of westernization on diabetes development; the Pima Indian studies are the most frequently cited of these. The Pima Indians of Arizona have the highest reported worldwide prevalence of type 2 diabetes [23]. Ravussin et al. [24] compared the prevalence of type 2 diabetes in Pima Indians living in Arizona to members of a population of Pima ancestry living in rural Mexico; the two genetically related populations had very different prevalence of diabetes. The Pima Indians living in Mexico were found to have a prevalence of 6 and 11%, for men and women, respectively, as compared to the frequency of 54 and 37% reported in the Pima Indians living in Arizona [24]. Investigations of the environmental factors that may be responsible for this markedly different prevalence between two populations who share the same genetic background have recognized parallel differences in obesity and body fat accumulation (including central obesity) between these traditional and migrant communities [25] and propose that they are a product of significantly reduced physical activity [26] and higher fat diets amongst the US Pimas than the Mexican group [27]: features of 'Westernization'. These studies and others [28] provide compelling evidence that changes in lifestyle associated with Westernization play a major role in the development of type 2 diabetes.

Epidemiological studies performed in North America, Europe and Australia have identified that ethnic minority groups (South Asian, Black African, Chinese) experience a higher risk of diabetes at lower levels of obesity than Whites [29–31]. This suggests that conventional clinical definitions for obesity that were derived from populations of White European descent (BMI ≥ 30 kg/m^2; waist circumference ≥ 88 cm in women and ≥ 102 cm in men) may not be appropriate for identifying diabetes risk in non-white groups. In response the World Health Organization (WHO) and International Diabetes

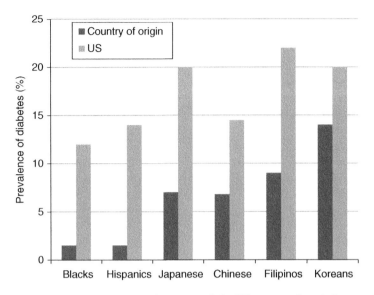

Figure 8.1.2 Prevalence of diabetes for ethnic groups of the US compared to their countries of origin. (Reproduced from Abate and Chandalia, *J. Diabetes Complications* **17** (2003) 39–58)

Federation (IDF) have proposed Asian specific thresholds in which overweight is defined as a BMI >23 kg/m^2 and obesity >27.5 kg/m^2, with waist circumference cut-offs of 80 cm for Asian women and 90 cm for Asian men [32,33]. At the time of publication there were insufficient data to derive specific cut-offs for Black men and women and European thresholds were recommended for use in these communities. In recent data from the UK Biobank, Ntuk et al. have demonstrated that compared to White men and women with a BMI of 30 kg/m^2, diabetes prevalence was equivalent in Black men and women with a BMI of 26 kg/m^2 [34].

Figure 8.1.2 summarizes the different prevalence of diabetes within the same ethnic group under different environmental conditions. The process of urbanization/westernization is clearly associated with a progressive increase in the prevalence of type 2 diabetes across all ethnic groups. However, there are differences in the reported prevalence of diabetes among various ethnic groups, suggesting that there is an ethnic susceptibility to diabetes. Epidemiological observations conducted in multi-ethnic populations highlight a different predisposition of various ethnic groups to develop diabetes when exposed to similar environmental challenges (Figure 8.1.3).

8.1.4 Pathogenesis

The pathogenesis of type 2 diabetes involves both insufficient insulin secretion and tissue insulin resistance. It was originally proposed that the principal abnormality in the development of type 2 diabetes was that of insulin resistance. This resistance would subsequently lead to hypersecretion of insulin in order to maintain normoglycaemia and only when the β-cells failed to secrete sufficient insulin to counteract the tissue resistance would hyperglycaemia result. However, it is now evident that there is a large variation in the relationship between insulin sensitivity and insulin secretion. A given individual may be severely insulin resistant but maintain normal glucose tolerance if β-cell secretory capacity matches the degree of insulin resistance. On the other hand, an individual may have a low β-cell secretory functional capacity but maintain normoglycaemia if insulin sensitivity is maintained to match the low β-cell function. The predominant mechanism leading to impaired glucose tolerance and diabetes appears to differ between different ethnicities. Whilst insulin resistance and β-cell dysfunction characterize the development of type 2 diabetes in Pima Indians [35], it is interesting to note that people

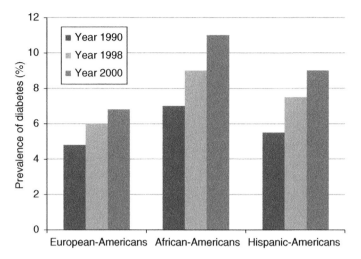

Figure 8.1.3 Prevalence of diabetes in various US ethnic groups (Mokdad et al., 2000, 2001). (Reproduced from Abate and Chandalia, *J. Diabetes Complications* **17** (2003) 39–58)

of African ancestry with diabetes have been reported to have relatively low rates of insulin resistance. Banerji and Lebovitz demonstrated that 50% of African-American patients with diabetes were insulin sensitive and the predominant mechanism leading to hyperglycaemia appeared to be β-cell dysfunction [36]. A number of studies in non-diabetic children and adults of African ancestry support these findings of hyperinsulinaemia. In the UKPDS study, South Asian diabetic patients were shown to be the most insulin-resistant ethnic group, compared to white-European and black African-Caribbean [37].

Insulin resistance is associated with the development of a clustering of metabolic abnormalities, now termed metabolic syndrome, which includes hyperinsulinaemia, increased plasma very low density lipoprotein (VLDL), triglyceride and small dense low density lipoprotein (LDL) and low high-density lipoprotein (HDL) concentrations, increased clotting activity (PAI-1) and hypertension as well as dysglycaemia [38]. These abnormalities contribute to the high prevalence of cardiovascular disease (CVD) in metabolic syndrome and type 2 diabetes [39,40]. South Asian and Hispanic populations commonly exhibit multiple features of the metabolic syndrome in the pre-diabetic and diabetic state, however, African ancestry groups have a different presentation: whilst they are characteristically

insulin resistant [41–45], they develop marked and early hypertension [44], with a cardioprotective lipid profile (low total and LDL-cholesterol, high HDL-cholesterol and low triglycerides) [41,45]. They do have high rates of CVD, at least in the diaspora [46] but their outcomes are different, with lower rates of myocardial infarction but high rates of stroke (and renal failure) [47–49] relating to their hypertension [44]. It must be noted that, in the US, a changing mortality profile in African-American populations is already evident with increasing levels of myocardial infarction in younger populations [50], a marker of advanced 'Westernization'.

Studies performed in a number of ethnic groups have shown that increasing body fat content is linearly and inversely related to insulin resistance [51–53], however, only 50% of the variability of insulin sensitivity is explained by obesity. It is now accepted that fat distribution, particularly abdominal/visceral fat, is a more sensitive predictor of insulin sensitivity than BMI. Several studies have demonstrated that when fat is distributed preferentially in the visceral area, insulin-mediated glucose disposal is reduced, independent of overall degree of adiposity [51–53]. Ethnic groups such as Hispanics and South Asians are more prone to developing visceral obesity and have more insulin resistance than African-ancestry groups or white-Europeans, who develop less visceral obesity for a similar BMI. Lovejoy et al. assessed visceral fat accumulation in a group of African-American and European-American women, matched for BMI and age, and showed that the African-American women had significantly less visceral fat than the European-American women, even though they were markedly more insulin resistant [54]. Such differences persisted after weight gain [55] and weight loss [56] and, furthermore, these differences have been recognized in African-American youths, indicating that these differences manifest early in life [57].

Ectopic fat is defined by the deposition of triglycerides within cells of non-adipose tissue that normally contain only small amounts of fat. Visceral fat has been the most widely researched ectopic fat depot but other depots of importance include the liver (intrahepatocellular lipid, IHCL), muscle (intramyocellular lipid, IMCL) and pancreatic cells. These are believed to be important in the development of insulin resistance [58], however, ethnicity specific patterns have not been well investigated. In European populations, IMCL has been shown to be consistently correlated with measures of insulin resistance; studies in South Asian populations have consistently shown elevated IMCL [59,60] and IHCL [61,62]. Ingram et al. have assessed IMCL in individuals of European and African ancestry and recognized that in people of African ancestry IMCL varies in a manner that is independent of insulin resistance [63]. Giday et al. report lower prevalence of hepatic steatosis in African-Americans compared with Euro-Americans, with Hispanics having markedly higher prevalence than any other group [64]. These findings of lower IHCL accumulation in African-American people are likely explained by the lower visceral fat accumulation that is observed. Overall, studies of ectopic fat accumulation show that these features identify a subset of individuals at increased risk of type 2 diabetes and CVD, although these relationships are affected by ethnicity. Data from across different ethnicities highlight differences in the pathogenesis of insulin resistance. Importantly, while IMCL and IHCL accumulation is linked to insulin resistance in European, South Asian and Hispanic groups, studies of people of African ancestry indicate that ectopic fat is not an indispensable feature of insulin resistance in these populations.

8.1.5 Conclusion

Migrant populations across the world exhibit remarkably high prevalence of type 2 diabetes that appears to be associated with an underlying genetic predisposition coupled with adoption of 'Westernized' lifestyles. The mechanisms by which diabetes develops in minority ethnic groups is not well understood and much work is needed. However, we know that South Asian and Hispanic groups develop visceral obesity and insulin resistance, which is accompanied by a detrimental lipid profile, whilst diabetes in people of African ancestry appears to be more strongly driven by β-cell exhaustion following prolonged hyperinsulinaemia and is accompanied by a cardioprotective lipid profile but marked hypertension.

> ## Key points
>
> - Ethnic minority populations are disproportionately affected by type 2 diabetes.
> - Changes in lifestyle associated with 'Westernization' (e.g. sedentariness, excess energy, fat and sugar intakes) play a major role in the development of type 2 diabetes in migrant populations.
> - Diabetes risk occurs at lower levels of adiposity (body mass index) in ethnic minority populations.
> - The predominant pathological mechanism leading to impaired glucose tolerance and diabetes appears to differ between ethnic groups; insulin resistance drives diabetes development in South Asian communities whilst β-cell dysfunction appears to be more important in African ancestry groups.
> - The metabolic syndrome presents classically in South Asian populations but atypically in African populations, in which lower levels of central adiposity are seen alongside lower triglycerides and higher HDL-cholesterol.
> - Ectopic fat accumulation, principally liver, muscle and pancreatic fat, show ethnic specific patterns.

References

1. Bhopal R. Glossary of terms relating to ethnicity and race: for reflection and debate. *J Epidemiol Community Health* 2004; **58**(6): 5.
2. Cruickshank JK, Beevers DG. *Ethnic Factors in Health and Disease*. Oxford: Butterworth-Heinemann Ltd, 1989.
3. National diabetes factsheet: national estimates and general information on diabetes and prediabetes in the United States, 2011. Atlanta, GA: U.S. Department of Health and Human Services, Centers for Disease Control and Prevention, 2011.
4. Lee ET, Howard BV, Savage PJ, Cowan LD, Fabsitz RR, Oopik AJ, et al. Diabetes and impaired glucose tolerance in three American Indian populations aged 45-74 years. The Strong Heart Study. *Diabetes Care* 1995; **18**(5): 599–610.
5. *Health Survey for England 2004: The Health of Minority Ethnic Groups*. Health and Social Care Information Group, 2006.
6. Dunstan DW, Zimmet PZ, Welborn TA, De Courten MP, Cameron AJ, Sicree RA, et al. The rising prevalence of diabetes and impaired glucose tolerance – The Australian diabetes, obesity and lifestyle study. *Diabetes Care* 2002; **25**(5): 829–834.
7. Colagiuri R, Thomas M, Buckley A. Preventing type 2 diabetes in culturally and linguistically diverse communities in NSW. Sydney: NSW Department of Health, 2007.
8. McCulloch B, McDermott R, Miller G, Leonard D, Elwell M, Muller R. Self-reported diabetes and health behaviors in remote in idigenous communities in Northern Queensland, Australia. *Diabetes Care* 2003; **26**(2): 397–403.
9. Ehtisham S, Kirk J, McEvilly A, Shaw N, Jones S, Rose S, et al. Prevalence of type 2 diabetes in children in Birmingham. *BMJ* 2001; **322**(7299): 1428.
10. Ehtisham S, Crabtree N, Clark P, Shaw N, Barrett T. Ethnic differences in insulin resistance and body composition in United Kingdom adolescents. *J Clin Endocrinol Metab* 2005; **90**(7): 3963–3969. doi: 10.1210/jc.2004-2001.
11. Dabelea D, Mayer-Davis EJ, Saydah S, Imperatore G, Linder B, Divers J, et al. Prevalence of type 1 and type 2 diabetes among children and adolescents from 2001 to 2009. *JAMA* 2014; **311**(17): 1778–1786. doi: 10.1001/jama.2014.3201.
12. Nsiah-Kumi PA, Lasley S, Whiting M, Brushbreaker C, Erickson JM, Qiu F, et al. Diabetes, pre-diabetes and insulin resistance screening in Native American children and youth. *Int J Obes (Lond)* 2013; **37**(4): 540–545. doi: 10.1038/ijo.2012.199.
13. Winter WE, Maclaren NK, Riley WJ, Clarke DW, Kappy MS, Spillar RP. Maturity-onset diabetes of youth in black Americans. *N Engl J Med* 1987; **316**(6): 285–291. doi: 10.1056/NEJM198702053160601.
14. Tan KC, Mackay IR, Zimmet PZ, Hawkins BR, Lam KS. Metabolic and immunologic features of Chinese patients with atypical diabetes mellitus. *Diabetes Care* 2000; **23**(3): 335–338.
15. Tanaka K, Moriya T, Kanamori A, Yajima Y. Analysis and a long-term follow up of ketosis-onset Japanese NIDDM patients. *Diabetes Res Clin Pract* 1999; **44**(2): 137–146.
16. Imran SA, Ur E. Atypical ketosis-prone diabetes. *Can Fam Physician* 2008; **54**(11): 1553–1554.
17. Mckeigue PM, Miller GJ, Marmot MG. Coronary Heart-Disease in South Asians Overseas - a Review. *J Clin Epidemiol* 1989; **42**(7): 597–609.
18. Ramachandran A, Snehalatha C, Dharmaraj D, Viswanathan M. Prevalence of Glucose-Intolerance in Asian Indians - Urban-Rural Difference and Significance of Upper-Body Adiposity. *Diabetes Care* 1992; **15**(10): 1348–13455.
19. Carter JS, Pugh JA, Monterrosa A. Non-insulin-dependent diabetes mellitus in minorities in the United States. *Ann Intern Med* 1996; **125**(3): 221–232.
20. Erasmus RT, Fakeye T, Olukoga O, Okesina AB, Ebomoyi E, Adeleye M, et al. Prevalence of Diabetes-Mellitus in a Nigerian Population. *Trans R Soc Trop Med Hyg* 1989; **83**(3): 417–418.
21. Harris MI, Flegal KM, Cowie CC, Eberhardt MS, Goldstein DE, Little RR, et al. Prevalence of diabetes, impaired fasting glucose, and impaired glucose tolerance in U.S. adults. The Third National Health and Nutrition Examination Survey, 1988–1994. *Diabetes Care* 1998; **21**(4): 518–524.
22. Rotimi CN, Cooper RS, Okosun IS, Olatunbosun ST, Bella AF, Wilks R, et al. Prevalence of diabetes and impaired glucose tolerance in Nigerians, Jamaicans and US blacks. *Ethn Dis* 1999; **9**(2): 190–200.
23. King H, Aubert RE, Herman WH. Global burden of diabetes, 1995–2025: prevalence, numerical estimates, and projections. *Diabetes Care* 1998; **21**(9): 1414–1431.
24. Ravussin E, Valencia ME, Esparza J, Bennett PH, Schulz LO. Effects of a traditional lifestyle on obesity in Pima Indians. *Diabetes Care* 1994; **17**(9): 1067–1074.
25. Schulz LO, Bennett PH, Ravussin E, Kidd JR, Kidd KK, Esparza J, et al. Effects of traditional and western environments on prevalence of type 2 diabetes in Pima Indians in Mexico and the U.S. *Diabetes Care* 2006; **29**(8): 1866–1871. doi: 10.2337/dc06-0138.
26. Esparza J, Fox C, Harper IT, Bennett PH, Schulz LO, Valencia ME, et al. Daily energy expenditure in Mexican and USA Pima indians: low physical activity as a possible cause of obesity. International journal of obesity and related metabolic disorders. *J Int Assoc Study Obes* 2000; **24**(1): 55–59.

27. Smith CJ, Nelson RG, Hardy SA, Manahan EM, Bennett PH, Knowler WC. Survey of the diet of Pima Indians using quantitative food frequency assessment and 24-hour recall. Diabetic Renal Disease Study. *J Am Diet Assoc* 1996; **96**(8): 778–784.

28. Stern MP, Gonzalez C, Mitchell BD, Villalpando E, Haffner SM, Hazuda HP. Genetic and environmental determinants of type II diabetes in Mexico City and San Antonio. *Diabetes* 1992; **41**(4): 484–492.

29. Gray LJ, Yates T, Davies MJ, Brady E, Webb DR, Sattar N, et al. Defining obesity cut-off points for migrant South Asians. *PLoS ONE* 2011; **6**(10): e26464. doi: 10.1371/journal.pone.0026464.

30. Razak F, Anand SS, Shannon H, Vuksan V, Davis B, Jacobs R, et al. Defining obesity cut points in a multiethnic population. *Circulation* 2007; **115**(16): 2111–2118. doi: 10.1161/CIRCULATIONAHA.106.635011.

31. Chiu M, Austin PC, Manuel DG, Shah BR, Tu JV. Deriving ethnic-specific BMI cutoff points for assessing diabetes risk. *Diabetes Care* 2011; **34**(8): 1741–1748. doi: 10.2337/dc10-2300.

32. Expert Consultation WHO. Appropriate body mass index for Asian populations and its implications for policy and intervention strategies. *Lancet* 2004; **363**: 157–163.

33. International Diabetes Federation. The IDF consensus worldwide definition of the metabolic syndrome. 2005.

34. Ntuk UE, Gill JM, Mackay DF, Sattar N, Pell JP. Ethnic-specific obesity cutoffs for diabetes risk: cross-sectional study of 490,288 UK biobank participants. *Diabetes Care* 2014; **37**(9): 2500–2507. doi: 10.2337/dc13-2966.

35. Weyer C, Bogardus C, Mott DM, Pratley RE. The natural history of insulin secretory dysfunction and insulin resistance in the pathogenesis of type 2 diabetes mellitus. *J Clin Invest* 1999; **104**(6): 787–794. doi: 10.1172/JCI7231.

36. Banerji MA, Lebovitz HE. Insulin action in black Americans with NIDDM. *Diabetes Care* 1992; **15**(10): 1295–1302.

37. UK Prospective Diabetes Study. XII: Differences between Asian, Afro-Caribbean and white Caucasian type 2 diabetic patients at diagnosis of diabetes. UK Prospective Diabetes Study Group. *Diabet Med* 1994; **11**(7): 670–677.

38. Reaven GM. Banting lecture 1988. Role of insulin resistance in human disease. *Diabetes* 1988; **37**(12): 1595–1607.

39. Reaven GM. Syndrome X: 6 years later. *J Intern Med Suppl* 1994; **736**: 13–22.

40. Reaven GM. Pathophysiology of insulin resistance in human disease. *Physiol Rev* 1995; **75**(3): 473–486.

41. Zoratti R, Godsland IF, Chaturvedi N, Crook D, Stevenson JC, McKeigue PM. Relation of plasma lipids to insulin resistance, nonesterified fatty acid levels, and body fat in men from three ethnic groups: relevance to variation in risk of diabetes and coronary disease. *Metabolism* 2000; **49**(2): 245–252.

42. Osei K, Cottrell DA. Minimal model analyses of insulin sensitivity and glucose-dependent glucose disposal in black and white Americans: a study of persons at risk for type 2 diabetes. *Eur J Clin Invest* 1994; **24**(12): 843–850.

43. Haffner SM, D'Agostino R, Saad MF, Rewers M, Mykkänen L, Selby J, et al. Increased insulin resistance and insulin secretion in nondiabetic African-Americans and Hispanics compared with non-Hispanic whites. The Insulin Resistance Atherosclerosis Study. *Diabetes* 1996; **45**(6): 742–748.

44. Chaturvedi N, McKeigue PM, Marmot MG. Resting and ambulatory blood pressure differences in Afro-Caribbeans and Europeans. *Hypertension* 1993; **22**(1): 90–96.

45. Chaturvedi N, McKeigue PM, Marmot MG. Relationship of glucose intolerance to coronary risk in Afro-Caribbeans compared with Europeans. *Diabetologia* 1994; **37**(8): 765–772.

46. Clark LT, Ferdinand KC, Flack JM, Gavin 3rd JR, Hall WD, Kumanyika SK, et al. Coronary heart disease in African Americans. *Heart Dis* 2001; **3**(2): 97–108.

47. Singh GK, Siahpush M. Ethnic-immigrant differentials in health behaviors, morbidity, and cause-specific mortality in the United States: an analysis of two national data bases. *Hum Biol* 2002; **74**(1): 83–109.

48. Wild S, McKeigue P. Cross sectional analysis of mortality by country of birth in England and Wales, 1970-92. *BMJ* 1997; **314**(7082): 705–710.

49. Tillin T, Forouhi NG, McKeigue PM, Chaturvedi N. The role of diabetes and components of the metabolic syndrome in stroke and coronary heart disease mortality in U.K. white and African-Caribbean populations. *Diabetes Care* 2006; **29**(9): 2127–2129. doi: 10.2337/dc06-0779.

50. Jolly S, Vittinghoff E, Chattopadhyay A, Bibbins-Domingo K. Higher cardiovascular disease prevalence and mortality among younger blacks compared to whites. *Am J Med* 2010; **123**(9): 811–8118.

51. Abate N, Garg A, Peshock RM, Stray-Gundersen J, Grundy SM. Relationships of generalized and regional adiposity to insulin sensitivity in men. *J Clin Invest* 1995; **96**(1): 88–98. doi: 10.1172/JCI118083.

52. Goodpaster BH, Thaete FL, Simoneau JA, Kelley DE. Subcutaneous abdominal fat and thigh muscle composition predict insulin sensitivity independently of visceral fat. *Diabetes* 1997; **46**(10): 1579–1585.

53. Karter AJ, Mayer-Davis EJ, Selby JV, D'Agostino Jr. RB, Haffner SM, Sholinsky P, et al. Insulin sensitivity and abdominal obesity in African-American, Hispanic, and non-Hispanic white men and women. The Insulin

Resistance and Atherosclerosis Study. *Diabetes* 1996; **45**(11): 1547–1555.

54. Lovejoy JC, de la Bretonne JA, Klemperer M, Tulley R. Abdominal fat distribution and metabolic risk factors: effects of race. *Metabolism* 1996; **45**(9): 1119–1124.

55. Lara-Castro C, Weinsier RL, Hunter GR, Desmond R. Visceral adipose tissue in women: longitudinal study of the effects of fat gain, time, and race. *Obes Res* 2002; **10**(9): 868–874. doi: 10.1038/oby.2002.119.

56. Weinsier RL, Hunter GR, Gower BA, Schutz Y, Darnell BE, Zuckerman PA. Body fat distribution in white and black women: different patterns of intraabdominal and subcutaneous abdominal adipose tissue utilization with weight loss. *Am J Clin Nutr* 2001; **74**(5): 631–636.

57. Gower BA, Nagy TR, Goran MI. Visceral fat, insulin sensitivity, and lipids in prepubertal children. *Diabetes* 1999; **48**(8): 1515–1521.

58. Gastaldelli A, Basta G. Ectopic fat and cardiovascular disease: what is the link? Nutrition, metabolism, and cardiovascular diseases. *NMCD* 2010; **20**(7): 481–490. doi: 10.1016/j.numecd.2010.05.005.

59. Sinha S, Misra A, Rathi M, Kumar V, Pandey RM, Luthra K, et al. Proton magnetic resonance spectroscopy and biochemical investigation of type 2 diabetes mellitus in Asian Indians: observation of high muscle lipids and C-reactive protein levels. *Magn. Reson. Imaging* 2009; **27**(1): 94–100. doi: 10.1016/j.mri.2008.06.001.

60. Misra A, Sinha S, Kumar M, Jagannathan NR, Pandey RM. Proton magnetic resonance spectroscopy study of soleus muscle in non-obese healthy and Type 2 diabetic Asian Northern Indian males: high intramyocellular lipid content correlates with excess body fat and abdominal obesity. *Diabet Med* 2003; **20**(5): 361–367.

61. Shah A, Hernandez A, Mathur D, Budoff MJ, Kanaya AM. Adipokines and body fat composition in South Asians: results of the Metabolic Syndrome and Atherosclerosis in South Asians Living in America (MASALA) study. *Int J Obes (Lond)* 2011. doi: 10.1038/ijo.2011.167.

62. Anand SS, Tarnopolsky MA, Rashid S, Schulze KM, Desai D, Mente A, et al. Adipocyte hypertrophy, fatty liver and metabolic risk factors in South Asians: the Molecular Study of Health and Risk in Ethnic Groups (mol-SHARE). *PLoS ONE* 2011; **6**(7): e22112. doi: 10.1371/journal.pone.0022112.

63. Ingram KH, Lara-Castro C, Gower BA, Makowsky R, Allison DB, Newcomer BR, et al. Intramyocellular lipid and insulin resistance: differential relationships in European and African Americans. *Obesity (Silver Spring)* 2011; **19**(7): 1469–1475. doi: 10.1038/oby.2011.45.

64. Giday SA, Ashiny Z, Naab T, Smoot D, Banks A. Frequency of nonalcoholic fatty liver disease and degree of hepatic steatosis in African-American patients. *J Natl Med Assoc* 2006; **98**(10): 1613–1615.

Clinical management of diabetes in ethnic groups

Mohammed S. B. Huda
Barts Health NHS Trust, London, UK

8.2.1 Introduction

The worldwide explosion in the number of people with diabetes continues with total numbers projected to increase from 171 million in 2000 to 366 million in 2030 [1]. South Asians (Indian, Pakistani, Bangladeshi and Sri Lankan descent) have particularly high rates of type 2 diabetes with India alone containing 32 million of the 285 million cases estimated worldwide in 2010 [2].

Much of our current knowledge is based on traditional classification of diabetes into type 1 and type 2 diabetes, and the evidence base for clinical management is primarily centred on Caucasian populations of European descent. As the above epidemiological projections indicate, management of diabetes in other ethnic groups is increasing in importance. Different ethnic groups have atypical forms of diabetes, present in varying ways and have different rates of complications.

This chapter will focus on the presentation and clinical management of various aspects of diabetes, and review the current evidence base.

8.2.2 Classification and atypical presentation

Standard classification of diabetes into type 1, an autoimmune driven insulin-deficient state that often presents as an emergency, and type 2,

a predominantly insulin-resistant state that often presents incidentally or with chronic symptoms, is likely to be inadequate. The most recent American Diabetes Association (ADA) classification, which also includes gestational diabetes and diabetes secondary to other medication conditions, identifies idiopathic diabetes as a subgroup of type 1 but otherwise there is little formal recognition of atypical presentations in different ethnic groups [3].

From the 1950s there have been reports of patients of African or African-Caribbean origin presenting acutely with hyperglycaemic symptoms, weight loss, evidence of ketosis or frank diabetic ketoacidosis (DKA) [4]. They are treated with insulin but unlike in classical type 1 diabetes, patients are able to discontinue insulin a few months after the acute episode and can remain on diet or minimal oral hypoglycaemics for many years before relapsing [5]. These patients have been described with various synonyms from different centres, including 'periodic insulin deficiency', 'flatbush diabetes', 'atypical ketosis prone diabetes' and 'idiopathic type 1 diabetes' and 'ketosis-prone type 2 diabetes' [5–7]. The term atypical ketosis prone diabetes (AKPD) will be used for the remainder of this chapter.

Patients with AKPD are usually obese, aged over 40, autoantibody negative and of Black African or African-Caribbean origin [5]. However this phenomenon has been described in other ethnic groups including Caucasian [8], Pakistani

Table 8.2.1 Retrospective studies in atypical ketosis prone diabetes in different ethnic groups

Year	Authors	Ethnic group	No. of patients	% of cohort	Follow up
1995	Aizawa et al.	Japanese	5	Case series	2.8 years
1997	Wilson et al.	Apache Indian	17	2% (724 type 2 pts)	None
1997	Pinhas-Hamiel et al.	African-American	12	17% (70 type 2 pts)	2 years
1999	Balasubramanyam et al.	Hispanic/African-American/white	55	39% (114 DKA pts)	None
2000	Tan et al.	Chinese	11	Case series	None
2000	Pitteloud et al.	White	7	16% (43 DKA pts)	None
2004	Jabber et al.	Pakistani	57	50% (114 DKA pts)	None

DKA: diabetic ketoacidosis.

[9], Hispanic [10], Native American [11] and Chinese patients [12]. Table 8.2.1 shows some of the studies in AKPD in different ethnic groups. Patients can remain in near normoglycaemic remission for many years before relapse to insulin dependence, which may be permanent or, again, temporary [5].

In stark contrast to AKPD, another atypical presentation is patients with a lean, ketosis resistant phenotype. Patients are typically very lean, with a history of previous malnutrition and usually under 30 years of age. Other typical features are shown in Box 8.2.1. They present with marked hyperglycaemia, catabolic symptoms and yet do not develop significant ketosis or DKA. They improve with insulin therapy but then can remain off insulin therapy for many years. They have relapses with hyperglycaemia but, unlike type 1 diabetes, do not develop DKA. Patients with this clinical syndrome present from parts of Asia [13] and Africa [14]. This syndrome also has a long history and was described under a different name – 'protein deficient pancreatic diabetes' – which originally was a sub-category of 'malnutrition-related diabetes' [15]. This term was later discontinued and there only now remains the term 'fibrocalculous pancreatic diabetes' within the WHO classification. This is likely to refer to a different clinical entity – these patients have chronic calculous pancreatopathy, exocrine pancreatic deficiency and abdominal pain – but there are some overlapping features with lean, ketosis resistant diabetes. It has also been named tropical diabetes, J type, ketosis

> **Box 8.2.1** Clinical features of lean ketosis resistant phenotype
>
> Aged < 30 years
> Features of pancreatic exocrine insufficiency
> Lean or underweight at presentation
> Malnourished or previous history of malnutrition
> Low socio-economic status
> Absence of ketones at presentation or after insulin withdrawal
> Some populations have increased frequency of type 1 diabetes associated human leukocyte antigen (HLA)
> Usually lower frequency of islet cell autoantibodies than seen in type 1 diabetes.

resistant diabetes of the young and malnutrition modulated diabetes [16].

Recent data from Ethiopia confirm that there are a large number of patients with diabetes, often needing insulin but surviving without insulin for long periods and who are slim (body mass index (BMI) around 20 kg/m²), show a male preponderance and 61% have low fasting c-peptide and 35% positive glutamic acid decarboxylase (GAD) antibodies [17]. This was also seen in another large survey in Ethiopia showing large numbers of insulin-treated patients with low BMI and from poor socio-economic background [14]. Large numbers of malnutrition-related diabetes have also been reported in Korea and India, with differing associations with islet cell antibodies and human leukocyte antigen (HLA) genes typical of type 1 diabetes [18,19].

The clinical management of these patients is often dependent on resources. Patients are treated with insulin when available but can remain off any treatment for long periods of time. The pathophysiology is unclear but, as mentioned above, many have evidence of auto-immunity and a background of chronic under-nutrition can lead to this particular phenotype.

8.2.3 Assessing glycaemic control

Glycated haemoglobin (HbA1c) is the universal method for the assessment of glycaemic control in diabetic patients. More recently, HbA1c has been recommended as a diagnostic test for diabetes [20]. However, there is ongoing debate about the interpretation of HbA1c values amongst patients of African-Caribbean and South Asian ethnicity and the possible need for ethnic specific targets and cut points [21,22]. African-Caribbean and South Asian people are known to have higher HbA1c values than White Caucasian people in both normal and hypergly-caemic states [23,24]. It is unclear whether these disparities stem from ethnic differences in fasting or post-load glycaemia, the tendency of haemo-globin to undergo glycation, erythrocyte turno-ver or erythrocyte permeability to glucose [22].

8.2.4 Glycaemic control management

The United Kingdom (UK) is an increasingly multi-ethnic society, and the UK Prospective Diabetes Study (UKPDS) provides useful evidence of ethnic diversity with regards to diabetes risk factors and outcomes [25]. This was a large cohort study that randomised over 5000 newly diagnosed type 2 diabetic patients to intensive glycaemic control over standard care. The ethnicity breakdown in the study was 82% white Caucasian, 10% (South Asian including Indian, Pakistani, Bangladeshi and Sri-Lankan) and 8% African-Caribbean.

At diagnosis African-Caribbean patients had a higher fasting plasma glucose and HbA1c than white Caucasian and South Asian patients. Of interest, South Asian patients were more insulin resistant than white Caucasian patients, and African-Caribbeans were more insulin deficient (measured by HOMA %S and %B). These findings have been replicated by other studies in type 2 diabetes [26,27]. Recent data from a study of a large multi-ethnic cohort in North-West London followed over 20 years (the SABRE study) have confirmed that insulin resistance and truncal obesity increase the incidence of diabetes by two-fold in South Asian and African-Caribbean women, but did not account for the increased incidence in men – it may be that ectopic fat outside the abdomen and other unknown factors are more relevant in men [28].

In the UKPDS, progressive worsening in gly-caemic control over nine years was similar in all three groups, suggesting that, despite the initial group differences in insulin physiology, ethnicity did not play a large role in determining gly-caemic progression [29]. An early analysis of the UKPDS data suggested that African-Caribbean patients benefited more with metformin, but this was not borne out in the final analysis after adjustment for confounders [30]. Hence, although initial ethnic differences are noted, current guidelines on glycaemic control management are not different between ethnic groups.

Indeed, the most recent American Diabetes Association (ADA)/ European Association for the Study of Diabetes (EASD) guidelines suggest metformin and lifestyle measures for all patients with type 2 diabetes as the first-line, regardless of race, ethnicity or gender [31]. After metformin, the guidelines suggest that a number of anti-hyperglycaemic agents can be considered – including sulfonylureas, thiazolidinediones, gliptins and glucagon-like-peptide 1 (GLP-1) therapies. The choice of agent should involve a patient-centred approach and take into account weight gain and the risk of hypoglycaemia.

There are some small studies suggesting the benefit of thiazolidinediones in South Asian patients, but many are observational and no clear recommendations can be made [32]. Similar to insulin physiology, there are likely to be subtle differences in incretin response to a glucose load. One study suggests that African Americans have higher fasted GLP-1 and a larger GLP-1 response to glucose than white Caucasians [33]. Ethnic minorities are represented in the newer drug trials, but none are adequately powered or designed to answer whether any particular ethnic group is better suited to any particular therapy.

We know from the progressive nature of type 2 diabetes that many patients will eventually need insulin therapy. An interesting small subgroup analysis of the Veterans Affairs Cooperative Study in Type 2 Diabetes Mellitus (VA CSDM) showed that African Americans responded better to intensive therapy with insulin, than non-African Americans despite correcting for baseline characteristics and other confounders [34]. Nevertheless, African Americans tend to have worse outcomes, self-monitoring and glycaemic control, as well as significant cultural barriers to insulin therapy and poor adherence [35].

8.2.5 Clinical management of complications

Retinopathy

Diabetic retinopathy is the most common microvascular complication and still remains the leading cause of blindness in the working-age population in Western countries [36]. It is caused by prolonged exposure to poorly controlled diabetes, particularly glycaemic control, and damages the microvasculature of the retina. The prevalence of diabetic retinopathy (DR) is decreasing in developed countries, secondary to improved screening and surveillance and probably effective multiple risk factor modification [37].

In type 1 diabetes the prevalence of DR worldwide ranges from 10 to 15%. Type 1 diabetes remains a predominantly white northern European condition, but data from other non-white dominated countries are limited. Comparison of the prevalence of DR between countries is hampered by different methods of screening and recording health outcomes. The EURODIAB study showed prevalence ranged from 25 to 60% in 16 European countries, whereas the Asian Young Diabetes Research

(ASDIAB) found prevalence of 5.3–15.1% in a young type 1 population in four Asian countries [38,39]. However, the absolute numbers of people with type 1 diabetes were small in this study. Cross-sectional data have not shown any difference in prevalence of DR between South Asians, African-Caribbeans and white Caucasians type with 1 diabetes in the United States (US), South Africa or Brazil when corrected for glycaemic control and duration of diabetes [40].

The Diabetes Control and Complications Trial (DCCT) compared conventional with intensive therapy in type 1 diabetes on the incidence of microvascular and macrovascular complications and showed that intensive therapy, particularly during the first five years of therapy, can reduce the rates of retinopathy [41]. Another risk factor is blood pressure, and control of blood pressure, particularly with angiotensin converting enzyme (ACE) inhibition or angiotensin receptor blockade (ARB) therapies have been shown to be beneficial [42]. Again, these data contain small numbers of ethnic minority patients, and hence the effectiveness of glycaemic control and blood pressure control in these groups must be extrapolated. High salt and energy intake are a risk factor for DR progression in African-Caribbean patients, however, whilst other factors, such as BMI and smoking, are common to all ethnic groups [43].

Therefore, in type 1 diabetes there are variations in DR prevalence worldwide, which generally reflect prevalence of type 1, but other factors such as socio-economic circumstances may play a role.

In type 2 diabetes, consistent reports show an overall prevalence of DR of around 40% in Europe [44]. There are more multi-ethnic data available, and there are consistent data showing an increased prevalence of DR in South Asian in the UK compared to white patients [45], and UKPDS showed that 17.5% of South Asians have DR at diagnosis compared to 7.9% in whites [46]. There are also data from the US suggesting that African American and Hispanic populations have higher rates of DR compared to non-Hispanic whites [47]. However, access to healthcare in the US is inconsistent and patients may present late with increased severity of DR. By contrast, the prevalence of DR appears to be lower in India (around 20%) and 5–7% at diagnosis. There are also wide variations in retinopathy in mainland China, Taiwan, the Middle East, sub-Saharan Africa and Australasia. As with type 1 diabetes, these variations can be partially explained by different healthcare systems and different screening programmes, but variable insulin sensitivity and retinal vascular calibre are also potential factors.

Neuropathy and diabetic foot ulceration

Peripheral neuropathy is the most important contributor to diabetic foot ulceration, and yet the data on ethnicity and neuropathy have been limited until recently. The UKPDS and data from our group suggest that South Asians and African-Caribbeans have less neuropathy at diagnosis compared with white Caucasians [25,48]. More recent data from the UK confirmed that South Asian patients with type 2 diabetes have less large and small fibre neuropathy than white Caucasians, although this may, in part, be due to lower smoking rates and improved tissue oxygenation independent of smoking [44]. However, a large observational study from the same group showed that despite lower neuropathy in South Asians (14%) compared with white Caucasians (22%) and African-Caribbeans (21%), South Asians had significantly higher rates of painful diabetic neuropathy symptoms, regardless of neurological deficit [49].

Diabetic foot ulcer disease is also less prevalent in South Asians (1.8%) and African-Caribbeans (2.7%) compared to white Caucasians (5.5%) after adjusting for age [5]. In South Asians, reduced rates of peripheral arterial disease, neuropathy, foot deformities and lower insulin usage all contributed to less diabetic foot ulceration. Reduced neuropathy was the most significant protective factor for African-Caribbeans, although they also had less foot deformities than white Caucasians. Interestingly, abnormal vibration perception (utilising large Aβ fibres) was a particular risk factor for diabetic foot ulceration for all ethnicities, but more significantly for South Asians and African-Caribbeans [50].

The aetiology behind reduced neuropathy in South Asians is unclear. Traditional risk factors such as hyperglycaemia and dyslipidaemia are similar to their European counterparts [51], and although smoking and alcohol rates were lower in South Asians, statistically this does not account for the lower neuropathy rate, but does contribute to reduced amputation rates [52].

Nephropathy

UKPDS analysis showed that South Asians were twice as likely to develop micro-albuminuria, macro-albuminuria and doubling of serum creatinine, compared with European counterparts, independent of blood pressure, and this has been confirmed by several other studies [53]. UK and US data on African-Caribbeans and African Americans show that the risk of end-stage renal failure secondary to diabetes is six times higher than in white Caucasian patients [54].

Again, the reasons behind renal impairment in South Asians or excess renal replacement therapy in African-Caribbeans/African Americans remain unclear. Access to renal replacement therapy may be improved in African-Caribbeans in the UK due to living in inner city areas where referral to specialist centres takes place, but the contrary may be true of African Americans in the US where access to health care may be restricted.

Macrovascular disease

Blood pressure is lower in South Asians at diagnosis compared to white Caucasians and African-Caribbeans, whereas African-Caribbeans have higher diastolic blood pressure than white Caucasians and evidence of left ventricular hypertrophy on electro-cardiogram (a marker of end-organ damage from hypertension) [25], but not all groups have found this [55]. Plasma lipid profiles are similar in white Caucasian and South Asian patients with type 2 diabetes at diagnosis whereas African-Caribbean patients have higher high-density lipoprotein

(HDL) cholesterol and lower plasma triglycerides [25]. This is corroborated by other groups and may be secondary to lower truncal obesity and greater insulin sensitivity in African-Caribbean patients compared with white Caucasians [55].

A recent analysis of long-term vascular outcomes in the UKPDS cohort has demonstrated significantly lower myocardial infarction rates in African-Caribbean patients with type 2 diabetes compared to South Asians and white Caucasians [56] that corroborates earlier reports of such patterns [55,57]. Furthermore, a population study of African-Caribbean, Hispanics and Chinese found lower coronary calcification in African-Caribbeans after adjustment for confounders [58]. US population studies have also found increased rates of stroke in patients of Black or Hispanic origin compared with white Caucasians [59], which is also true of African-Caribbean patients in the UK [56]. There are also data suggesting increased cerebral small vessel disease in Black patients with stroke [60]. In contrast, rates of peripheral vascular disease are markedly lower in both African-Caribbeans and South Asian patients compared to white Caucasians [56].

The aetiology of these differences is not known. Genetic, cultural or lifestyle factors may influence the racial disparities in macrovascular outcomes but other vascular biomarkers, such as C-reactive protein, fibrinogen, lipoprotein (a) and homocysteine could be important [61].

There is a perception that African-Caribbean patients have low plasma renin activity, and hence derive less benefit from blockade of the renin-angiotensin-aldosterone system [62]. However, most trials are underpowered to clearly confirm benefits of ARB and in diabetic patients use of ARB or ACE inhibitors remains the first line for the treatment of hypertension, regardless of ethnicity [63].

8.2.6 Summary

Presentation with atypical forms of diabetes is more common in certain ethnic groups, and the early clinical management may be very different to conventional management. By contrast, glycaemic control and progression of type 2 diabetes appears to be similar amongst all ethnic groups and management is not specific to ethnicity. Also, although there are few data in type 1 diabetes, there is currently little to suggest different clinical progression between ethnic groups. However, in both type 1 and type 2 diabetes differences in genetic, social, economic and cultural circumstances, as well as differing access to healthcare, will impact on clinical management.

There is considerable disparity in the prevalence of various complications amongst different ethnic groups, but as most clinical trials have not been powered to examine this, the recommended clinical management remains the same as for their European counterparts.

In conclusion, clinicians should be aware of the potential differences between ethnic groups in the presentation and complications of diabetes when determining clinical management.

Key points

- Rates of type 2 diabetes are disproportionately high in ethnic minority groups.
- Atypical forms of diabetes, such as atypical ketosis prone diabetes, present more commonly in ethnic minority groups.
- HbA1c values are higher in South Asian and African-Caribbean groups but at present there are no ethnic specific diagnostic cut-offs for HbA1c.
- There is only limited evidence for ethnic specific approaches to the management of glycaemia and at present no ethnic specific guidelines.
- Ethnic patterns in microvascular complications are recognised; diabetic retinopathy and nephropathy is more common in ethnic minority patients but neuropathy is less common.
- Ethnic patterns in macrovascular disease are recognised; hypertension and stroke are more common amongst patients of African ancestry, whilst myocardial infarction rates are low in these patients. Peripheral vascular disease rates are low in African-Caribbean and South Asian patients.

References

1. Wild S, Roglic G, Green A, Sicree R, King H. Global prevalence of diabetes: estimates for the year 2000 and projections for 2030. *Diabetes Care* 2004; **27**(5): 1047–1053.
2. International Diabetes Federation. *Diabetes Atlas*, 4th edn. Brussels, Belgium: International Diabetes Federation, 2009.
3. American Diabetes Association. Diagnosis and classification of diabetes mellitus. *Diabetes Care* 2006; **29** (Suppl. 1): S43–S48.
4. Hugh-Jones P. Diabetes in Jamaica. *Lancet* 1955; **269**(6896): 891–897.
5. Mauvais-Jarvis F, Sobngwi E, Porcher R, Riveline JP, Kevorkian JP, Vaisse C, et al. Ketosis-prone type 2 diabetes in patients of sub-Saharan African origin: clinical pathophysiology and natural history of beta-cell dysfunction and insulin resistance. *Diabetes* 2004; **53**(3): 645–653.
6. Pinero-Pilona A, Litonjua P, Aviles-Santa L, Raskin P. Idiopathic type 1 diabetes in Dallas, Texas: a 5-year experience. *Diabetes Care* 2001; **24**(6): 1014–1018.
7. Umpierrez GE, Casals MM, Gebhart SP, Mixon PS, Clark WS, Phillips LS. Diabetic ketoacidosis in obese African-Americans. *Diabetes* 1995; **44**(7): 790–795.
8. Pitteloud N, Philippe J. Characteristics of Caucasian type 2 diabetic patients during ketoacidosis and at follow-up. *Schweiz Med Wochenschr* 2000; **130**(16): 576–582.
9. Jabbar A, Farooqui K, Habib A, Islam N, Haque N, Akhter J. Clinical characteristics and outcomes of diabetic ketoacidosis in Pakistani adults with Type 2 diabetes mellitus. *Diabet Med* 2004; **21**(8): 920–923.
10. Maldonado MR, Otiniano ME, Cheema F, Rodriguez L, Balasubramanyam A. Factors associated with insulin discontinuation in subjects with ketosis-prone diabetes but preserved beta-cell function. *Diabet Med* 2005; **22**(12): 1744–1750.
11. Wilson C, Krakoff J, Gohdes D. Ketoacidosis in Apache Indians with non-insulin-dependent diabetes mellitus. *Arch Intern Med* 1997; **157**(18): 2098–2100.
12. Tan KC, Mackay IR, Zimmet PZ, Hawkins BR, Lam KS. Metabolic and immunologic features of Chinese patients with atypical diabetes mellitus. *Diabetes Care* 2000; **23**(3): 335–338.
13. Ahuja MM, Sharma GP. Serum C-peptide content in nutritional diabetes. *Horm Metab Res* 1985; **17**(5): 267–268.
14. Alemu S, Dessie A, Seid E, Bard E, Lee PT, Trimble ER, et al. Insulin-requiring diabetes in rural Ethiopia: should we reopen the case for malnutrition-related diabetes? *Diabetologia* 2009; **52**(9): 1842–1845.
15. World Health Organisation 1985 Diabetes Mellitus: Report of a WHO study group. Geneva. WHO Technical Report Series 727, 1985.
16. Hoet JJ, Tripathy BB. Report of the International Workshop on types of Diabetes Peculiar to the Tropics. *Diabetes Care* 1996; **19**(9): 1014.
17. Gill GV, Tekle A, Reja A, Wile D, English PJ, Diver M, et al. Immunological and C-peptide studies of patients with diabetes in northern Ethiopia: existence of an unusual subgroup possibly related to malnutrition. *Diabetologia* 2011 Jan; **54**(1): 51–7.
18. Huh KB, Lee HC, Kim HM, Cho YW, Kim YL, Lee KW, et al. Immunogenetic and nutritional profile in insulin-using youth-onset diabetics in Korea. *Diabetes Res Clin Pract* 1992; **16**(1): 63–70.
19. Sanjeevi CB, Seshiah V, Moller E, Olerup O. Different genetic backgrounds for malnutrition-related diabetes and type 1 (insulin-dependent) diabetes mellitus in south Indians. *Diabetologia* 1992; **35**(3): 283–286.
20. World Health Organisation (2011). Use of Glycated Haemoglobin (HbA1c) in the Diagnosis of Diabetes Mellitus. http://www.who.int/diabetes/publications/report-hba1c_2011.pdf
21. Likhari T, Gama R. Glycaemia-independent ethnic differences in HbA(1c) in subjects with impaired glucose tolerance. *Diabet Med* 2009; **26**(10): 1068–1069.
22. Selvin E, Steffes MW, Ballantyne CM, Hoogeveen RC, Coresh J, Brancati FL. Racial difference in glycaemic markers: a cross-sectional analysis of community-based date. *Ann Intern Med* 2011; **154**: 303–309.
23. Likhari T, Gama R. Ethnic differences in glycated haemoglobin between white subjects and those of South Asian origin with normal glucose tolerance. *J Clin Pathol* 2010; **63**(3): 278–280.
24. Herman WH, Dungan KM, Wolffenbuttel BH, Buse JB, Fahrbach JL, Jiang H, et al. Racial and ethnic differences in mean plasma glucose, hemoglobin A1c, and 1,5-anhydroglucitol in over 2000 patients with type 2 diabetes. *J Clin Endocrinol Metab* 2009; **94**: 1689–1694.
25. UK Prospective Diabetes Study. XII: Differences between Asian, Afro-Caribbean and white Caucasian type 2 diabetic patients at diagnosis of diabetes. UK Prospective Diabetes Study Group. *Diabet Med* 1994; **11**(7): 670–677.
26. Chaiken RL, Banerji MA, Pasmantier R, Huey H, Hirsch S, Lebovitz HE. Patterns of glucose and lipid abnormalities in black NIDDM subjects. *Diabetes Care* 1991; **14**(11): 1036–1042.
27. Mohan V, Sharp PS, Cloke HR, Burrin JM, Schumer B, Kohner EM. Serum immunoreactive insulin responses to a glucose load in Asian Indian and European type 2 (non-insulin-dependent) diabetic patients and control subjects. *Diabetologia* 1986; **29**(4): 235–237.
28. Tillin T, Hughes AD, Godsland IF, Whincup P, Forouhi NG, Welsh P, et al. Insulin Resistance and Truncal Obesity as Important Determinants of the Greater Incidence of Diabetes in Indian Asians and

African Caribbeans Compared With Europeans: The Southall and Brent Revisited (SABRE) cohort. *Diabetes Care* 2013; **36**(2): 383–393.

29. Davis TM, Cull CA, Holman RR. Relationship between ethnicity and glycemic control, lipid profiles, and blood pressure during the first 9 years of type 2 diabetes: U.K. Prospective Diabetes Study (UKPDS 55). *Diabetes Care* 2001; **24**(7): 1167–1174.

30. Davis TME, Cull C, Holman R, Turner R. Effects of ethnicity on metabolic control during the first six years of NIDDM. *Diabetologia* 1997; **40**(Suppl. 1): A642.

31. Inzucchi SE, Bergenstal RM, Buse JB, Diamant M, Ferrannini E, Nauck M, et al. Management of hyperglycemia in type 2 diabetes: a patient-centered approach: position statement of the American Diabetes Association (ADA) and the European Association for the Study of Diabetes (EASD). *Diabetes Care* 2012; **35**(6): 1364–1379.

32. Barnett AH, Grant PJ, Hitman GA, Mather H, Pawa M, Robertson L, et al. Rosiglitazone in Type 2 diabetes mellitus: an evaluation in British Indo-Asian patients. *Diabet Med* 2003; **20**(5): 387–393.

33. Velasquez-Mieyer PA, Cowan PA, Umpierrez GE, Lustig RH, Cashion AK, Burghen GA. Racial differences in glucagon-like peptide-1 (GLP-1) concentrations and insulin dynamics during oral glucose tolerance test in obese subjects. *Int J Obes Relat Metab Disord* 2003; **27**(11): 1359–1364.

34. Agrawal L, Emanuele NV, Abraira C, Henderson WG, Levin SR, Sawin CT, et al. Ethnic differences in the glycemic response to exogenous insulin treatment in the Veterans Affairs Cooperative Study in Type 2 Diabetes Mellitus (VA CSDM). *Diabetes Care* 1998; **21**(4): 510–515.

35. Campbell JA, Walker RJ, Smalls BL, Egede LE. Glucose control in diabetes: the impact of racial differences on monitoring and outcomes. *Endocrine* 2012; **42**(3): 471–482.

36. Congdon NG, Friedman DS, Lietman T. Important causes of visual impairment in the world today. *JAMA* 2003; **290**(15): 2057–2060.

37. Brown JB, Pedula KL, Summers KH. Diabetic retinopathy: contemporary prevalence in a well-controlled population. *Diabetes Care* 2003; **26**(9): 2637–2642.

38. Microvascular and acute complications in IDDM patients: the EURODIAB IDDM Complications Study. *Diabetologia* 1994; **37**(3): 278–285.

39. Rema MM, Mohan V. Retinopathy at diagnosis among young Asian diabetic patients: the ASDIAB Study Group. *Diabetes* 2002; **51**(Suppl. 2): A206–A207.

40. Arfken CL, Salicrup AE, Meuer SM, Del Priore LV, Klein R, McGill JB, et al. Retinopathy in African Americans and whites with insulin-dependent diabetes mellitus. *Arch Intern Med* 1994; **154**(22): 2597–2602.

41. White NH, Sun W, Cleary PA, Tamborlane WV, Danis RP, Hainsworth DP, et al. Effect of prior intensive therapy in type 1 diabetes on 10-year progression of retinopathy in the DCCT/EDIC: comparison of adults and adolescents. *Diabetes* 2010; **59**(5): 1244–1253.

42. Chaturvedi N, Porta M, Klein R, Orchard T, Fuller J, Parving HH, et al. Effect of candesartan on prevention (DIRECT-Prevent 1) and progression (DIRECT-Protect 1) of retinopathy in type 1 diabetes: randomised, placebo-controlled trials. *Lancet* 2008; **372**(9647): 1394–1402.

43. Roy MS, Janal MN. High caloric and sodium intakes as risk factors for progression of retinopathy in type 1 diabetes mellitus. *Arch Ophthalmol* 2010; **128**(1): 33–39.

44. Sivaprasad S, Gupta B, Crosby-Nwaobi R, Evans J. Prevalence of diabetic retinopathy in various ethnic groups: a worldwide perspective. *Surv Ophthalmol* 2012; **57**(4): 347–370.

45. Stolk RP, van Schooneveld MJ, Cruickshank JK, Hughes AD, Stanton A, Lu J, et al. Retinal vascular lesions in patients of Caucasian and Asian origin with type 2 diabetes: baseline results from the ADVANCE Retinal Measurements (AdRem) study. *Diabetes Care* 2008; **31**(4): 708–713.

46. Kohner EM, Aldington SJ, Stratton IM, Manley SE, Holman RR, Matthews DR, et al. United Kingdom Prospective Diabetes Study, 30: diabetic retinopathy at diagnosis of non-insulin-dependent diabetes mellitus and associated risk factors. *Arch Ophthalmol* 1998; **116**(3): 297–303.

47. Emanuele N, Moritz T, Klein R, Davis MD, Glander K, Khanna A, et al. Ethnicity, race, and clinically significant macular edema in the Veterans Affairs Diabetes Trial (VADT). *Diabetes Res Clin Pract* 2009; **86**(2): 104–110.

48. Winkley K, Sivaprasad S, Stahl D, Thomas S, Ismail K, Amiel SA. Complication status of patients with a new diagnosis of type 2 diabetes in south London, UK. *Diabet Med* 2012; **29**(Suppl. 1): 16–17.

49. Abbott CA, Malik RA, van Ross ER, Kulkarni J, Boulton AJ. Prevalence and characteristics of painful diabetic neuropathy in a large community-based diabetic population in the U.K. *Diabetes Care* 2011; **34**(10): 2220–2224.

50. Abbott CA, Garrow AP, Carrington AL, Morris J, Van Ross ER, Boulton AJ. Foot ulcer risk is lower in South-Asian and african-Caribbean compared with European diabetic patients in the U.K.: the North-West diabetes foot care study. *Diabetes Care* 2005; **28**(8): 1869–1875.

51. Abbott CA, Chaturvedi N, Malik RA, Salgami E, Yates AP, Pemberton PW, et al. Explanations for the lower rates of diabetic neuropathy in Indian Asians versus Europeans. *Diabetes Care* 2010; **33**(6): 1325–1330.

52. Chaturvedi N, Abbott CA, Whalley A, Widdows P, Leggetter SY, Boulton AJ. Risk of diabetes-related

amputation in South Asians vs. Europeans in the UK. *Diabet Med* 2002; **19**(2): 99–104.

53. Retnakaran R, Cull CA, Thorne KI, Adler AI, Holman RR. Risk factors for renal dysfunction in type 2 diabetes: U.K. Prospective Diabetes Study 74. *Diabetes* 2006; **55**(6): 1832–1839.

54. Roderick PJ, Raleigh VS, Hallam L, Mallick NP. The need and demand for renal replacement therapy in ethnic minorities in England. *J Epidemiol Community Health* 1996; **50**(3): 334–339.

55. Chaturvedi N, Jarrett J, Morrish N, Keen H, Fuller JH. Differences in mortality and morbidity in African Caribbean and European people with non-insulin dependent diabetes mellitus: results of 20 year follow up of a London cohort of a multinational study. *BMJ* 1996; **313**(7061): 848–852.

56. Davis TME, Coleman RL, Holman RR; UKPDS Group. Ethnicity and long-term vascular outcomes in Type 2 diabetes: a prospective observational study (UKPDS 83) *Diabet Med* 2014; **31**: 200–207.

57. UK Prospective Diabetes Study Group. Ethnicity and cardiovascular disease. The incidence of myocardial infarction in white, South Asian, and Afro-Caribbean patients with type 2 diabetes (U.K. Prospective Diabetes Study 32). *Diabetes Care* 1998; **21**(8): 1271–1277.

58. Bild DE, Detrano R, Peterson D, Guerci A, Liu K, Shahar E, et al. Ethnic differences in coronary calcification: the Multi-Ethnic Study of Atherosclerosis (MESA). *Circulation* 2005; **111**(10): 1313–1320.

59. Zhang H, Rodriguez-Monguio R. Racial disparities in the risk of developing obesity-related diseases: a cross-sectional study. *Ethn Dis* 2012; **22**(3): 308–316.

60. Markus HS, Khan U, Birns J, Evans A, Kalra L, Rudd AG, et al. Differences in stroke subtypes between black and white patients with stroke: the South London Ethnicity and Stroke Study. *Circulation* 2007; **116**(19): 2157–2164.

61. Allison MA, Criqui MH, McClelland RL, Scott JM, McDermott MM, Liu K, et al. The effect of novel cardiovascular risk factors on the ethnic-specific odds for peripheral arterial disease in the Multi-Ethnic Study of Atherosclerosis (MESA). *J Am Coll Cardiol* 2006; **48**(6): 1190–1197.

62. Creditor MC, Loschky UK. Incidence of suppressed renin activity and of normokalemic primary aldosteronism in hypertensive Negro patients. *Circulation* 1968; **37**(6): 1027–1031.

63. National Institute for Health and Care Excellence (2009) Type 2 diabetes: the management of type 2 diabetes. https://www.nice.org.uk/guidance/cg87

Chapter 8.3

Lifestyle management of diabetes in ethnic groups

Baldeesh Rai[1] and Louise Goff[2]
[1]London North West Healthcare NHS Trust, London, UK
[2]King's College London, London, UK

8.3.1 Introduction

Lifestyle intervention forms the cornerstone of diabetes management. Patients of all ethnicities often find it difficult to change their lifestyle in response to a diagnosis of a chronic disease, but environmental, economic and personal barriers, all of which impede the ability to make lifestyle change, are often greater in minority groups who have a higher burden of disease and fewer resources [1]. The healthcare professional's awareness of the wider cultural influences demonstrates cultural competency [2] that has been shown to increase patient satisfaction and adherence to healthcare management [3].

8.3.2 Nutritional considerations in ethnic groups

Traditional lifestyles and acculturation

Dietary acculturation is the process by which diasporic racial/ethnic groups adopt the dietary patterns of the host country [4]. It is associated with poor dietary choices over generations, including surplus intakes of sweetened beverages, animal products, refined, processed and energy-dense foods, and suboptimal intakes of pulses and grains, fruits and vegetables [5]. This results in excess intakes of energy, fat, saturated fat and sugar and low intakes of fibre in younger migrant generations [6] and an increased risk of chronic disease [7], highlighting an important area where healthcare professionals may affect the development of health problems among minority populations. It is, therefore, important for healthcare professionals to be aware of the varying levels of acculturation that exist in any ethnic minority community.

Overview of traditional diets of minority ethnic groups

South asians

The collective term 'South Asian' [8] usually refers to populations originating from the Indian subcontinent, with the main sub-groups being Indians, Pakistanis, Bangladeshis and Sri Lankans; significant heterogeneity is recognised between these sub-cultures.

Generally, the basis of a traditional South Asian diet is starchy foods, including various types of flat breads (e.g. chapatti, roti, naan, pitta bread), rice and potatoes; butter and margarines may or may not be used liberally on flat breads. Flat bread is often eaten with vegetables, including okra, aubergines, cauliflower, peas prepared as curries (many vegetable curries would also include potatoes, a further source of starch), beans and pulses in the form of dahls and meat or fish in a curry. South Asian cuisine is well known for the wide range of herbs and spices

Advanced Nutrition and Dietetics in Diabetes, First Edition. Edited by Louise Goff and Pamela Dyson.
© 2016 John Wiley & Sons, Ltd. Published 2016 by John Wiley & Sons, Ltd.

that are used. Oily, sweet or salty pickles and natural yoghurt are commonly served with main meals. Fried snacks, such as Bombay mix and crisps are commonly consumed. High fat foods, including samosas, pakoras and Indian sweets, formerly reserved for special occasions, are now eaten more frequently as they are widely available and affordable. Fat intake may be high and can be difficult to assess due to traditional cooking practices where ingredients are not measured, cooking oil is poured directly from a container and butter is added to cooked dahls *ad libitum* [9].

African Caribbean

The traditional Caribbean diet includes large portions of highly seasoned vegetable-based soups with stewed meat (goat, lamb and beef), chicken and fish (tilapia, saltfish and snapper), called 'one pot meals'. Meals are usually based on more than one portion of starchy carbohydrate (rice, potato, plantain) and there are multiple sources of protein in one meal (pulses, meat and fish). Fruit and vegetable consumption is high, vegetables are often processed and tropical fruits are eaten in season (mango, papaya, avocado, pineapple, breadfruits). Traditional Caribbean diets are high in starchy carbohydrate, protein and fibre and low in total and saturated fat. Migrant communities have been shown to commonly adopt host foods and dishes into the diet, including take-away meals, sugar-sweetened beverages and confectionary, and to reduce their intake of fruit and vegetables, which results in an increasing intake of fat and saturated fat and reduced starchy carbohydrate and fibre intake [10]. Excess sodium intakes in migrant diets are related to flavouring dishes with salt and the heavy use of pre-prepared seasonings. Snacks that are commonly eaten include patties, salt fish fritters and dumplings that are fried and high in fat [11].

The traditional African diet contains little variation and, similarly to the Caribbean diet, is often based on 'one-pot' soups and stews that are tomato-based with added fish or meat and are usually cooked with palm oil as the main source of fat. The consumption of large portions of starchy staples, including maize, cassava, fu-fu (made by boiling cassava or yam and then pounding them into a dense dough), rice, yams and plantain is also characteristic of the traditional African diet. As with people of Caribbean ancestry, the nutritional composition of the diet is high in starchy carbohydrate and fibre and low in total and saturated fat [12].

Latinos

The traditional Mexican diet is low in fat and high in fibre and foods such as corn, tortillas, rice and beans are staples [13]. Many Hispanics still retain core elements of the traditional diet, including a reliance on grains and beans [14]. In the United States, the American Dietetic Association and American Diabetes Association have conducted studies showing that it is important for healthcare teams working with these communities to assess the level of acculturation to mainstream American practices [15]. In recent work from the Multiethnic Cohort, Sharma et al. have described important foods in the diets of American Latino adults demonstrating the importance of 'Western' foods, such as sugar-sweetened beverages, beer, potato chips, burgers and ice cream [16]. Nutrition education programmes aimed at improving the quality of the Hispanic diet are currently based on a combination of preserving some elements of the traditional diet (including a reliance on beans, rice and tortillas) and change in others, such as reduced consumption of high fat dairy foods and less use of fat in cooking [15].

Chinese descent

This ethnic group includes mainly people from China, Taiwan and Hong Kong. There is large variation in the traditional diet of people of Chinese descent from region to region. In Southern China rice is staple, whilst in Northern China wheat products (such as noodles), maize and corn are commonly consumed as a staple food. Communal dining is usual and a Chinese main meal consists of rice or Chinese bread plus several dishes cooked by different methods and using different ingredients to produce a variety of textures and flavours. Chinese dishes often have an abundance of green, leafy vegetables (e.g. pok choi, and choi sum). Vegetables are often quick fried and served with a sweet and sour or soy sauce. There is also heavy reliance on soya milk and other soya products. Chinese food is not highly spiced, but salt and soy sauce are used in abundance [17]. Additionally, traditional health remedies are important in these cultures [15].

Specific dietary issues in relation to diabetes in ethnic groups

Religion and fasting

Religious laws and practices have a significant impact on the diets and eating patterns of some ethnic groups and food is an important part of many religious festivals and celebrations; it is beyond the scope of this chapter to give an overview of these but such information can be found in the *Multicultural Handbook of Food, Nutrition and Dietetics* by Thaker and Barton [18].

Fasting is an important aspect of many religions, particularly Islam, Hinduism, Jainism and Buddhism. For example, some members of the Hindu community fast regularly throughout the year with some fasting once a week. It is important to ascertain what 'fasting' entails in each community, in some groups fasting allows or excludes certain foods and food groups, whilst for others it involves complete abstinence from food [19,20]. The Islamic month of Ramadan is one of the longest periods of fasting. Ramadan takes place twice a year (in the 9th month of the Islamic year) and involves abstaining from food from dawn to sunset. Muslims will rise before sunrise (*sehri*) to have a meal similar to breakfast and break their fast at sunset (*iftari*) with a meal of abundance and high sugar/high fat foods. Both meal times and meal composition change significantly during Ramadan, which has important considerations for blood glucose control and medication requirements. Educating patients with diabetes to prepare for Ramadan and other periods of fasting is vital in order to prevent hypoglycaemia or hyperglycaemia. Patients should be advised to consume low glycaemic index carbohydrates (e.g. basmati rice, pitta bread, chapattis and daal) to keep their blood glucose levels more consistent during their fast. Additionally patients should be counselled to minimise the amount of sugary and fatty foods (e.g. Indian sweets, cakes, samosas, puris) that are consumed when they break their fast at sunset. There is a range of information available on the Diabetes UK website and The Department of Health publication of *Ramadan Health Guide* (Communities in Action 2007).

Therapeutic foods, herbal and traditional remedies

South Asian cultures commonly practise and believe in ayurvedic (traditional) medicine, of which food is an important component. Particular foods are classified as 'hot' (e.g. mangoes and ginger) and 'cold' (e.g. potatoes), which may be recommended or avoided in certain diseases and circumstances. Sour foods (e.g. lemon or taramind) are believed to exacerbate joint pain and may be avoided in older generations. Herbal and traditional preparations are important in South Asian and East Asian communities; some have hypoglycaemic effects and patients may take them on their own or in conjunction with other therapeutic agents. Fenugreek seeds contain trigonelline, an alkaloid known to reduce blood glucose levels. South Asian patients may take fenugreek preparations in many different ways (e.g. as a powder incorporated into daal or chapattis, or as seeds). Kerala (bitter gourd) is commonly consumed in the form of a vegetable juice, capsules or eaten raw for its hypoglycaemic effects. The active components of kerala are thought to be charantin, vicine and polypeptide-p. To have a clinical effect kerala needs to be taken on a daily basis, but most people eat it on an *ad hoc* basis, which has implications for diabetes control. Other traditional remedies include jamun juice and cinnamon. Assessment of the use of these remedies is an important part of management of patients with diabetes [21].

Caribbean cultures often exhibit a strong desire for natural remedies, with a distrust of conventional medicine. 'Bush teas' (e.g. cerassie, annatto, periwinkle, dandelion, vervine, guaco, cashew bark, coconut shell, aloe vera) are commonly used amongst Caribbean patients with diabetes for their hypoglycaemic effects. Hibiscus tea (sorrel) is also commonly consumed amongst Caribbean patients for the blood pressuring lowering effects it is believed to exhibit.

Factors affecting dietary choices

Dietary habits are complex and influenced by many factors:

- *Availability and affordability of traditional and host foods* – traditional foods may not be available or may be expensive [22].
- *Income* – a low income may restrict food choice by limiting selection to cheaper foods that are often more energy-dense and of poorer quality [23].
- *Food beliefs,* such as the concept of 'hot' and 'cold' foods, may determine meal structure. A balance between the two is considered necessary for good health in Chinese, Mexican American and South Asian people [23].
- *Generation* – older generations are more likely to follow traditional diets whilst younger generations may eat more Western foods.
- *Gender roles* – meals are usually prepared by women in the South Asian cultures and are based on family preferences, as the husband and children are seen as the priority [19,20].

8.3.3 Cultural barriers to lifestyle modifications

Cultural expectations around food can make behaviour change challenging. Ethnic minority patients often complain about the dietary advice they receive, finding the recommended diet expensive, lacking taste and traditional foods, and recommendations to limit or avoid traditional or preferred foods are challenging for patients to adhere to [24]. The importance of the family unit and mealtime enjoyment can often mean that there is a lack of family support for lifestyle change, particularly for females who feel that preparing and eating foods that the family prefer is more important than adhering to dietary guidelines for the management of their diabetes [25]. This often means that women living with diabetes neglect their own diets or spend less time managing their condition and lifestyle [25]. Work carried out with United Kingdom (UK) Muslim women found there was a broad awareness and knowledge of healthy eating, however, when attempting to eat healthy food, the main obstacles they encountered were the cost of goods, limited knowledge of how to prepare healthy, yet tasty meals and complex social relationships meaning it was the foods appearance, price and availability that determined choices about what to eat rather than a focus on health [26]. Furthermore, patients from minority ethnic groups are likely to seek information and dietary advice from many informal sources, including relatives, other diabetic patients, traditional healers, Christian faith healers and herbalists [24] and express a distrust of formal healthcare professional advice [27].

The importance of economic barriers in lifestyle adherence has been recognised. These barriers include limited access to healthy foods and supermarkets, which shape meal possibilities for families, along with food insecurity and insufficiency [1]. Financial constraints also impact on adherence to physical activity interventions; patients from minority backgrounds often state a lack of time, multiple caregiving responsibilities and lack of facilities and safe areas for exercise, as barriers to taking up physical activity interventions. In addition to financial considerations, ethnic minority patients often report a lack of information from healthcare professionals regarding the benefits of physical activity, perhaps due to language difficulties; family members inhibiting activity or being overprotective; females, in particular, feeling uncomfortable exercising alone; belief systems relating to fate and a general attitude that sedentariness is a normal part of ageing; a lack of culturally sensitive facilities e.g. same gender classes or instructors; and a lack of time related to people's obligations to others and contribution to community activities as barriers to physical activity and reasons for not adhering to physical activity advice [28].

With this in mind, activities that focus on the social context, for example incorporating family and friends into exercise programmes have been found to increase motivation in all ethnic groups, and walking is frequently identified as the preferred form of physical activity by most minority ethnic groups. Undertaking physical activity in conjunction with blood-glucose self-monitoring, thus providing an instant sense of achievement and understanding of the benefits of exercise, is also recommended [28].

Overweight and obesity drive a significant proportion of diabetes risk in ethnic minority groups and therefore weight management is a principal focus of prevention and management strategies. It is important to consider cultural influences and attitudes towards body weight when working with or targeting ethnic minority populations. Many ethnic populations see the larger body as a source of power, prestige and financial status compared to Caucasian cultures where the emphasis is on thinness [29]. Ethnic populations are more likely to underestimate their weight than White populations, and this is particularly marked in men [30]. African and Middle-Eastern Arab cultures particularly value bigger body sizes, with African women reporting greater acceptance or satisfaction with their body size and expressing less negativity towards obesity than women from other ethnic groups. However, whilst the negative perception of obesity in White European women is focused on emotional and social consequences, Black women are more likely to concentrate on health implications and, therefore, it is important to approach weight loss with a health promotion focus with these patients [31].

8.3.4 Designing lifestyle interventions for ethnic minority groups

'Culturally sensitive' is a term used to describe interventions that have been tailored to increase their appropriateness for ethnic minority groups. To work effectively with ethnic minority patients and communities it is essential that all healthcare professionals achieve an in-depth knowledge of the targeted population's culture, for example become knowledgeable on cultural influences on food consumption, including differences by ethnicity and between first and later generations. Additionally it is important that the healthcare professional has an awareness of their personal biases and examines their competency at working with individuals whose cultural backgrounds differ from that of their own.

In the absence of a detailed literature base for specific ethnic minority initiatives culturally sensitising interventions usually equates to adapting existing interventions [32]. Resnicow et al. have distinguished between interventions adapted at a 'surface structure', such as language, and those adapted at 'deep structure', including cultural, social, environmental and psychological forces that influence health behaviour [33]. It is also essential to consider the impact of deep-rooted influences, such as lower socio-economic status, on health and behaviours [34–36] when planning initiatives aimed specifically at minority populations.

A systematic review by Netto et al. that evaluated interventions related to reducing the main causes of mortality for specifically South Asian and South-East Asian communities identified five key principles of adaptations for behavioural interventions aimed at minority ethnic groups [32]:

(1) Use community resources to increase intervention accessibility by, for example using ethnic-specific media and networks, local community leaders and community events.
(2) Identify and address barriers to access and participation in interventions, for example providing transport or keeping costs of participation low addresses the disadvantaged socio-economic status of many target groups. Providing creche facilities overcomes barriers related to the gendered nature of caring responsibilities.
(3) Develop communication strategies that address language use and differential information requirements. Conventionally, bilingual facilitators can be employed to overcome language barriers, additionally

consider that the participants may be able to speak but not read their native language or have varying levels of literacy, furthermore, participants may be better able to express their health concerns in their native language.

(4) Identify and work with cultural or religious values that either motivate or inhibit behavioural change. Ma et al. [37] recognises the importance of supporting participants in making behavioural or attitudinal changes by highlighting the compatibility of health promotion messages with their beliefs, for example using the value attached to persistence among Chinese-American participants to encourage them to persist in their attempts to stop smoking [37]. Other cultural values hinder the adoption of healthier lifestyles, for example fatalistic views amongst some South Asian communities discourage them from taking preventative actions.

Accommodate degrees of cultural affiliation in the planning and evaluation of targeted interventions. The need to take account of varying degrees of cultural identification and acculturation among the target population, for example *Sun* et al. suggested that Chinese-American youth who held both traditional Chinese and mainstream American values need longer exposure to health measures [38].

Di Noia et al. have reviewed the literature specifically for designing dietary interventions for African-American populations [39]. Their review provides an in-depth discussion of the cultural influences that need to be considered and describes a range of strategies or recommendations for the development of culturally sensitive interventions for communities of African ancestry:

(1) Establish and maintain trust, for example conduct formative research to explore potential suspicions among community members regarding motives for the planned work. Acknowledge historical influences on trust, and appreciate that concerns are based in historical reality. Design interventions to give back to the community through

long-term sustainability and broader diffusion. Community forums and partnerships with local organisations are vital for identifying local priorities and concerns as well as the intervention strategies. Participatory approaches are essential for building and maintaining trust with community members, nurturing community strengths and problem-solving abilities, and increasing social capital, community capacity, and ownership of health programs. By design, they ensure a 'do with' rather than a 'do to' approach to programme development that is essential to individual and community empowerment.

(2) Acknowledge the cultural meanings of food. Traditional food practices are often an important component of cultural identity, and maintaining these practices is seen as a way of sustaining this identity. Explore connotative meanings of food, particularly those that may inhibit or facilitate change.

(3) Improve access to healthy food – host events where only healthy food is offered and provide transportation and free food as incentives to participation.

(4) Adapt materials for individuals with low literacy and numeracy skills – simplify language and use delivery modalities that show promise for reaching low-literature groups, for example audiovisual materials and interactive media.

(5) Use cultural targeting and tailoring to enhance programme relevance and impact. Several strategies are recommended: incorporation of pictures of group members, images and colours familiar to and preferred by group members; evidential strategies or the presentation of statistics on the health problem and its impact on the group; linguistic strategies or the use of the dominant or native language in communication materials; constituent-involving strategies or the identification of key roles for audience members in programme planning and decision-making; and sociocultural strategies or the discussion of health-related issues in the context of core values and characteristics.

(6) Raise awareness of links between beliefs and behaviours. Increase understanding of the potential for perceptions about ideal weight to raise risk for obesity or to limit the extent to which efforts to eat healthily are sustained.

(7) Target influential role models. Include women as a key focus of intervention and incorporate their unique needs and perspectives on dietary change. Encourage the involvement and support of extended family members, particularly those who occupy a central role in food-related decisions and who may be unreceptive to dietary change.

(8) Use preferred delivery settings and modalities – the centrality of the church in African American culture suggests that it is an important venue for implementing interventions. Church-based interventions can improve access to hard-to-reach populations or those who may view traditional healthcare with distrust. Nurture the values of collectivism by using group versus individual modalities.

(9) Incorporate strategies that resonate with cultural values and learning styles. Adapt theoretical models and intervention approaches with evidence of effectiveness.

Peer leaders have been identified as an effective strategy for promoting lifestyle change in many ethnic minority communities [26,40]. The Eat Well Live Well Programme to combat obesity-related chronic disease in African-American women has utilised peer leaders and was more effective compared to non-peer-led interventions that have previously been reported as being 'inherently biased towards the needs and values of Caucasian middle-class women' [41]. The Khush Dil project in South Asian communities based in the UK has additionally demonstrated the positive impact of peer leaders and educators [42]. Diabetes UK 'Community Champions' is an initiative to educate and raise awareness of diabetes to people from Black, Asian and minority ethnic communities, which uses volunteers and figure heads from minority communities to act as peer leaders to improve engagement. In a review of the evidence for the effectiveness of interventions to improve glycaemic control in ethnic minority groups, Lirussi concluded that strategies adopted in community-gathering places, family-based, multifaceted, and those tackling the social context were likely to be more effective. Self-management education was successful if culturally tailored and involving community leaders [40].

8.3.5 Culturally tailored care in practice

In 2008, Hawthorne et al. published a Cochrane systematic review and meta-analysis of the effects of culturally appropriate health education for type 2 diabetes in ethnic minority groups [43]; reviewing 11 studies the authors concluded that there are short-term positive effects of culturally appropriate diabetes health education on glycaemic control and knowledge of diabetes and healthy lifestyles. Their review included 11 trials, of which 5 focused on African-Americans, 3 on South Asians in the UK, 1 on Surinam Asians in the Netherlands and 3 on Hispanic populations in the USA and Canada. The cultural tailoring of the South Asian interventions mainly focused on the delivery of education by educators and link workers with relevant language skills (e.g. Punjabi or Urdu speaking), separate sessions for women and men, and the use of culturally relevant picture flashcards that have been shown to be effective in improving knowledge and self-management practices amongst South Asian patients. The studies amongst African-Americans mainly focused on group-based interventions and community settings that nurture the sense of collectivism to promote behaviour change through theories of social learning. These interventions have demonstrated greater benefit in glycaemic control and self-management practices compared to the usual care, and confirm the recommendations set out by Lirussi that community-based interventions are appropriate for ethnic minority groups.

Healthcare professionals working with individual patients/clients from ethnic minority cultures should focus on the healthy components of

Table 8.3.1 Glycaemic index of South Asian foods

Food	Glycaemic index
Pulses and lentils	
Chickpeas	28
Mung beans	31
Red lentils	21
Chana dal	12
Kidney beans	29
Bengal gram	47
Green gram	48
Black gram	48
Cereals	
Chapatti	60
Basmati rice	58
Potato	70
Breakfast snacks	
Pongal	55
Pasarattu	60
Upma	75
Idli	80
Chola	65
Vegetables	
Karela	65
Saag (spinach)	0
Fruit	
Banana	51
Mango	56
Water melon	72
Dates (dried)	45

Ref: Thaker and Barton [18].

traditional cultural diets. The traditional South Asian diet, whether Gujarati, Punjabi or Pakistani, is based on starchy carbohydrates, rich in vegetables, beans and pulses and is relatively low in fat. Patients should be encouraged to consume traditional dishes and educated about their benefits (e.g. low glycaemic index of basmati rice, pulses and daals (see Table 8.3.1)) whilst being advised on the detrimental effects of increasing fat and sugar in the diet through the introduction of 'westernised' processed foods and increased consumption of traditional South Asian foods (e.g. Indian sweets and deep fried snacks) that were historically only consumed occasionally (see Table 8.3.2).

Similarly, patients of Caribbean and African culture should be educated on the healthy properties of a traditional African and Caribbean diet that is high in carbohydrate and low in fat and be encouraged to consume traditional foods, for example yam and pulses that are used within traditional 'soups' have a low glycaemic index. Overweight and obesity may be particularly problematic amongst African and Caribbean patient groups and advice on portion sizes, particularly relating to starchy carbohydrate foods, can be particularly important (see Table 8.3.3).

There are a range of resources available for healthcare professionals working with ethnic minority groups. In the UK the 'DESMOND' structured education programme has been adapted for South Asian communities and can be delivered by interpreters or healthcare professionals in Punjabi, Gujarati, Urdu and Bengali, with use of culturally-sensitive resources and images to avoid reliance on written information (Ref http://www.desmond-project.org.uk/bmefoundationnewlydiagnosed-279.html). The American Diabetes Association (ADA) has a wide range of programs that target raising awareness of diabetes amongst all its minority communities, such as Project POWER a faith-based program targeting the African-American community (http://www.diabetes.org/in-my-community/awareness-programs/african-american-programs/project-power.html), and the Office for Minority Health has a wide range of information and resources to assist healthcare professionals working with minority groups. Culturally tailored information sources are available for use by healthcare professionals, for example 'O Taste & See Recipes' from the ADA for African-American patients, 'Traditional Foods – Healthy Dishes' and 'Taste of South Asia' from the British Heart Foundation for African Caribbean and South Asian patients, respectively, and 'Enjoy Food' for African and Caribbean patients from Diabetes UK. The *Ismaili Nutrition Centre* is a website featuring a library of recipes of foods with African, Central and South Asian and Middle Eastern origin, which are supported with nutritional information and healthy eating tips. The website recipe finder allows users to input their dish preferences with

Table 8.3.2 Dietary modification of South Asian diet for diabetes

Food group	Encourage	Discourage
Carbohydrates	Wholemeal/wholegrain bread, wholegrain cereals, chapatti made with wholemeal flour, boiled rice	Parathas, puri, fried toast
Protein	Meat or chicken curry, daal (using small amounts of oil). Fish curry using oily and white fish. Boiled eggs. Boil/steam/grill meat/fish.	Fried egg/omelette. Fatty meats and fried meat/fish.
Dairy	Semi-skimmed or skimmed milk.	Full-fat milk, cream, evaporated milk.
Desserts	Fresh or tinned fruit in natural juice Rice pudding or vermicelli (made with semi-skimmed milk) Fruit salad Fruit yoghurt	Halwa (made with carrots or semolina), Zarda (sweet rice)
Snacks	Oven-baked samosas. Chana (chickpeas) and/or potato chaat, fruit chaat. Muthiya, dhokra, khaman. Grilled kebab with pitta/naan bread with salad. Fruit and vegetables.	Fried samosas, pakoras, chips. Bombay mix, chevdo, sev, ghatiya, crisps. Asian sweets (jalebi, halwa, burfi)
Drinks	Water, unsweetened fruit juices. Diet or sugar-free soft drinks. Lassi.	Sugar sweetened fizzy and soft drinks and juices.
Fats and oils	Reduce all fats and oils. Avoid deep-frying and adding fat to chapattis/flat breads.	Ghee, butter. Oily pickles.

Ref: Thaker and Barton [18].

Table 8.3.3 Dietary modification of African-Caribbean diet for diabetes

Food group	Encourage
Starchy foods / root vegetables Sweet potato, yam, dasheen, coco, potato, bammy, breadfruit, cassava, fufu, kenkey, cornmeal, oats, green banana, rice, plantain, bread, dumplings	Include a starchy food at each meal. Choose lower GI starches (e.g. yam, cassava, green banana). Limit portion sizes of starches.
Vegetables and fruits Pumpkin, callaloo, cho-cho, okra, sweetcorn, carrots, ackee, avocado. Mango, pineapple, grapefruit, melon, banana, paw-paw	Add plenty of vegetables to soups and one-pot meals. Aim for 5 portions of fruit and vegetables per day. Have fruit for snacks and desserts. If consuming tinned fruit, avoid syrup.
Meat, fish and pulses Beef, chicken, goat, mutton, pork, turkey, offal. Snapper, bream, mullet, jackfish, mackerel, sardines, pilchards. Black-eyed beans, red kidney beans, gunga peas.	Remove skin before cooking. Reduce oil in cooking. Reduce portion size. Steam or bake fish rather than fry. Aim to have two portions of oily fish per week. Use more beans, pulses and lentils and less meat in dishes. Add beans/lentils/pulses to soups and stews.
Milk and dairy Fresh milk, condensed milk, evaporated milk, butter, cheese.	Use lower fat milks and avoid sweetened evaporated and condensed milks. Have low fat yoghurt and reduced fat cheese.
Sugary foods and drinks Honey, molasses, brown sugar, ginger beer, fruit punch, carrot juice. Cakes, buns, biscuits, sweets, chocolate.	Choose diet or sugar-free drinks. Add less sugar to cereals and drinks. Limit sweet snacks to small amounts.

Ref: Thaker and Barton [18].

regard to their ingredients and nutritional values according to the UK FSA traffic light system (www.theismaili.org/nutrition).

8.3.6 Recommendations for future research, policy and practice

The FSA review [26] made six recommendations for the evaluation of future dietary interventions in minority ethnic groups.

(1) Evaluations of dietary interventions in black and minority ethnic groups should use rigorous and appropriate research methodologies.
(2) To collaborate with other agencies or groups to increase the funding for good evaluations of dietary interventions.
(3) Evaluations of dietary interventions for the general population should consider increasing the numbers of black and minority ethnic participants so that conclusions can be made relating to these groups.
(4) To develop and validate evaluation tools for specific minority groups (e.g. food intake measurement techniques and various terminology used for dishes).
(5) Any future evaluations of dietary interventions to include the theoretical bases, for example behaviour change models, to structure the intervention.
(6) Cost-effectiveness and sustainability of evaluations of dietary interventions should be assessed.

8.3.7 Conclusion

People from minority ethnicities are disproportionately affected by diabetes, particularly type 2 diabetes. Diet and lifestyle education forms the cornerstone of diabetes management, however, specific cultural barriers may limit healthcare access and contribute to poorer outcomes for minority patients. Culturally-tailored care improves diabetes management and is identified as a priority by patient groups. Traditional diets may change because of acculturation,

therefore, the needs of different generations are likely to vary. The recommendations and outcomes of the various reviews and reports highlighted in this chapter demonstrate the crucial importance of tailoring lifestyle and nutritional interventions that emphasize patients' ethnic preferences and traditions (for example adapting ethnic recipes to meet dietary goals), the use of available community resources for exercise, and should be delivered utilising appropriate strategies and materials in order to have any hope of modifying traditional eating patterns and effectively treating type 2 diabetes.

Key points

- It is important that healthcare professionals working with ethnic minority groups have an in-depth knowledge and understanding of the traditional, cultural dietary practices of their patient groups.
- Many traditional, cultural dietary practices are healthy and should be promoted.
- Fasting and religious food practices are important in many ethnic minority groups, which may impact on their diabetes management.
- Ethnic minority groups may have a strong belief in traditional or herbal remedies for the management of their diabetes.
- It is important that healthcare professionals working with ethnic minority groups have an in-depth knowledge and understanding of cultural barriers and motivations to lifestyle change.
- Culturally sensitive diet and lifestyle interventions are those that have been adapted in some way to target/engage specific cultural groups; culturally sensitive lifestyle advice has been shown to be more effective in the management of diabetes than standard care.

References

1. Orzech KM, Vivian J, Huebner Torres C, Armin J, Shaw SJ. Diet and exercise adherence and practices among medically underserved patients with chronic disease: variation across four ethnic groups. *Health Educ Behav* 2013; **40**(1): 56–66.

2. Leonard BJ, Plotnikoff GA. Awareness: the heart of cultural competence. *AACN Clin Issues* 2000; **11**(1): 51–59.

3. Beach MC, Price EG, Gary TL, Robinson KA, Gozu A, Palacio A, et al. Cultural competence: a systematic review of health care provider educational interventions. *Med Care* 2005; **43**(4): 356–373. Epub 2005/03/22.

4. Corral I, Landrine H. Acculturation and ethnic-minority health behavior: a test of the operant model. *Health Psychol* 2008; **27**(6): 737–745.

5. Gilbert PA, Khokhar S. Changing dietary habits of ethnic groups in Europe and implications for health. *Nutr Rev* 2008; **66**(4): 203–215.

6. Luke A, Cooper RS, Prewitt TE, Adeyemo AA, Forrester TE. Nutritional consequences of the African diaspora. *Annu Rev Nutr* 2001; **21**: 47–71.

7. Klurfeld DM, Kritchevsky D. The Western diet: an examination of its relationship with chronic disease. *J Am Coll Nutr* 1986; **5**(5): 477–485.

8. Leung G, Stanner S. Diets of minority ethnic groups in the UK: influence on chronic disease risk and implications for prevention. *Br Nutr Bull* 2011; **36**: 161–198.

9. Wyke S, Landman J. Healthy Eating? Diet and cuisine amongst Scottish South Asian people. *Br Food J* 1997; **99**: 27–34.

10. Goff LM, Timbers L, Style H, Knight A. Dietary intake in Black British adults; an observational assessment of nutritional composition and the role of traditional foods in UK Caribbean and West African diets. *Public Health Nutr* 2014: 1–11.

11. Sharma S, Cruickshank JK. Cultural differences in assessing dietary intake and providing relevant dietary information to British African-Caribbean populations. *J Hum Nutr Diet* 2001; **14**(6): 449–456.

12. Owusu M, Thomas J, Wiredu E, Pufulete M. Folate status of Ghanaian populations in London and Accra. *Br J Nutr* 2010; **103**(3): 437–444.

13. Kulkarni KD. Food, culture and diabetes in the United States. *Clin Diabetes* 2004; **22**(4): 190–192.

14. Aldrich L, Variyam JN. Acculturation erodes the diet quality of U.S. Hispanics. *Food Rev* 2000; **23**: 51–55.

15. Educators AAoD. Cultural sensitivity: definition, application and recommendations for diabetes educators. *Diabetes Educ* 2002; **28**: 922–927.

16. Sharma S, Wilkens LR, Shen L, Kolonel LN. Dietary sources of five nutrients in ethnic groups represented in the Multiethnic Cohort. *Br J Nutr* 2013; **109**(8): 1479–1489.

17. Chau CM. Health experiences of Chinese people in the UK. London: 2008.

18. Thaker A, Barton A. Multicultural handbook of food, nutrition and dietetics. Chichester, UK: 2012.

19. Simmons D, Williams R. Dietary practices among Europeans and different South Asian groups in Coventry. *Br J Nutr* 1997; **78**(1): 5–14.

20. Group SADRW. Background information for health professionals. Canada: 2007.

21. Pawa M. Use of traditional/herbal remedies by Indo-Asian people with type 2 diabetes. *Pract Diabetes Int* 2005; **22**(8): 292–294.

22. Lawrence JM, Devlin E, Macaskill S, Kelly M, Chinouya M, Raats MM, et al. Factors that affect the food choices made by girls and young women, from minority ethnic groups, living in the UK. *J Hum Nutr Diet* 2007; **20**(4): 311–9.

23. Lip GY, Malik I, Luscombe C, McCarry M, Beevers G. Dietary fat purchasing habits in whites, blacks and Asian peoples in England–implications for heart disease prevention. *Int J Cardiol* 1995; **48**(3): 287–293.

24. Nthangeni G, Steyn NP, Alberts M, Steyn K, Levitt NS, Laubscher R, et al. Dietary intake and barriers to dietary compliance in black type 2 diabetic patients attending primary health-care services. *Public Health Nutr* 2002; **5**(2): 329–338.

25. SADRW Group. Background information for health professionals. Canada: 2007.

26. Stockley L. Review of Dietary intervention models for Black and Minority Ethnic Groups. Wales, UK: 2009.

27. Stone MA. Making education in diabetes culturally appropriate for patients. *Pract Nurs* 2006; **17**(12): 5.

28. Horne M, Tierney S. What are the barriers and facilitators to exercise and physical activity uptake and adherence among South Asian older adults: a systematic review of qualitative studies. *Prev Med* 2012; **55**(4): 276–284.

29. Bush HM, Williams RG, Lean ME, Anderson AS. Body image and weight consciousness among South Asian, Italian and general population women in Britain. *Appetite* 2001; **37**(3): 207–215.

30. Dorsey RR, Eberhardt MS, Ogden CL. Racial/ethnic differences in weight perception. *Obesity (Silver Spring)* 2009; **17**(4): 790–795.

31. Shoneye C, Johnson F, Steptoe A, Wardle J. A qualitative analysis of black and white British women's attitudes to weight and weight control. *J Hum Nutr Diet* 2011; **24**(6): 536–542.

32. Netto G, Bhopal R, Lederle N, Khatoon J, Jackson A. How can health promotion interventions be adapted for minority ethnic communities? Five principles for guiding the development of behavioural interventions. *Health Promot Int* 2010; **25**(2): 248–257.

33. Resnicow K, Baranowski T, Ahluwalia JS, Braithwaite RL. Cultural sensitivity in public health: defined and demystified. *Ethn Dis* 1999; **9**(1): 10–21.

34. McAllister G, Farquhar M. Health beliefs: a cultural division? *J Adv Nurs* 1992; **17**(12): 1447–1454.

35. Pasick R, Onofrio C, Otero-Sabogal R. Similarities and differences across cultures: questions to ifnorm a

third generation for health promotion research. *Health Educ Q* 1996; **23**: 142–1161.

36. Greenhalgh T, Helman C, Chowdhury AM. Health beliefs and folk models of diabetes in British Bangladeshis: a qualitative study. *BMJ* 1998; **316**(7136): 978–983.

37. Ma GX, Shive SE, Tan Y, Thomas P, Man VL. Development of a culturally appropriate smoking cessation program for Chinese-American youth. *J Adolesc Health* 2004; **35**(3): 206–216.

38. Sun WY, Sangweni B, Chen J, Cheung S. Effects of a community-based nutrition education program on the dietary behaviour of Chinese-American college students. *Health Promot Int* 1999; **14**: 214–249.

39. Di Noia J, Furst G, Park K, Byrd-Bredbenner C. Designing culturally sensitive dietary interventions for African Americans: review and recommendations. *Nutr Rev* 2013; **71**(4): 224–238.

40. Lirussi F. The global challenge of type 2 diabetes and the strategies for response in ethnic minority groups. *Diabetes Metab Res Rev* 2010; **26**(6): 421–432.

41. Williams JH, Auslander WF, de Groot M, Robinson AD, Houston C, Haire-Joshu D. Cultural relevancy of a diabetes prevention nutrition program for African American women. *Health Promot Pract* 2006; **7**(1): 56–67.

42. Farooqi A, Bhavsar M. Project Dil: a coordinated primary care and community health promotion programme for reducing risk factors for coronary heart disease amongst the south Asian community of Leicester - experiences and evaluation of the project. *Ethn Health* 2001; **6**(3): 265–270.

43. Hawthorne K, Robles Y, Cannings-John R, Edwards AG. Culturally appropriate health education for type 2 diabetes mellitus in ethnic minority groups. *Cochrane Database Syst Rev* 2008; (3): CD006424. Epub 2008/07/23.

SECTION 9

Complications and comorbidities of diabetes

Chapter 9.1

Microvascular disease (renal) and diabetes

Thushara Dassanayake
Imperial College Healthcare NHS Foundation Trust, London, UK

9.1.1 Introduction

Diabetic nephropathy is currently the leading cause of chronic kidney disease (CKD) in people starting renal replacement therapy [1]. In those with type 2 diabetes, worldwide estimates of CKD prevalence are 5–30% [2].

Diabetes-related diet and lifestyle modification is of benefit across the CKD disease spectrum. Dietary modification contributes to CKD prevention; minimising disease progression in early CKD; blood glucose management and malnutrition prevention in dialysis (CKD 5) and risk factor management for optimal graft survival in transplant recipients. The chronic and evolving nature of CKD complications calls for the fostering of a positive and collaborative therapist–client relationship to help create a personal nutrition care agenda that enhances client autonomy and coping ability while improving health outcomes and quality of life.

9.1.2 Early diabetic CKD (stages 1–3) management

Diabetic nephropathy is characterised by a progressive increase in urinary albumin excretion and blood pressure leading to a decline in glomerular filtration rate (GFR) (Table 9.1.1). Clinical practice guidelines for diabetes and CKD suggest that screening for diabetic nephropathy

should begin 5 years after the diagnosis of type 1 diabetes and at the diagnosis of type 2 diabetes [4].

The primary medical management aims for people with diabetic nephropathy involve cardiovascular risk management and CKD progression minimisation [5]. The aim of dietary management is to achieve optimal blood sugar and blood pressure control within a moderate-protein, cardio-protective diet.

Cardiovascular risk management

People with diabetic nephropathy have a 20–40-fold increase in cardiovascular disease risk [6]. This increased risk begins very early, on detection of microalbuminuria even with normal GFR [7]. There is a strong association between abnormal blood lipid profiles and progression and severity of cardiovascular disease in type 2 diabetes [8]. Risk factor control through cardio-protective diet and lifestyle modification, including smoking, weight reduction and exercise, therefore remains relevant in CKD prevention and for risk factor management once CKD has become established.

Glycaemic control

Hyperglycaemia, the defining feature of diabetes, is a fundamental cause of vascular target organ complications, including diabetic kidney

---

Advanced Nutrition and Dietetics in Diabetes, First Edition. Edited by Louise Goff and Pamela Dyson.
© 2016 John Wiley & Sons, Ltd. Published 2016 by John Wiley & Sons, Ltd.

Table 9.1.1 Chronic kidney disease classification [3]

Stage	GFR (ml/min/1.73m^2)	Description
1	>90	Normal or increased GFR with other evidence of kidney damage
2	60–89	Slight decrease in GFR with other evidence of kidney damage
3a	45–59	Moderate decrease in
3b	30–44	GFR with or without other evidence of kidney damage
4	15–29	Severe decrease in GFR with or without other evidence of kidney damage
5	<15	Established renal failure

GFR: glomerular filtration rate.

disease [9]. Therefore minimising renal disease progression through tight blood glucose control is a primary management aim in early diabetic nephropathy. Clinical trials on type 1 diabetes and type 2 diabetes patients have consistently demonstrated that HbA1c levels below 53 mmol/mol (7%) are associated with decreased risk of clinical and structural manifestations of diabetic nephropathy [4]. In the Diabetes Control and Complications Trial (DCCT), intensive treatment of diabetes reduced the incidence of microalbuminuria by 39% [10]. The UK Prospective Diabetes Study (UKPDS) data showed that reducing glucose exposure [HbA1c 53 mmol/mol (7.0 %) versus 63 mmol/mol (7.9 %) over median 10.0 years], with sulfonylurea or insulin therapy, reduced the risk of "any diabetes-related endpoint" by 12% and microvascular disease by 25% [11]. A recent 5-study systematic review of intensive versus conventional glycaemic control in type 2 diabetic CKD and non-CKD patients concluded that intensive glucose control reduced the risk of new onset micro- and macro-albuminuria, however, it also resulted in a 2.5-fold increased risk of severe hypoglycaemia [12]. These issues are reflected

in the 2012 update of the KDOQI clinical practice guidelines [9] for diabetes and CKD, guideline 2, which recommends:

- A target HbA1c averaging 7.0% to prevent or delay progression of the microvascular complications of diabetes, including diabetic kidney disease.
- Not treating to an HbA1c target of <7.0% in patients at risk of hypoglycaemia
- Extending target HbA1c above 7.0% in individuals with comorbidities or limited life expectancy and risk of hypoglycaemia.

Diabetes medication in ckd

Table 9.1.2 presents a summary of the 2012 KDOQI Diabetes Guidelines Update [9].

Blood pressure control

There is much evidence demonstrating that hypertension is the single most important factor that accelerates the progression of microvascular disease, including diabetic nephropathy [13]. In an embedded study, the UKPDS showed that microvascular endpoints, including microalbuminuria development, were reduced by 37% in an intensive blood pressure control group compared to the less tightly managed controls [14].

Due to large inter-individual variation in blood pressure response to sodium restriction, individual studies relating dietary sodium restriction to blood pressure improvements have been inconclusive. However meta-analyses do demonstrate population reductions in blood pressure achieved by salt restriction [15]. A meta-analysis of 11 studies showed that reduced sodium intake was as effective as antihypertensive medication in maintaining good blood pressure control [16]. Similarly in the CKD stages 1–3 population, a multi-centred crossover randomised controlled trial of 52 subjects showed that, with a background of angiotensin converting enzyme (ACE) inhibition, a low sodium diet reduced proteinuria more effectively than did an angiotensin receptor blockade (ARB) [17].

People with diabetic nephropathy are thus advised to reduce dietary salt to at least 5–6 g/day

Table 9.1.2 Summary of the 2012 KDOQI Diabetes Guidelines

Name	Recommendation	Rationalle for recommendation
Metformin	Restrict in CKD Re-evaluate at GFR <45 ml/min/1.73m². Stop at GFR <30 ml/min/1.73m². (British National Formulary, BNF)	Cleared by the kidney. Lactic acidosis (rare but serious side effect)
Thiazolidinediones Pioglitazone	Limit use in advanced CKD	Fluid Retention (side effect) Linked to increased fracture rates and bone loss
Acarbose (disaccharidease inhibitor)	Nor recommended at GFR <26 ml/min/1.73m²	Serum levels of drug and metabolites increase significantly with reduced kidney function.
Dipeptidyl peptidase (DPP-4) inhibitors - the 'gliptins'	Suitable in CKD but some require downward dose adjustments	Decrease the breakdown of incretin hormones and improve both fasting and post-prandial glucose levels.
Injectable incretin mimetics Exenatide Liraglutide	Exenatide: stop use at GFR <30 ml/min/1.73m² Liraglutide Not recommended at GFR <60 ml/min/1.73m²	Exenatide is excreted by the kidneys. Case report associations with acute kidney injury. Liraglutide is not excreted by the kidney, however, limited long-term data available.

(80–100 mmol/d) [18]. This restriction should occur alongside drug therapies such as ACE inhibition and/or renin-angiotensin blockers to achieve blood pressure targets [19]. From CKD-3 onward, potassium lowering dietary management may also be necessary if serum potassium increases following the addition or dose increase of medications such as potassium-sparing diuretics, ACE inhibitors, ARBs or non-steroidal anti-inflammatory medications.

Protein restriction

Although much evidence exists to demonstrate the efficacy of low protein diets in delaying the onset of dialysis through uraemic symptom management [20], the effect of protein restriction in delaying diabetic nephropathy progression is not so well defined. One meta-analysis of eight randomised controlled trials of low protein diets in diabetic nephropathy showed a small 3 mmol/mol decrease (0.3%) in HbA1c, but not in GFR [21]. Another review based on 12 studies concluded that protein restriction marginally slowed CKD progression [22].

Epidemiological evidence exists to show that high protein diets lead to kidney damage and to the development of microalbuminuria in people with diabetes and hypertension [23]. A 2009 Cochrane meta-analysis, demonstrated that complying with a low-protein intake modestly slows the progression of diabetic nephropathy and extrapolated that this can delay dialysis by, on average around 1–2 months [22]. Although improvement in GFR was greater with increasingly tighter protein restriction, many studies were confounded by difficulties with dietary adherence, which worsened with the severity of the protein restriction.

The optimum level of protein intake in practice would therefore require a compromise between efficacy and achievability of protein restriction in a population who are already likely to be following other dietary restrictions relating to diabetes and CVD. The National Kidney Foundation/Kidney Dialysis Outcomes Quality Initiative (KDOQI) clinical practice guidelines for diabetes and CKD recommend a dietary protein intake at the lower end of the normal range (0.8 g/kg body weight/day), as an achievable goal for minimising CKD progression [4]. This can be achieved by reducing intake and portion size of high biological value protein sources while keeping low biological value protein quantities unchanged. When dietary protein intake is restricted, an adjustment to carbohydrates and/or fats intake is required to keep the diet isocaloric. Due to possible increased risk of malnutrition, care should be taken when advising protein restrictions below 0.8 g/kg body weight.

9.1.3 Nutritional requirements

Few specific guidelines exist for macronutrient intake (apart from protein) for diabetes-related CKD or dialysis. The reader should refer to standard dietetic textbooks for dietary recommendations regarding macronutrient and micronutrient guidelines for renal patients [24,25]. Table 9.1.3 summarises the main internationally recognised nutrition-related targets in CKD stages 1–5.

9.1.4 Nutritional assessment

Nutritional assessment of people with diabetes and CKD stages 1–4 does not differ from standard nutritional assessment protocols. Table 9.1.4 contains information about the dietetic assessment of CKD stage 5 patients with or without diabetes.

9.1.5 Late diabetic CKD (stages 4–5) management

The use of HbA1c in CKD

Kalantar-Zadeh et al. [26] demonstrated an association between increasing HbA1c and higher mortality rates in a study of 83 000 dialysis patients, mirroring general population outcomes in the UKPDS [14] and DCCT trials [27]. Current National Institute for Health and Clinical Excellence (NICE) guidelines for diabetes recommend management including diet and lifestyle advice to achieve a reduction in HbA1c towards 48 mmol/mol (6.5%) or less where feasible [8], however, KDOQI guidelines

recommend moderation for those with CKD. Individual targets should be set in conjunction with the patient and take into consideration lifestyle, comorbidity and hypoglycaemic history.

Although HbA1c remains the most commonly used indicator of long-term diabetic control, its validity in the haemodialysis (HD) population is questioned. Due to decreased metabolism, anaemia, shorter red cell life, transfusions, haemolysis, assay interferences from uraemia and increased glucose variability on HD, it is suggested that HbA1c may not be adequately representative of actual glycaemic control in this group [28]. Alternative parameters such as glycated serum protein (albumin corrected fructosamine – acF), have been investigated, although their validity also remains unproven. Thus, KDOQI suggest that currently HbA1c remains the best clinical marker of long-term glycaemic control, particularly if combined with blood glucose self-monitoring [9].

Validity aside, it should be noted that neither spot capillary blood glucose nor HbA1c accurately reflect the inter-day variations or the inter-dialytic excursions in glycaemia experienced by the HD patient. Kazempour et al. [29], using continuous glucose monitors found that 24-h mean glucose values were significantly lower on dialysis days compared to dialysis-free days, with risk of asymptomatic hypoglycaemia highest within 24 hours of dialysis.

Therefore, when formulating dietary advice, inter-day symptom variation in appetite, food intake, access to food and snacking frequency should be regarded. Modification of HD dialysate glucose concentrations, which vary from 1–2 g/L, could also be considered. A lower hypoglycaemic agent dose on dialysis days and/or a higher glucose concentration dialysate (2 g/L compared to the standard 1g/L) could be used to ameliorate glucose variability in patients who frequently experience post-dialysis hypoglycaemia.

Haemodialysis

Caplin et al. [30] who surveyed 550 HD patients to quantify dialysis-associated symptoms found fatigue (82%), intradialytic hypotension (76%), cramps (74%), dizziness (63%) and headaches

Table 9.1.3 Nutritional targets in CKD based upon NKF/KDOQI (2007), Renal Association Guideline (2011) [6], NICE Guidelines (2008) and British Dietetic Association Renal Nutrition Group (2011)

CKD Stage	HbA1c	BP	BMI	Total cholesterol	LDL	Protein	Energy
All stages	48–58 mmol/mol, (6.5–7.5%) [7] <7 [4]			<4 or 25% reduction from baseline [7]	Fasting level <2 or 30% reduction from baseline [7]		30–35 kcal/ kg IBW/d [7]
1–3	<48 mmol/mol (6.5%) (NICE 2008) <53 mmol/mol (7%)	130/80 mmHg [4,7]	General population guidelines	<4 (NICE 2008)	<2 (NICE 2008). Target LDL <100 mg/ dL [4]	0.8 g/kg/d IBW [4] Stage 1–4	
4			General population guidelines		Target LDL <100 mg/ dL [4]	0.8 g/kg/d IBW [4] Stage 1–4 0.75 g/kg IBW /d [7] Stage 4	
5 (HD)		Recommendations vary depending on multiple dialysis factors	>23			>1.0 g/kg/d IBW (BDA RNG 2011) >1.2 g/kg/d [7]	
5 (CAPD)						1.0–1.2 g/kg/d IBW (BDA RNG 2011) Minimum 1.2 g/kg/d [7]	
Transplant & diabetes	Achieve normoglycaemia		Health eating if BMI 20–25 or 10% weight reduction if overweight				

BDA: British Dietetic Association;
RNG: Renal Nutrition Group

Table 9.1.4 The dietetic assessment of CKD stage 5 patients with or without diabetes

Assessment	Parameter	Description
Anthropometrics	Dry weight	Dry weight should be measured after HD. PD fluid weight should be subtracted from total weight as appropriate. Ensure that the dialysis patient is neither fluid overloaded nor clinically dry. In practice dry weight is assessed by the nephrologists in association with the renal multidisciplinary team.
	SGA	A tool based on clinical, physical and subjective measures that is used to assess malnutrition. Beware of masking of anthropometric parameters due to fluid overload. The Renal Association suggests Subjective Global Assessment (SGA) <3 (on 7-point scale) is a risk factor for malnutrition.
		The Renal Association 2011 guidelines for malnutrition risk screening in CKD: BMI <20 kg/m^2, weight loss >5% in 3 months or >10% in 6 months.
	Anthropometry	In HD patients this should be assessed immediately after dialysis, when the patient is not fluid overloaded. Mid-arm circumference, mid-arm muscle circumference and 4-site skinfold thickness should be performed by the same individual. Arm measurements should be performed on the non-fistula arm [5].
Biochemistry	Pre-dialysis blood results	Refer to local normal renal reference ranges. A serial decline in pre-dialysis serum urea, creatinine, potassium & phosphate may be indicative of lean muscle mass loss rather than an improvement in renal function.
	nPCR	Normalised protein catabolic rate (nPCR), also known as nPNA (normalised protein nitrogen appearance), is an indirect marker of protein intake in stable dialysis patients. Aim for >1.2 g/kg/day in HD patients and >1.3 g/kg/day in CAPD patients [3].
Clinical	Under dialysis	Can result in elevated serum biochemical parameters & blood pressure and fluid overload. Associated uraemia can cause decreased appetite.
	Gastroparesis	Can result in abdominal distension, vomiting and early satiety. See Chapter 9.6 for management details.
	Dialysis related losses	1 HD session results in 6–12g amino acid losses Daily protein losses on CAPD 5–15g Peritonitis protein can greatly increase protein losses.
	Insulin & blood sugars	As CKD progresses insulin clearance by the kidney usually decreases. This may lead to progressively decreased insulin requirements until dialysis initiation. Hypoglycaemic agent doses thereby may require titrating during the transition from early CKD to dialysis.
Diet	Dietary assessment	The usual methods for assessing dietary intake can be used, however, variations in nutritional intake of HD patients on dialysis day versus non-dialysis days should be considered. In CAPD the energy contribution from absorption of glucose-containing dialysate should be considered.
	Under-nutrition	Dialysis-related poor intake can be due to uraemia, inadequate dialysis, missing meals due to travelling to dialysis or being on dialysis during mealtimes, taste disturbances, satiety & abdominal distension from CAPD fluids in peritoneal cavity.
	Over-nutrition	This can result in elevated serum urea, potassium, phosphate, and sodium and fluid levels in the dialysis patient. Dietary and psychosocial modification should incorporate a patient-centred approach and include educational, motivational and behavioural components.

(54%) to be the most commonly reported. This illustrates that the typical symptoms of hyperglycaemia are also recognisable as common side-effects of routine dialysis. This side-effect duality can mask hyperglycaemic symptoms, thereby making it difficult for patients to manage their diabetes based on symptom recognition.

The effects of hyperglycaemia can also have additional repercussions in dialysis. For example, if excessive thirst caused by hyperglycaemia was addressed by drinking more, this could result in large inter-dialytic weight gain, pulmonary oedema and hypertension. Similarly, severe hyperglycaemia can also lead to hyperkalaemia and subsequent associated life-threatening effects.

Diabetes education should aim to be inclusive of an individual's renal dietary adaptations and lifestyle restrictions and address the patient's particular issues relating to balancing both conditions. It should also focus on helping patients to recognise, understand and address their body signals in relation to both diabetes and dialysis and teach people how to convey these signals to the relevant healthcare professional [31].

Peritoneal dialysis

Energy requirements for peritoneal dialysis (PD) patients are partially met from dialysate glucose of which approximately 70% is absorbed [32]. Depending on the dialysate glucose concentration and volume, energy from glucose can provide 120–1200 kcal per day. Absorption of PD dialysate glucose may increase the requirement of hypoglycaemic agents [33]. If weight maintenance is the desired therapeutic outcome, then dietary advice to compensate for dialysate energy by reducing energy from food is suggested. In obese patients, weight reduction can result in a lower concentration and volume of dialysate glucose required to achieve an adequate dialysis, thereby further reducing energy burden. Fluid and salt management will also help limit PD dialysate requirements.

There is growing evidence that regular use of hypertonic glucose dialysate solutions is associated with weight gain, poor diabetic control, delayed gastric emptying, hyperinsulinaemia

and acceleration of detrimental peritoneal membrane changes [34]. An alternative osmotic agent could be considered to lessen glucose load; or when glucose-based dialysates result in inadequate dialysis. Icodextrin, a starch-derived, high molecular weight glucose polymer has been shown to promote sustained ultrafiltration, equivalent to that achieved with hypertonic glucose dialysates. A multi-centred RCT of 201 PD patients showed that substituting 2.5% glucose dialysate solutions with 7.5% icodextrin reduced the energy load, alleviated fluid overload by improving ultrafiltration and reduced blood cholesterol but did not affect fasting blood glucose levels [35].

Short-term studies have shown that amino acid-based peritoneal dialysis solutions, despite having a relatively short effective ultrafiltration duration, may be of benefit in supplementing amino acids during dialysis while also reducing glucose load. Solutions with an adequate lactate buffer, a high percentage of essential amino acids with glucose, used in malnourished patients have been associated with improved results [36], however, a few small studies have associated amino acid dialysate with culture negative peritonitis [37]. If used, the patient should be encouraged to consume a carbohydrate-based snack to ensure maximum protein utilisation from dialysate.

Intraperitoneal insulin administration has been used in PD patients, as insulin passes directly into the portal vein and is thus absorbed more rapidly and evenly than subcutaneous insulin. However, reports of intraperitoneal insulin as a risk factor in the pathogenesis of hepatic subcapsular steatosis have led to a decline in this mode of administration [38].

Malnutrition and diabetes in renal disease

Chronic, low-grade inflammation is implicated in the pathogenesis of diabetes. Inflammation, confounded by protein energy malnutrition (PEM) is common in the dialysis population and is consistently linked to increased morbidity and mortality. Interrelated and concurrent conditions associated with both inflammation and PEM, such as poor appetite, hypercatabolism, nutrient losses via dialysis, oxidative stress, hyperphosphataemia, uraemia and fluid overload have led to the term 'malnutrition-inflammation complex syndrome' (MICS).

In addressing MICS, there is evidence that conventional cardiovascular risk factors that reflect over-nutrition may need to be modified for use in the renal patient population. For example, although in the general population obesity confers an increased cardiovascular risk; in the renal population, obesity is associated with protection from MICS and offers a survival advantage [26]. The use of standard body mass index (BMI) thresholds for determining cardiovascular risk should therefore be used with caution in this patient population. The European Best Practice Guidelines recommend that HD patients should maintain a BMI >23 kg/m² [39], however. no upper BMI limit has been advised.

Food fortification methods and nutritional supplements should be considered to help combat malnutrition and meet nutritional requirements. In dialysis patients, intra-dialytic parenteral nutrition can be considered if food fortification and other nutrition support routes are unsuccessful. There are no guidelines regarding specific macronutrient recommendations in diabetic CKD, however, KDOQI recommend a protein intake of 1.0–1.3 g/kg/d with energy requirements being the same as for the general population [4].

Transplantation

New-onset diabetes after organ transplantation (NODAT) has emerged as an increasingly important determinant of outcome and survival in transplant recipients [40]. With a prevalence of approximately 20%, NODAT is caused by a combination of insulin resistance and deficient insulin production [41]. Patients are initially at greatest risk during the first 6 months post-transplant after which time the number of patients developing diabetes increases progressively [42]. Early detection and appropriate treatment can lessen the long-term complications of the condition [40].

Key modifiable risk factors in the development of NODAT are type of immuno-suppression (particularly steroid therapy and tacrolimus) and obesity [41]. In the absence of robust studies to inform the nutritional management of diabetes in kidney transplant recipients, general population advice for diet in diabetes prevention and cardiovascular protection in high risk groups should be followed [43]. Additionally, because organ transplant recipients are considered to be more susceptible to food-borne infections, Australian Guidelines [44] recommend that it is prudent to incorporate general food safety guidelines into any advice given.

9.1.6 Future developments

Worldwide CKD rates are increasing in line with diabetes prevalence. Also an aging population and improvements in healthcare mean that the time span over which this population lives with CKD is lengthening. There remains limited research conducted into the impact of these two chronic conditions and their interactions on people's daily lives.

It is known that, currently, patient concordance with complex treatment regimes in diabetic CKD is poor, and that the effectiveness of diabetic CKD education programmes is often not sufficiently evaluated [45]. Thus, it seems there is need for further research into the lived experience of people with diabetes-induced CKD, to help establish patient-identified needs that will contribute to developing more interactive, responsive and effective dietetic management strategies.

Key points

- Diabetic nephropathy is the leading cause of chronic kidney disease.
- Risk factors for the development of renal disease include poor glycaemic control and hypertension.
- Standard nutritional assessment procedures can be used in people with diabetes.
- Nutritional management is similar to that of people without diabetes.
- Management of glycaemia can be challenging in those receiving dialysis.

References

1. Bethesda M. US Renal Data System: USRDS 2003 Annual Data Report: Atlas of End-Stage Renal Disease in the United States. 2003.
2. Chadban S, Howell M, Twigg S, Thomas M, Jerums G, Cass A, et al. Caring for Australians with Renal Impairment (CARI) guidelines for the prevention and management of chronic kidney disease in type 2 diabetes. *Nephrology* 2010; **15**: S162–S194.
3. National Centre for Health and Clinical Excellence. Chronic kidney disease: early identification and management of. 2008.
4. National Kidney Foundation/Kidney Dialysis Outcomes Quality Initiative. NKF/KDOQI clinical practice guidelines and clinical practice recommendations for diabetes and chronic kidney disease. *Am J Kidney Dis* 2007; **49**(2): Suppl 2.
5. Bain S, Karla P, Frankel A, Brake J, Wilkinson I, Jacques N, et al. Addressing kidney damage in type 2 diabetes. *DiabetesPrimary Care* 2011; **13**(2), supplement.
6. Alzaid A. Microalbuminuria in patients with NIDDM: an overview. *Diabetes Care* 1996; **19**: 79–89.
7. The Renal Association. The Renal Association UK eCKD Guide. www.renal.org. 2011.
8. Royal College of Physicians. Type 2 Diabetes: National Institute for Health & Clinical Excellence guideline for management in primary and secondary care (update). 2008.
9. National Kidney Foundation. KDOQI clinical practice guidelines for diabetes and CKD: 2012 update. *Am J Kidney Dis* 2012; **60**(5): 850–886.
10. The DCCT Research Group. Effects of intensive therapy on the development and progression of diabetic nephropathy in the Diabetes Control & Complications Trial. *Kidney Int* 1995; **47**: 1703–1720.
11. Intensive blood-glucose control with sulphonylureas or insulin compared with conventional treatment and risk of complications in patients with type 2 diabetes. *Lancet* 1998; **352**(9131): 837–853.
12. Slinin Y, Ishani A, Rector T, Fitzgerald P, MacDonald R, Tacklind J, et al. Management of hyperglycemia, dyslipidemia, and albuminuria in patients with diabetes and CKD: A systematic review for a KDOQI clinical practice guideline. *Am J Kidney Dis* 2012; **60**(5): 747–769.
13. Levin N. Blood pressure in chronic kidney disease stage 5D; report from a Kidney Disease: Improving Global Outcomes Controversies Conference. 2009.
14. UKPDS Group (38). UKPDS Group; Tight blood pressure control and risk of macrovascula and microvascular complications in Type 2 diabetes. *BMJ* 1998; **317**: 703.
15. Midgley J, Matthew A, Greenwood C, Logan A. Effect of reduced dietary sodium on blood pressure: a meta-analysis of randomized controlled trials. *JAMA* 1996; **275**: 1590–1597.
16. Hooper L, Bartlett C, Smith G, Ebrahim S. Systematic review of long term effects of advice to reduce dietary salt in adults. *BMJ* 2002; **325**(7365): 628–636.
17. Slagman MC, Waanders F, Hemmerlder MH, Woittiez AJ, Janssen WM, Heerspink HJ, et al. Moderate dietary sodium restriction added to ACE inhibition compared with dual blockade in lowering proteinurea & blood pressure randomised controlled trial. HONEST Nephrology Study Group. *BMJ* 2011; **343**: 4366.
18. National Kidney Foundation/Kidney Dialysis Outcomes Quality Initiative. Clinical Practice Guidelines on Hypertension and Antihypertensive Agents in Chronic Kidney Disease Guideline 6. 2002.
19. Suckling R. Altered dietary salt intake for preventing and treating diabetic kidney disease. *Cochrane Database Syst Rev* Issue 12; 2010 CD006763. doi: 10.1002/14651858.CD006763.pub2
20. Fouque D, Laville M. Low protein diets for chronic kidney disease in non diabetic adults (Review). *Cochrane Database Syst Rev* 2009 Jul 8; (3): CD001892. doi: 10.1002/14651858.CD001892.pub3.
21. Pan Y, Guo LL, Jin HM. Low protein diet for diabetic nephropathy: a meta –analysis of randomised controlled trials. *Am J Clin Nutr* 2008; **88**: 660–666.
22. Waugh N, Robertson A. Protein Restriction for Diabetic Renal Disease; *Cochrane Database Syst Rev* CD002181; 2007, Issue 4. doi: 10.1002/14651858. CD002181.pub2
23. Brenner B, Meyer T, Hostetter T. Dietary protein intake and the progressive nature of kidney disease: The role of hemodynamically mediated glomerular injury in the pathogenesis of progressive glomerular sclerosis in aging, renal ablation, and intrinsic renal disease. *N Engl J Med* 1982; **307**: 652–659.
24. Kopple JD, Massry SG, ed. *Kopple and Massry's Nutritional Management of Renal Disease*. 2nd edn, Philadelphia: Lippincott Williams & Wilkins, 2004.
25. Thomas B, Bishop J, ed. *Manual of Dietetic Practice*, 4th edn. Kent: Blackwell, 2007.
26. Kalantar-Zadeh K. Recent advances in understanding the malnutrition-inflammation-cachexia syndrome in chronic kidney disease patients. *Semin Dial* 2005; **18**(5): 365–369.
27. DCCT Research Group. The effect of intensive treatment of diabetes on the development and progression of long-term complications in insulin-dependent diabetes mellitus. *N Engl J Med* 1993; **329**(14): 977–986.
28. Marshal S. Recent advances in diabetic nephropathy. *Postgrad Med J* 2004; **80**: 624–633.
29. Kazempour-Ardebili S, Lecamwasam V, Dassanayake T, Frankel A, Tam F, Dornhorst A, et al. Assessing glycaemic control in maintenance HD patients with Type 2 diabetes. *Diabetes Care* 2009; **32**(7): 1137–1142.

30. Caplin B, Kumar S, Davenport A. Patients' prespective of haemodialysis-associated symptoms. *Nephrol Dial Transplant* 2011; **26**: 2656–2663.

31. Schipper K, Abma T. Coping, family and mastery: Top priorities for social science research with CKD. *Nephrol Dial Transplant* 2011; **26**: 3189–3195.

32. Grodstein G, Blumenkrantz M, Kopple J, Moran J, Coburn J. Glucose absorbtion during continuous ambulatory peritoneal dialysis. *Kidney Int* 1981; **19**: 564–567.

33. National Kidney Foundation/Kidney Dialysis Outcomes Quality Initiative. NKF/KDOQI clinical practice guidelines for cardiovascular disease in dialysis patients. *Am J Kidney Dis* 2005; **45**(4): Suppl. 3.

34. Woodrow G, Davies S. Renal Association Clinical Practice Guidelines on Peritoneal Dialysis. *Nephron Clin Pract* 2011; **118**(Suppl. 1): c287–c310.

35. Lin A, Qian J, Yu X, Liu W, Chen N, Mei C, et al. Icodextrin National Multi-centre Cooperation Group; Randomised controlled trial of icodextrin versus glucose containing PD fluid. *Clin J Am Soc Nephrol* 2009; **4**(11): 1799–1804.

36. Lindholm B, Park MS, Bergstrom J. Supplemented dialysis: amino acid based solutions in PD. *Contrib Nephrol* 1993; **103**: 168–182.

37. Os I, Gudmundsdottir H, Draganov B, Von der Lippe E. Sterile peritonitis associated with amino-acid containing dialysate. *Perit Dial Int* 2011; **31**(1): 103.

38. Torun D, Oguzkurt L, Sezer S, Zumrutdal A, Singan M, Adam F, et al. Hepatic subcapsular steatosis is a complication associated with intraperitoneal insulin treatment in diabetic peritoneal dialysis patients. *Perit Dial Int* 2005; **25**(6): 596–600.

39. Fouque D. European best practice guidelines on nutrition. *Nephrol Dial Transplant* 2007; **22**(2): ii45–ii87.

40. Miles AM, Sumrani N, Horowitz R, Homel P, Maursky V, Markell MS, et al. Diabetes mellitus after renal transplantation: As deleterious as non-transplant-associated diabetes? *Transplantation* 1998; **65**(3): 380–384.

41. Chadban S, Chan M, Fry K, Patwardhan A, Ryan C, Trevillian P, et al. Caring for Australians with Renal Impairment (CARI) guidelines for the nutritional management of diabetes mellitus in adult kidney transplant recipients. *Nephrology* 2010; **15**: S37–S39.

42. Davidson J. New-onset diabetes after transplant: 2003 International consensus guidelines 1. *Transplantation* 2003; **75**(10): SS3–SS24.

43. Kasiske B, Cosio F, Beto B, Bolton K, Chavers B, Grimm Jr. R, et al. NKF/KDOQI clinical practice guidelines for managing dyslipidemias in kidney transplant patients: A report from the Managing Dyslipidemias in Chronic Kidney Disease Work Group of the National Kidney Foundation Kidney Disease Outcomes Quality Initiative. *Am J Transplant* 2004; **4**(S7): 13–53.

44. Chadban S, Chan M, Fry K, Patwardhan A, Ryan C, Trevillian P, et al. Caring for Australians with Renal Impairment (CARI) guidelines for food safety recommendations for adult kidney transplant recipients. *Nephrology* 2010; **15**: S35–S36.

45. Li T, Wu H, Wang F, Huang C, Yang M, Dong BR, et al.; Education programmes for people with diabetic kidney disease. *Cochrane Database Syst Rev* 2011, Issue 6. doi: 10.1002/14651858.CD007374.pub2

Chapter 9.2

Macrovascular disease and diabetes

Nicola Tufton and Mohammed S. B. Huda

Barts Health NHS Trust, London, UK

Since the advent of insulin in the early part of the last century, the cause of mortality in patients with diabetes has shifted from insulin deficiency causing metabolic complications of ketoacidosis, to the long-term effects of cardiovascular sequelae [1]. Cardiovascular disease (CVD) accounts for the majority of deaths in diabetic patients and diabetes is an independent risk factor for CVD [2]. Although CVD is not specific to patients with diabetes, it is more prevalent amongst patients with type 1 or 2 diabetes than the general population. Macrovascular disease, characterised by damage to large blood vessels and the development of atherosclerosis, is highly prevalent amongst the diabetic population and is responsible for higher rates of mortality and morbidity than within the non-diabetic population from coronary heart disease (CHD), cerebrovascular disease and peripheral vascular disease [3,4].

9.2.1 Epidemiology of macrovascular disease in diabetes

The Framingham cohort demonstrated that the incidence of CVD was approximately twice for men (3.1 vs 19.1 per 1000 persons at risk) and three times for women (27.2 vs 10.2 per 1000 persons at risk) in the diabetic population compared to their non-diabetic counterparts [1]. In a study that collated glucose exposure data from 52 countries, it was found that cardiovascular mortality increased continuously with blood glucose levels greater than 4.9 mmol/L, including levels below traditional thresholds for the diagnosis of diabetes. These data show that in 2001, 950 000 deaths were directly attributed to diabetes; but a further 1 490 000 fatal coronary events (21% of all deaths) and 709 000 fatal stroke events (13% of all deaths) were attributable to high blood glucose [5,6]. The relative risk for ischaemic heart disease for 1 mmol/L increase in fasting plasma glucose was 1.424, 1.196 and 1.196, respectively in age groups <60 years, 60–69 years and >70 years [6]. In the UKPDS trial (United Kingdom Prospective Diabetes study) 5102 patients with newly diagnosed diabetes aged 25–65 years were recruited and followed up to establish whether, in patients with type 2 diabetes, intensive blood-glucose control reduced the risk of macrovascular or microvascular complications, and whether any particular therapy was advantageous. The highest rate of mortality (51.5%) was attributable to CVD, followed by 24.2% related to cancer [7,8]. The annual rate of macrovascular events has been reported to be 2.2–3.0% [9].

Type 1 diabetes is associated with at least a 10-fold increase in CVD compared to an age-matched non-diabetic population [1]. In the Epidemiology of Diabetes Interventions and Complications trial (EDIC), 143 cardiovascular events occurred in 83 patients over 17 years follow-up, of 1394 patients in the original Diabetes Control and Complications Trial (DCCT) (97%); with event rates of 0.38–0.8 per 100 patient years (intensive vs standard insulin

Advanced Nutrition and Dietetics in Diabetes, First Edition. Edited by Louise Goff and Pamela Dyson.

© 2016 John Wiley & Sons, Ltd. Published 2016 by John Wiley & Sons, Ltd.

treatment) [3]. There were 12 deaths from all CVD, 6 non-fatal cerebrovascular events occurred and 51 non-fatal or silent myocardial infarctions (MIs) [1]. In a 30 year follow-up observational study there was a cumulative incidence of 9–14% CVD (intensive insulin therapy versus conventional therapy) and less than 1% required an amputation [10].

Cardiovascular death accounts for 51–55% of all-cause mortality in diabetic patients [2,5]. In the Multiple Risk Factor Intervention Trial (MRFIT) 347 978 men aged 35–57 years were followed up over 12 years; the risk of cardiovascular death in men with diabetes was five times higher compared to men without diabetes; with a relative risk of 3.0. The relative risk in diabetic compared to non-diabetic men was 3.2 for CHD (65.91 vs 17.05 per 10 000 person years) [2]. Clinically manifest CHD has a worse prognosis in diabetic patients than non-diabetic patients [11].

In a Finnish study of patients with type 2 diabetes, there was a similar incidence of MI amongst the non-diabetic patients who had experienced a prior event, compared to the diabetic patients who had not [12]. A prior history of MI was associated with increased incidence of MI, stroke and death from cardiovascular causes [6], suggesting that diabetes is as strong a risk factor for future cardiovascular event as having experienced a previous cardiac event. In the diabetic population in this study the incidence of MI was 45% in those with prior MI and 20.2% in those without prior MI [6]. This was further investigated some years later, in a cohort of 4045 men aged 60–79 years, demonstrating that both diabetes and prior MI increase the risk of future major cardiovascular event, regardless of duration of diabetes. However, only those with longer duration of diabetes (average 16.7 years) showed a similar relative risk of vascular events to men with a prior history of MI [13]. In the OASIS registry, an unstable angina outcome study, diabetes increased mortality by 57% [14,15].

Similarly, diabetes increases the risk of stroke. In a subset of the UKPDS study 3776 patients aged 25–65 years with newly diagnosed type 2 diabetes, without known CVD, were followed up for a median of 7.9 years. Of the 3776 patients,

2.6% (99 patients) had a stroke. In addition to diabetes, other significant risk factors for stroke were age, male sex, hypertension and atrial fibrillation [16]. In the MRFIT study [2] of nearly 350 000 individuals there was a three-fold risk in diabetic patients; the relative risk of stroke in diabetic men was 2.8 compared to non-diabetic men (6.72 vs 1.75 per 10 000 person years). Stroke risk was 10-fold in the Baltimore-Washington Cooperative Young Stroke Study in patients < 44 years old [17]. Absolute excess risk of cardiovascular death (CHD and stroke) was progressively higher with increasing age, serum cholesterol level, systolic blood pressure and cigarette smoking for diabetic compared to non-diabetic men [2].

Peripheral arterial disease (PAD) has a similar underlying pathophysiology and as a result prevalence is also increased in the diabetic population. Diabetic PAD often affects distal limb vessels, such as the tibial and peroneal arteries, limiting the potential for collateral vessel development and reducing options for revascularisation. Therefore, these patients are more likely to develop symptomatic disease, such as intermittent claudication and critical limb ischaemia, and undergo amputation [17]. In an analysis of data from the 1999–2000 National Health and Nutrition Examination Survey in the United States of individuals over the age 40 years, the prevalence of PAD (based on measurements of ankle-brachial index <0.9) in the diabetic population was 10.8% compared to 3.6% in individuals who did not have diabetes, and increased with age in both groups [18]. In the Framingham cohort, there was a three- and eightfold increase in symptomatic claudication in diabetic men and women, respectively, compared to non-diabetic individuals [19].

9.2.2 Effects of intervention on glycaemic control

Type 1 diabetes

Although there is now clear evidence of the benefit of intensive glycaemic control on the development and progression of microvascular complications, this has not been as clear for macrovascular complications.

In the Diabetes Control and Complications Trial (DCCT); the original study investigating the progression of long-term complications in 1441 patients aged 13–39 years with type 1 diabetes (evidenced by deficit of C-peptide secretion); demonstrated a non-significant trend of reducing the risk of CVD in the intensive treatment group (0.5 vs 0.8 events per 100 patient years) [4]. Intensive therapy reduced the development of hypercholesterolaemia by 34% ($p=0.02$) [4]. The subsequent Epidemiology study of Diabetes Interventions and Complications (EDIC) followed up 1394 patients (97% of original cohort) from the DCCT for 17 years on an intention to treat basis, investigating the effects on macrovascular disease. A total of 144 cardiovascular events occurred in 83 patients; 46 among 31 patients originally assigned to the intensive treatment group and 98 among 52 patients originally assigned to the conventional treatment. Event rates were 0.38 and 0.80 per 100 patient years ($p=0.007$) [3]. This gave a prevalence of 5.95% of at least one cardiovascular event within the 17 year follow-up period, regardless of treatment group.

Intensive insulin therapy reduced albuminuria and microalbuminuria by 54% and 39% in the DCCT study [2] and a history of microalbuminuria or albuminuria was associated with a significant increase in the risk of CVD by a factor of > 2.5 [3,10].

Cumulative incidence of the first cardiovascular event showed that intensive treatment was associated with a 42% relative reduction in risk compared to the conventional treatment group ($p=0.02$); and the risk of the first occurrence of non-fatal MI, stroke or death from CVD was reduced by 57% with intensive treatment [3]. This suggests that intensive insulin treatment from the outset in patients with type 1 diabetes is protective against future cardiovascular events. Further analysis of the EDIC trial showed that an HbA1c of 10% (86 mmol/mol) or lower was associated with a hazard ratio of 0.80, equating to a 20% relative reduction in the risk of cardiovascular event [3]. The DCCT/EDIC trials demonstrated that a 6.5 year period of intensive insulin therapy had sustained effects on development of microvascular and macrovascular complications, even after the intensive treatment period had

finished [3]. Intensive as compared with conventional therapy reduced the progression of atherosclerosis, and the prevalence of coronary-artery calcification, due to improvements in endothelial function, platelet function and reduced formation of glycoslyated end products with plaque formation [3].

Type 2 diabetes

The UKPDS was associated with a reduction of 16% in the relative risk of MI, but this effect was not significant ($p=0.052$) [7]. However, there was a significant relative risk reduction of 39% in the obese patients, primarily treated with metformin ($p=0.01$) [7]. There was no difference between the two groups in all-cause mortality. The ten year follow-up study to UKPDS found no difference in the proportion of patients that experienced a silent MI, cardiomegaly or evidence of PVD [7]. However, within the 10 year post-trial monitoring study, not only were significant risk reductions maintained for microvascular end points, but post-trial risk reductions emerged for any diabetes-related death and MIs (17% vs 15%, respectively, at $p=0.01$) despite the loss of difference between HbA1c after one year post-trial, referred to as the legacy or metabolic memory effect [8]. However, no significant risk reduction was observed in the post-trial period for stroke or PVD [8]. In the overweight group treated with metformin the relative risk reductions for any diabetes-related death and MI (30% and 33%, respectively) were maintained at 10 years follow-up [8], but there were no significant risk reductions for stroke or PVD in this group.

In contrast to this, the ACCORD study (Action to Control Cardiovascular Risk in Diabetes) was terminated after 3.5 years due to an increase in all-cause death rates in the intensive therapy group [20]. This trial randomised 10 251 diabetic patients, aged 40–79 years with either previous CVD or at least two high cardiovascular risk factors, to intensive therapy aimed at lowering the HbA1c <6%, or standard therapy to target HbA1c 7.0–7.9% (53–63 mmol/mol). There were 257 and 203 deaths in the intensive therapy group and standard group, respectively, suggesting harm of intensive glucose control in these high risk individuals. It did also demonstrate, however, that the rate of non-fatal MI was lower in the intensive treatment group (3.6% vs 4.6%) but found no significant difference between the intensive therapy group and standard therapy group for rate of non-fatal stroke [20].

The ADVANCE study followed up 11 140 people with type 2 diabetes over the age of 55 years, with at least one additional risk factor, for five years, from 20 countries across Asia, Europe, North America and Australasia. They also found no significant difference in rates of cardiovascular and cerebrovascular events in the intensive blood glucose-lowering arm (using Gliclazide modified release (MR) and other glucose-lowering medication as needed to achieve HbA1c <6.5%) [21].

Although the ACCORD and ADVANCE trials dispute the UKPDS finding of a protective cardiovascular effect of intensive glycaemic control, it is worth noting that the populations in ADVANCE and ACCORD had more advanced diabetes than UKPDS participants with longer duration of diabetes (mean duration 8–11 years), and either known CVD or multiple cardiovascular risk factors [22].

The Veterans Affairs Diabetes Trial (VADT) randomised 1791 military veterans with poorly controlled type 2 diabetes to intensive therapy (aiming for a target absolute reduction of 1.5% in HbA1c) or standard therapy and followed them over a median of 5.6 years. They observed no difference between the two groups in the rates of macrovascular or microvascular complications, although there was an increase in sudden death in the intensive arm [23].

To overcome the uncertainty regarding intensive glucose-lowering on cardiovascular outcomes, the trial investigators from ADVANCE, ACCORD, VADT and UKPDS collaborated to facilitate a meta-analysis [24]. A total of 27 049 participants with type 2 diabetes were included, and a total of 2370 major cardiovascular events occurred. The analysis demonstrated a modest reduction in major cardiovascular events with greater glucose-lowering; with a relative risk reduction by 9% of major cardiovascular event, and relative risk of MI was reduced by 15%. They found a non-significant reduction in risk of stroke and no difference for hospitalised fatal

heart failure or cardiovascular death. An additional finding was that participants who did not have a prior history of macrovascular disease tended to benefit more from intensive glycaemic control, compared to those with a history of a macrovascular disease [24].

Table 9.2.1 shows the current American Diabetes Association (ADA), National Institute for Health and Clinical Excellence (NICE) and International Diabetes Federation (IDF) guidance on HbA1c targets and treatment interventions to achieve glucose control [22,25–28].

9.2.3 Effects of intervention on other cardiovascular risk factors

Blood pressure

Atherosclerosis is diffuse in diabetic patients and requires aggressive treatment to minimise cardiovascular risk [15]. There are numerous risk factors, both modifiable and non-modifiable, that contribute to CVD and these need to be addressed in diabetic patients in the same way as they are within the non-diabetic population. These primary preventions need to include addressing smoking, hypertension, raised lipids and obesity [3,15,29]. Targeted intervention at multiple risk factors reduces the risk of cardiovascular events, as well as microvascular events, by approximately 50% in patients with type 2 diabetes [15,30].

The UKPDS trial demonstrated a 32% relative reduction in risk of death related to diabetes (p=0.019), a 44% reduction in stroke (p=0.013) and a 56% reduction in risk of heart failure (p=0.0043) in the tight blood pressure control group (targeting BP <150/85mmHg) compared to the less intensive blood pressure control group (targeting BP <180/105mmHg) [31]. Every 10 mmHg decrease in systolic blood pressure resulted in an 11% relative reduction in risk of MI (p<0.001) [32]. These effects were equal in both the group treated with beta receptor blockers and those with angiotensin converting enzyme inhibitors (ACE-i) [33]. There was a 21% non-significant trend in reduction of MI and a 49%

Table 9.2.1 Current guidance on HbA1c targets and treatment interventions to achieve glucose control

	American Diabetes Association [23,24]	NICE [20]	International Diabetes Federation [25,26]
HbA1c targets in non-pregnant adults	<7%	individualised goals	HbA1c below 7.0% / 53 mmol/mol to minimise the risk of complications
	More stringent goals for selected individuals such as those with short duration of diabetes, no underlying CVD and long life expectancy and less stringent goals for those with multiple comorbidities, advanced micro- or macrovascular complications, history of severe hypoglycaemia and limited life expectancy	No target should be < 6.5%, and many will need to be higher than this based on side effects and comorbidities	
Treatment of type 1 diabetes	Multiple daily injections or continuous subcutaneous insulin infusion with matching carbohydrate intake with prandial insulin	Multiple daily injections or continuous subcutaneous insulin infusion with matching carbohydrate intake with prandial insulin	
Treatment of type 2 diabetes	Early intervention with lifestyle interventions and metformin; with timely augmentation of treatment as needed	Start metformin treatment in a person who is overweight or obese, whose glucose is poorly controlled with lifestyle measures and add another agent (usually a sulfonylurea) if glucose is inadequate (see Figure 9.1 in NICE guideline for full details of augmentation strategy)	Begin oral glucose lowering medications when lifestyle interventions alone are unable to maintain blood glucose control at target levels and review at 3 months. First line therapy is with metfomin, then sulfonylurea can be added. Other options include an a-glucosidase inhibitor, a dipeptidyl (see page 57 of guideline for algorithm) peptidase 4 (DPP-4) inhibitor or a thiazolidinedione or rapid-acting insulin secretagogue

non-significant trend in reduction in amputations [30]. However in the 10 year follow-up study these significant reductions were not maintained after loss of the blood pressure difference between the original intensive control group and the standard treatment group [34]. The exception to this was the effect on the development of PVD, although only a small number of these patients developed this complication (21 in each original group). There was a significant reduction in amputations of at least one digit or death from PVD at year 10 of 50% (p=0.02) [34].

The ADVANCE trial demonstrated additional benefit of further lowering systolic blood pressure to less than 145mmHg in diabetic patients; showing an 18% reduction in cardiovascular deaths, 9% reduction in major vascular events and 14% reduction in total coronary events. In contrast to the ACCORD trial there was no evidence of increased risk of death in the intensive treatment group [35].

The Heart Outcomes Prevention Evaluation (HOPE) study randomised 3577 people over the age of 55 years with diabetes who had had a previous cardiovascular event or at least one other cardiovascular risk factor to ramipril (an ACE inhibitor) or placebo. The HOPE study demonstrated a clear benefit of ramipril versus placebo on reducing cardiovascular events and was stopped six months early because of this clear protective benefit. Ramipril lowered the relative risk of MI by 22%, stroke by 33% and cardiovascular death by 37%. These benefits were evident in both the type 1 and type 2 diabetic populations (albeit the actual number of patients with type 1 diabetes was small) and were maintained during follow-up over 4.5 years. They also demonstrated the benefit of ramipril on nephropathy, with a reduction of 24% in the treatment group above and beyond that expected by the effects on blood pressure alone [36], this renal benefit is likely to further protect against CVD.

The HOT study (hypertension optimal treatment) investigated the benefit of lowering diastolic blood pressure in over 19 000 patients across 26 countries in Europe, North and South America and Asia [37]. They randomised approximately 500 patients with diabetes into each of the diastolic blood pressure groups and demonstrated that the rate of cardiovascular events decreased with the diastolic blood pressure. The risk of major cardiovascular events was halved in the target blood pressure group <80 mmHg compared to the group <90 mmHg. They also demonstrated a relative risk reduction of 30% of stroke in the lowest blood pressure group compared to the highest [37].

Table 9.2.2 shows the current ADA, (NICE) and IDF guidance blood pressure targets and treatment regimens [22,25–28].

In type 1 diabetes, hypertension is usually the result of underlying nephropathy and this therefore needs to be addressed as a priority [26].

Lipids

Serum lipid abnormalities in patients with type 2 diabetes are characterised by decreased high-density lipoprotein (HDL) and elevated total cholesterol, low-density lipoprotein (LDL), very low-density lipoprotein (VLDL) and triglycerides levels [11,15,38] and these are positively associated with coronary artery disease [39]. In the Scandinavian Simvastatin Survival Study (4S) [38] 4444 patients with angina or previous MI and cholesterol of 5.5–8.0 mmol/L were randomised to simvastatin or placebo. Lipid-lowering therapy produced a greater reduction in the rate of coronary events in diabetic subjects than in non-diabetic subjects (55% vs. 32%). However, in the Cholesterol and Recurrent Events study (CARE), there were similar reductions in diabetic and non-diabetic subjects (27% and 25%, respectively) [40]. They demonstrated that the benefits of lipid-lowering in cardiovascular events, extends to patients with coronary artery disease and cholesterol levels within the normal range [40]. In a meta-analysis of 14 studies an approximately linear relationship was identified between the absolute reductions in LDL-cholesterol and the reduction in the incidence of coronary and other major vascular events. They identified a 0.75 risk reduction in cardiovascular events per mmol/l reduction in LDL cholesterol. There was a 19% reduction in CHD death, 23% reduction in incidence of first major coronary event (RR 0.75 $p<0.001$); 17% reduction in incidence of first stroke (RR 0.83 $p<0.001$) and 21% reduction in major vascular events [41].

In both CARE and 4S studies the lipid-lowering treatment groups had significant reductions in total cholesterol, LDL, triglycerides and increased HDL. The reduction in CHD mortality was not statistically significant, but the risk of a major CHD and cerebrovascular event was significantly reduced in both studies [11,38,40].

Fibrates have also been shown to be beneficial in diabetic patients. These are PPAR-α agonists

Table 9.2.2 Current guidance blood pressure targets and treatment regimens

	American Diabetes Association [23,24]	NICE [20]	International Diabetes Federation [25,26]
Blood Pressure targets	<130/80 mmHg	<140/80 mmHg and <130/80 mmHg in individuals with a raised microalbuminuria, retinopathy or with prior stroke or transient ischaemic attack	≤130/80 mmHg. Higher targets should be used in the elderly
Lifestyle intervention	Initial interventions for maximum of 3 months if BP< 140/90 mmHg. Sodium intake <1500 mg/day. Reduce excess body weight. Increase fruit and vegetable intake to 8–10 servings per day and low fat diary products 2–3 servings per day. Increase activity levels	Offer lifestyle advice if blood pressure is confirmed as being consistently above 140/80 mmHg (or above 130/80 mmHg if there is kidney, eye or cerebrovascular damage	Aiming to reduce energy intake, salt intake, alcohol intake and inactivity
Alcohol intake	No more than 2 servings/day in men and no more than 1 serving/day in women		
Pharmological treatment	If >140/90 mmHg start ACE-i or ARB2 immediately	First line treatment is ACEi unless African-Caribbean descent (start should be an ACE inhibitor plus either a diuretic or a generic calcium channel) or women planning pregnancy (start calcium channel blocker)	Any agent can be used of ACE-, ARB2, CCB or diuretic that is effective for individual patients

that raise HDL cholesterol levels and lower triglyceride levels. The Veterans Affairs High Density Lipoprotein Cholesterol Intervention Trial (VA-HIT) demonstrated a 24% reduction in death from CHD, non-fatal MI and stroke in both diabetic and non-diabetic patients [15]. In the FIELD study 9795 participants aged 50–75 years with type 2 diabetes were randomised to fenofibrate (200 mg daily) or placebo and effects on cardiovascular events were monitored over 5 years. They demonstrated a significant 24% relative reduction in non-fatal MIs (p=0.01), but no significant difference between the two groups in death from CVD [42].

Table 9.2.3 shows the current ADA, (NICE) and (IDF) guidance for lipid profile targets and treatment options [22,25–28].

Antiplatelet therapy

The HOT study demonstrated the benefit of treating patients with aspirin 75 mg per day with a reduction of 9% in cardiovascular events, including silent MI, and this benefit was similar between the diabetic and non-diabetic populations. However, there was no benefit in the prevention of stroke with aspirin [37].

Table 9.2.4 shows the current ADA, NICE and IDF guidance for antiplatelet therapy [22,25–28].

Lifestyle therapy

As demonstrated in the MRFIT study there is significant potential for the prevention of cardiovascular deaths if lifestyle aspects such as cigarette

Table 9.2.3 Current guidance for lipid profile targets and treatment options

	American Diabetes Association [23,24]	NICE [20]	International Diabetes Federation [25,26]
Lipid profile targets	LDL <100 mg/dl (2.6 mmol/l) if no CVD or LDL<70 mg/dl (1.8 mmol/l). HDL >40 mg/dl (1.0 mmol/l) in men and >50 mg/dl (1.3 mmol/l) in women	Total cholesterol level <4.0 mmol/l or LDL cholesterol level <2.0 mmol/l	LDL cholesterol <2.0 mmol/l (<80 mg/dl), triglyceride <2.3 mmol/l (<200 mg/dl), HDL cholesterol >1.0 mmol/l (>39 mg/dl), non-HDL cholesterol <2.5 mmol/l (<97 mg/dl). LDL cholesterol should be <1.8 mmol/l (<70 mg/dl) in established CVD.
Triglycerides targets	<150 mg/dl (1.7 mmol/l)	If cardiovascular risk is high, consider adding a fibrate if triglyceride levels remain in the range 2.3–4.5 mmol/l	Consider the addition of fenofibrate where serum triglycerides are >2.3 mmol/l (>200 mg/dl) and high density lipoprotein (HDL) cholesterol is low, especially when retinopathy is present. Combination of gemfibrizol with a statin is not recommended
Initial treatment	Lifestyle modification focusing on the reduction of saturated fat, *trans*-fat, and cholesterol intake; increase of omega-3 fatty acids, viscous fibre, and plant stanols/sterols; weight loss (if indicated); and increased physical activity	Simvastatin 40 mg in diabetic patients over the age of 40 years, unless the cardiovascular risk from non-hyperglycaemia-related factors is low, or under 40 years old, if the cardiovascular risk factor profile is poor (multiple features of the metabolic syndrome, presence of conventional risk factors, microalbuminuria, at-risk ethnic group, or strong family history of premature CVD).	Initial lifestyle measures. Treat high risk individuals with statins unless contraindicated.
Augmenting treatment	Add statin therapy if patients have overt cardiovascular disease, or >40 years that have one additional risk factor or if LDL remains >100 mg/dl (2.6 mmol/l).	See triglyceride treatment	See triglyceride treatment

smoking are addressed, as well as hypertension and cholesterol levels, as these factors all increase cardiovascular mortality more significantly in diabetic compared to non-diabetic patients [2].

The absolute excess risk of cardiovascular death for men with the highest daily cigarette use was more than double for diabetic patients compared to non-diabetic patients [2]. Cardiovascular death

Table 9.2.4 Current guidance for antiplatelet therapy

	American Diabetes Association [23,24]	NICE [20]	International Diabetes Federation [25,26]
Aspirin once daily as primary prevention	Aspirin 75–162 mg: all diabetic patients with increased cardiovascular risk (10 year risk >10%. eg. Men >50 years and women >60 years who have one additional risk factor	Aspirin 75 mg: diabetic patients >40 years of BP <145/90 mmHg and <50 years who have other cardiovascular risk factors	Anti-platelet therapy is not routinely recommended in high risk individuals who have not had a CVD event.
Aspirin as secondary prevention	All adults with diabetes and CVD	Offer low-dose aspirin, 75 mg daily, to a person who is 50 years old or over if blood pressure is below 145/90 mmHg	People with a previous CVD event should be treated with lifestyle modification, low-dose aspirin (or clopidogrel), statins and blood pressure lowering medications, unless contraindicated
Post ACS	Combination aspirin and clopidogrel 75 mg for up to 1 year and β-blockers for at least 2 years		

rates progressively increased with increasing number of major risk factors (hypertension, cholesterol levels and smoking) from 30.7 with no major risk factors to 125.2/10000 person years with the highest level of all three risk factors. However the effect of modifiable risk factors on the occurrence of stroke is less clear. In a sub-analysis of the UKPDS study of 3776 patients with newly diagnosed type 2 diabetes, male gender, increasing age and hypertension were positively associated with stroke, but obesity, lack of exercise, smoking, poor glycaemic control, hyperinsulinaemia, dyslipidaemia, and microalbuminuria were not significantly associated with the occurrence of stroke [16].

In the Steno-2 study multiple factor intensive intervention, including a 3 month initiation of diet (total daily intake of fat that was less than 30% and of saturated fatty acids that was less than 10% of the daily energy intake) and physical activity (light-to-moderate exercise for at least 30 minutes three to five times weekly), followed by a stepwise pharmacological approach to hyperglycaemia and blood pressure management if required, was compared to conventional therapy. A total of 118 cardiovascular events occurred; with 85 events in 35 patients (44%) in the conventional therapy group compared to 33

events among 19 patients (24%) in the intensive therapy group. This included 20 versus 3 non-fatal strokes, 14 versus 7 amputations and 12 versus 6 vascular surgical interventions for PAD for conventional therapy versus intensive therapy groups, respectively [30].

However, in the Look AHEAD trial, a large randomised control trial investigating solely lifestyle interventions on cardiovascular outcomes in type 2 diabetes, there were no significant differences in cardiovascular outcomes between the lifestyle intervention and control groups, despite significant differences in weight loss, HbA1c and other cardiovascular risk factors. These differences diminished over the course of the trial and the trial was stopped due to futility at 9.6 years [20,43] however the overall conclusions of this trial are a matter of debate as there were much lower than expected rates of major outcomes in both groups due to optimised CVD risk management. Furthermore, the control group were managed more aggressively with medication and therefore an alternative interpretation of the results is that the lifestyle group achieved the same rates of CVD as the control group despite significantly less use of medications for risk management.

Table 9.2.5 Current guidance for lifestyle interventions for patients at risk of diabetes

	American Diabetes Association [23,24]	NICE [20]	International Diabetes Federation [25,26]
Lifestyle interventions for patients at risk of diabetes	Individuals with diabetes or pre-diabetes should receive individualised medical nutrition therapy	Provide individualised and ongoing nutritional advice, sensitive to the individual's needs, culture and beliefs	Offer lifestyle advice to all people with type 2 diabetes around the time of diagnosis. Individualise advice on food/meals to match needs, preferences and culture
Physical acitivity	Minimum 150 min per week		Introduce exercise gradually; up to 30–45 min on 3–5 days per week or an accumulation of 150 min per week of moderate-intense aerobic activity (50–70% of maximum heart rate) and resistance training 3 times per week
Diet	Reduce energy intake and dietary fat intake with saturated fat intake of <7% of total energy	People who are overweight, an initial body weight loss of 5–10%. Encourage high-fibre, low glycaemic index sources of carbohydrate in the diet, such as fruit, vegetables, wholegrains and pulses; include low-fat dairy products and oily fish; and control the intake of foods containing saturated and trans-fatty acids.	Advise on reducing energy intake and control of foods with high amounts of added sugars, fats or alcohol.
Supplements	Routine supplementation with antioxidants, such as vitamins E and C and carotene, is not advised because of lack of evidence of efficacy		

Approximately 24% of men and 26% of women are now classified as obese (defined as a body mass index >30 kg/m^2) and 65% of men and 58% of women are overweight (defined as a body mass index 25–29.9 kg/m^2) in the United Kingdom [44]. The distribution of body fat is also important and excess fat stored around the waist is also a risk factor for diabetes. Regular physical activity lowers the risk of developing type 2 diabetes by increasing insulin sensitivity, and reduction in the risk of diabetes is independent of body weight [45]. Physical activity rates are low across the entire adult population – around six in ten men and seven in ten women are not sufficiently physically active [45].

Exercise therapy, specifically individualised programs, may greatly benefit many patients with diabetes by reducing hyperglycaemia, insulin resistance, dyslipidaemia and hypertension; these reductions may translate into an improved vascular disease risk profile, as well as benefits in weight loss and improved physical function [46]. Supervised exercise training in people with PAD has been shown to be highly beneficial in terms of walking distance and time, time to claudication and pain, and quality of life [46].

Table 9.2.5 shows the current ADA, NICE and IDF guidance for lifestyle interventions for patients at risk of diabetes [22,25–28].

9.2.4 Conclusions

Cardiovascular disease is more prevalent amongst patients with diabetes than the general population [3,4] and accounts for the majority of deaths in diabetic patients [2].

Optimising glycaemic and blood pressure control, with lifestyle interventions and/or pharmacological measures can reduce the risk of cardiovascular events. People with diabetes who develop CVD can benefit from secondary prevention measures, including treatment with low dose aspirin, β-blockers and lipid-lowering agents. People with diabetes, identified as being at increased risk of developing lower limb complications, can reduce this risk by participating in a foot care programme and prompt intervention can minimise their risk of subsequent disability and amputation [22,45].

Key points

- Macrovascular disease is the leading cause of death in people with diabetes.
- Diabetes increases the risk of cardiovascular disease by 2–4-fold.
- Meta-analyses suggest a moderate risk-reduction associated with improved glycaemic control.
- Management of cardiovascular risk factors, including blood pressure, dyslipidaemia, smoking and body weight improves outcomes.

References

1. Kannel W, McGee D. Diabetes and cardiovascular risk factors: The Framingham study. *Circulation* 1979; **59**(1): 8–13.

2. Stamler J, Vaxxaro O, Neaton J. Diabetes, other risk factors, and 12 year cardiovascular mortality for men screened in the multiple risk factor intervention trial. *Diabetes Care* 1993; **16**(2): 434–444.

3. The Diabetes Control and Complications Trial/Epidemiology of Diabetes Interventions and Complications (DCCT/EDIC) study Research group. Intensive diabetes treatment and cardiovascular disease in patients with type 1. *N Engl J Med* 2005; **353**(25): 2643–3764.

4. The Diabetes Control and Complications Trial Research group (DCCT). The effects of intensive treatment of diabetes on the development and progression of long term complications in insulin-dependant diabetes mellitus. *N Engl J Med* 1993; **329**(14): 977–986.

5. Danaei G, Lawes CM, Vander Hoorn S, Murray CJ, Ezzati M. Global and regional mortality from ischaemic heart disease and stroke attributable to higher-than-optimum blood glucose concentration: comparative risk assessment. *Lancet* 2006; **368**: 1651–1659.

6. Kengne AP, Turnbull F, MacMahon S. The Framingham Study, Diabetes Mellitus and Cardiovascular Disease: Turning Back the Clock. *Prog Cardiovasc Dis* 2010; **53**: 45–51.

7. UK Prospective Diabetes Study (UKPDS) Group. Intensive blood-glucose control with sulphonylureas or insulin compared with conventional treatment and risk of complications in patients with type 2 diabetes (UKPDS 33). *Lancet* 1998; **352**: 837–853. Erratum, *Lancet* 1999; **354**: 602.

8. Holman RR, Paul SK, Bethel MA, Matthews DR, Neil HAW. 10 year follow up on intensive glucose control in type 2 diabetes. *N Engl J Med* 2008; **359**: 1577–1589.

9. The ADVANCE Collaborative Group. Intensive blood glucose control and vascular outcomes in patients with type 2 diabetes. *N Engl J Med* 2008; **358**: 2560–2572.

10. Nathan D, Zinman B, Cleary PA, Backlund JY, Genuth S, Miller R, et al. Modern-day clinical course of type 1 diabetes mellitus After 30 years' duration: The Diabetes Control and Complications Trial/Epidemiology of Diabetes Interventions and Complications and Pittsburgh Epidemiology of Diabetes Complications Experience (1983–2005). *Arch Intern Med* 2009; **169**(14): 1307–1316.

11. Pyörälä K, Pedersen TR, Kjekshus J, Faergeman O, Olsson AG, Thorgeirsson G. Cholesterol lowering with simvastatin improves prognosis of diabetic patients with coronary heart disease: a subgroup analysis of the Scandinavian Simvastatin Survival Study (4S). *Diabetes Care* 1997; **20**: 614.

12. Haffner SM, Lehto S, Ronnemaa T, Pyorala K, Laakso M. Mortality from coronary heart disease in subjects with type 2 diabetes and in nondiabetic subjects with and without prior myocardial infarctions. *N Engl J Med* 1998; **339**(4): 229–234.

13. Wannsmethee SG, Shaper AG, Whincup PH, Lennon L, Sattar N. Impact of diabetes on cardiovascular disease risk and all cause mortality in older men. Influence of age at onset, diabetes duration and established and novel risk factors. *Arch Intern Med* 2011; **171**(5): 404–410.

14. Malmberg K, Yusuf S, Gerstein HC, Brown J, Zhao F, Hunt D, et al. Impact of diabetes on long-term prognosis in patients with unstable angina and non–Q-wave myocardial infarction: results of the OASIS (Organization to Assess Strategies for Ischemic Syndromes) Registry. *Circulation* 2000; **102**: 1014–1019.

15. Lüscher TF, Creager MA. Diabetes and vascular disease pathophysiology, clinical consequences, and medical therapy: Part II. *Circulation* 2003; **108**: 1655–1661.

16. Davis TM, Millns H, Stratton IM, Holman RR, Turner RC. Risk factors for stroke in type 2 diabetes mellitus: United Kingdom Prospective Diabetes Study (UKPDS) 29. *Arch Intern Med* 1999; **159**(10): 1097–1103.

17. Rohr J, Kittner S, Feeser B, Hebel JR, Whyte MG, Weinstein A, et al. Traditional risk factors and ischemic stroke in young adults: the Baltimore-Washington Cooperative Young Stroke Study. *Arch Neurol* 1996; **53**: 603–607.

18. Selvin E, Erlinger TP. Prevalence of and risk factors for peripheral arterial disease in the United States. Results from the National Health and Nutrition Examination Survey, 1999–2000. *Circulation* 2004; **110**: 738–743.

19. Kannel WB, McGee DL. Update on some epidemiologic features of intermittent claudication: the Framingham Study. *J Am Geriatr Soc* 1985; **33**: 13–18.

20. The Action to Control Cardiovascular Risk in Diabetes Study Group. Effects of intensive glucose lowering in type 2 diabetes. *N Engl J Med* 2008; **358**: 2545–2559. doi: 10.1056/NEJMoa0802743.

21. The ADVANCE Collaborative Group. Intensive blood glucose control and vascular outcomes in patients with type 2 diabetes. *N Engl J Med* 2008; **358**: 2560–2572.

22. National Collaborating Centre for Chronic Conditions. Type 2 diabetes. The Management of type 2 diabetes. National Institute for Health and Clinical Excellence. 2008. NICE clinical guideline 66.

23. Duckworth W, Abraira C, Moritz T, Reda D, Emanuele N, Reaven PD, et al. Glucose control and vascular complications in veterans with type 2 diabetes. *N Engl J Med* 2009; **360**: 129–139.

24. Turnbull FM, Abraira C, Anderson RJ, Byington RP, Chalmers JP, Duckworth WC, et al. Meta-analysis. Intensive glucose control and macrovascular outcomes in type 2 diabetes. *Diabetologia* 2009; **52**: 2288–2298.

25. American Diabetes Association Position Statement. Standards of Medical Care in Diabetes. 2012. *Diabetes Care* 2012; **35**(Suppl.1): S11–S63.

26. American Diabetes Association. Standards of Medical Care in Diabetes—2011. *Diabetes Care* 2011; **34** (Suppl. 1): S11–S61.

27. International Diabetes Federation. 2012. Clinical Guidelines Task force. Global Guideline for Type 2 Diabetes. www.idf.org

28. International Diabetes Federation. 2011. Global IDF/ISPAD Guideline for Diabetes in Childhood and Adolesence. www.idf.org

29. Garcia MJ, McNamara PM, Gordon T, Kannel WB. Morbidity and mortality in diabetics in the Framingham population sixteen year follow up study. *Diabetes* 1974; **23**: 105.

30. Gæde P, Vedel P, Larsen N, Jensen GVH, Parving H-H, Pedersen O. Multifactorial intervention and cardiovascular disease in patients with type 2 diabetes. *N Engl J Med* 2003; **348**: 383–393.

31. UK Prospective Diabetes Study Group. Tight blood pressure control and risk of macrovascular and microvascular complications in type 2 diabetes: UKPDS 38. *BMJ* 1998; **317**: 703–713.

32. UK Prospective Diabetes Study (UKPDS) Group. Association of systolic blood pressure with macrovascular and microvascular complications of type 2 diabetes (UKPDS 36). *BMJ* 2000; **321**: 412–419.

33. UK Prospective Diabetes Study Group. Efficacy of Atenolol and captopril in reducing risk of macrovascular and microvascular complications: UKPDS 39. *BMJ* 1998; **317**: 713–720.

34. Holman RR, Paul SK, Bethel MA, Neil HAW, Matthews DR. Long-term follow-up after tight control of blood pressure in type 2 diabetes. *N Engl J Med* 2008; **359**: 1565–1576.

35. Patel A. The ADVANCE Collaborative Group Effects of a fixed combination of perindopril and indapamide on macrovascular and microvascular outcomes in patients with type 2 diabetes mellitus (the ADVANCE trial): a randomised controlled trial. *Lancet* 2007; **370**(9590): 829–840.

36. Heart Outcomes Prevention Evaluation Study Investigators Effects of ramipril on cardiovascular and microvascular outcomes in people with diabetes mellitus: results of the HOPE study and MICRO-HOPE substudy. *Lancet* 2000; **355**: 253–259.

37. Hansson L, Zanchetti A, Carruthers SG, Dahlf B, Elmfeldt D, Julius S, et al. Effect of intensive blood-pressure lowering and lowdose aspirin in patients with hypertension: principal results of the hypertension optimal treatment (HOT) randomised trial. *Lancet* 1998; **351**: 1755–1762.

38. Scandinavian Simvastatin Survival Study Group. Randomised trial of cholerserol lowering in 4444 patient with coronary heart disease: the Scandinavian Simvsatatin Survival Study (4S). *Lancet* 1994; **344** (8934): 1383–1389.

39. Turner RC, Millns H, Neil HA, Stratton IM, Manley SE, Matthews DR, et al. Risk factors for coronary artery disease in non-insulin dependent diabetes mellitus: United Kingdom Prospective Diabetes Study (UKPDS: 23) *BMJ* 1998; **316**(7134): 823–828.

40. The Cholesterol and Recurrent Events Trial Investigators (CARE study). The effect of pravastatin on coronary events after myocardial infarction in patients with average cholesterol levels. *N Engl J Med* 1996; **335**: 1001–1009.

41. Baigent C, Keech A, Kearney PM, Blackwell L, Buck G, Pollicino C, et al. Efficacy and safety of cholesterol-lowering treatment: prospective meta-analysis of data from 90,056 participants in 14 randomised trials of statins. *Lancet* 2005; **366**(9493): 1267–1278.

42. The FIELD study investigators. Effects of long-term fenofibrate therapy on cardiovascular events in 9795 people with type 2 diabetes mellitus (the FIELD study): randomised controlled trial. *Lancet* 2005; **366**(9500): 1849–1861.

43. The Look AHEAD Research Group. Cardiovascular effects of intensive lifestyle intervention in type 2 diabetes. *N Engl J Med* 2013; **369**: 145–154.

44. NHS. Statistics on Obesity, Physical Activity and Diet: England, 2013. The Health and Social Care Information Centre

45. National Service Framework for Diabetes: Standards. National Service Framework. Department of Health. 2001.

46. Cade WT. Diabetes-related microvascular and macrovascular diseases in the physical therapy setting. *Phys Ther* 2008; **88**(11): 1322–1335.

Chapter 9.3

Coeliac disease and diabetes

Alyson Hill
University of Ulster, Londonderry, UK

9.3.1 Introduction

Coeliac disease (CD) is defined as a state of heightened immunological responsiveness to ingested gluten in genetically susceptible individuals [1]. It is considered to be a primarily digestive systematic disorder consisting of a common inflammatory disease of the small intestine triggered and maintained mainly by an immunological response following gluten exposure in the diet [2]. The characteristic clinical response is triggered by exposure to gluten, the name given to the proteins present in a group of cereals including mainly gliadin (wheat), secalin (rye), hordein (barley) and triticale (hybrid of wheat and rye) [2]. Individuals display various degrees of intestinal inflammation in the small intestinal mucosa, ranging from mild intraepithelial lymphocytosis to severe mononuclear infiltration resulting in total villous atrophy at the most evolved stages [3,4].

CD is frequently found in conjunction with other autoimmune diseases such as type 1 diabetes. Individuals with type 1 diabetes have been shown to have a 4–7% chance of having concomitant CD [5], which is significantly higher than the estimated prevalence of CD in the general United Kingdom (UK) population, which ranges from 0.8 to 1.9% [6]. There is no increased risk of CD in those with type 2 diabetes, with the frequency being similar to that of the general population [7].

The increased prevalence of CD in type 1 diabetes can partly be explained by the similar genetic background, with both sharing disease-specific alleles. The presence of the common HLA markers B8 and DR3 [8–10] and the DQB1 *0201 allele that encodes a particular heterodimer [11,12] are present in the majority of people with both type 1 diabetes and CD.

The diagnosis of CD should be made in people with diabetes as mucosal atrophy and inflammation can alter the absorption of nutrients affecting glycaemic control and body mass index and causing hypoglycaemia [13,14].

9.3.2 Clinical onset and symptoms

CD can develop at any age and is no longer regarded as a childhood disorder. Reported frequencies of CD among people with type 1 diabetes are generally higher in adults [15]. In most cases (90%) type 1 diabetes is diagnosed before CD [10]. However, the delay in diagnosis of CD is usually many years [16], making it difficult to specify the order in which diseases appear [17]. Evidence suggests that when CD is diagnosed before diabetes, the clinical presentation of diabetes is reported to be more severe and there is a higher prevalence of multiple autoimmune diseases [18].

Advanced Nutrition and Dietetics in Diabetes, First Edition. Edited by Louise Goff and Pamela Dyson.
© 2016 John Wiley & Sons, Ltd. Published 2016 by John Wiley & Sons, Ltd.

Most cases of CD with diabetes are reported to be asymptomatic (silent) or present with only mild symptoms detected by serologic screening [19]. Gastrointestinal symptoms may be present but are often mild and recognised retrospectively [20]. Severe malabsorption is unusual with most having few or no symptoms or consequences of malabsorption [20]. Iron or folic acid deficiency with or without anaemia is the most common laboratory abnormality [17]. Failure to grow in children has been reported in about one third of children with CD [10,12,21]; however, this has not been reported by others [22,23]. Recurrent and symptomatic hypoglycaemic episodes and a reduced insulin requirement and poor metabolic control have been reported prior to diagnosis of CD [13,24], possibly related to malabsorption.

In those detected by screening, evidence is controversial as to the effect of a gluten-free diet (GFD) on metabolic control and insulin requirements. Acerini et al. [25] reported no difference between coeliac and non-coeliac in terms of glycosylated haemoglobin or total insulin needs. However a study by Page et al. [7] found better metabolic control in those with CD than in those without. Others reported less hypoglycaemic episodes [12,26], which may be a reflection of the limited damage to the mucosa of the small intestine in subclinical CD [15]. In some cases, however, adherence to a GFD was not strict. However, Kaukinen et al. [27] observed that adherence to a strict coeliac diet had no detrimental effect on metabolic control of diabetes, suggesting that both conditions can be treated at the same time.

9.3.3 Diagnosis

CD is diagnosed by small intestinal (duodenal) biopsy that reveals characteristic morphological changes, typified by villous atrophy and intraepithelial lymphocytosis [5] that recover on a GFD. This remains the 'gold' standard test for diagnosis of CD, which requires the consumption of gluten-containing foods in more than one meal every day for a minimum of 6 weeks before testing [6].

Serological antibody testing is routinely used as a preliminary non-invasive screening test for those being investigated for CD. It is recommended that anyone with type 1 diabetes is screened for CD [6].

Tests for immunoglobulin A IgA endomysial antibodies (EMA) and IgA tissue transglutaminase antibodies (tTGA) are the preferred choice as they have a sensitivity and specificity of >90%. Test accuracy is dependent on normal levels of IgA antibody; therefore a false-negative test result will occur if the patient is IgA deficient. CD occurs more frequently in patients with IgA deficiency than in the general population [28]. However, a study on patients with type 1 diabetes reported none with IgA deficiency [29]. Patients with deficiency of IgA will require IgG class of tTGA and EMA testing.

Immunoglobulin G (IgG) and IgA anti-gliadin antibody (AGA) lack sensitivity by comparison with IgA EMA and are not recommended in the diagnosis of CD [6].

9.3.4 Treatment of coeliac disease

CD is treated by life-long adherence to a strict GFD that usually leads to resolution of symptoms and a reduction in the long-term risks of complications for most patients [30]. For many of those with diabetes, the additional dietary restrictions imposed by a GFD make adherence difficult.

Gluten is a generic term to encompass all the proteins derived from wheat, rye and barley. The specific proteins are gliadins in wheat, secalins in rye and hordeins in barley. Foods containing these proteins should be avoided. Table 9.3.1 indicates foods that must be avoided. Oats contain proteins called avenins and are not toxic, and most people with CD can eat oats. However, many oats are produced in the same place as wheat, barley and rye that makes them unsafe due to contamination. Trace amounts of gluten may provoke intestinal inflammation as individuals have variable sensitivity to gluten [5]. There are limited data available on the safe threshold for daily consumption of gluten; however, the

Table 9.3.1 Foods permitted and not permitted on a gluten free diet

	Foods suitable for GFD	Foods not suitable for GFD
Starches/grains	oats*, rice & wild rice, rice flour, rice bran, rice malt, rice rusk, corn (maize), corn starch, cornflour, polenta (cornmeal), potato flour, potato starch, soya, soya flour, bean flours chickpea flour, sago, tapioca, cassava, arrowroot, amaranth, buckwheat, chestnut flour, gram flour, millet, quinoa, sorghum, teff, modified starch, mustard flour	Wheat, rye, barley, barley flour, barley malt & malted barley, bulgar wheat, durum wheat, wheat flour, wheat bran, wheat protein, wheat starch, wheat rusk, rye flour, semolina, spelt, couscous, rusk, dinkel, einkorn, emmer wheat, kamut, triticale
Meat, poultry and fish and alternatives	Fresh meats, poultry, cured pure meats, plain cooked meats, smoked meats. Dried, fresh, kippered and smoked fish, fish canned in brine, oil, water, shellfish, game, eggs, plain tofu, peas, beans, lentils, plain nuts and seeds	Cooked/coated in batter or breadcrumbs, haggis, meat pies, meat puddings, sausages, sausage meat, faggots, rissoles, scotch eggs
Milk and milk products	All milk (liquid & dried), all cream (single, double, whipping, clotted, soured, crème fraiche, buttermilk, plain fromage frais, plain yoghurt, cheese	Yoghurts containing muesli or cereals
Fruits vegetables and potatoes	All canned, dried, fresh, frozen and pure fruit and vegetable juices; vegetables pickled in vinegar. Plain potatoes, baked, boiled or mashed	Battered, breadcrumbed or dusted with flour. Pies and pastries
Fats and oils	Butter, cooking oils, margarine, reduced and low fat spreads, ghee, lard	
Soups, sauces, seasonings	All vinegars (including barley, malt vinegar), garlic puree, ground pepper, herbs and spices, mint sauces, salt, tomato puree, Worcestershire sauce	Chinese soy sauce, stuffing and stuffing mixes
Savoury snacks	Home made popcorn, rice cakes, rice crackers	
Preserves, spreads and confectionary	Honey, sugar, glucose, golden syrup, jam, marmalade, glucose molasses, treacle, yeast extract, boiled sweets/jellies	Ice cream cones and wafers, communion wafers
Drinks	Clear fizzy drinks & fruit squash, fruit juice, mineral water, cocoa, coffee, tea, ginger beer, cider, spirits, port, sherry, wine	Barley waters/squash, malted drinks, beer, lager, stout
Home baking	Arrowroot, artificial sweeteners, bicarbonate of soda, cream of tarter, food colouring, gelatine, icing sugar, yeast (dried & fresh)	

Oats* uncontaminated oats are permitted.

Broad list of foods; Always check the food label and refer to your local Gluten-Free Food and Drink Directory (e.g. www.coeliac.org.uk).

safe daily limit is likely to be in the region of 10 mg each day [5]. The current threshold level of gluten permitted in gluten-free (GF) food as set by the Codex standard used in the UK and Europe (Codex Alimentarius Commission) suggests that food containing less than 20 ppm (parts per million) of gluten can be labelled as 'gluten free' and that foods containing between 21 and 100 ppm of gluten can be labelled as 'very low gluten'.

Given that all patients will be exposed to small amounts of gluten contamination within their diet adherence to a strict GFD is recommended [31].

9.3.5 Dietary sources of gluten

Table 9.3.1 summarises the main food sources of gluten that should be avoided with suggested GF alternatives. However, adherence also involves the elimination of any foods containing wheat, rye and barley, which are not always easily identifiable. Wheat flour is added as an ingredient, binder, filler or a carrier for flavourings and spices and can be present in almost any type of manufactured product and can vary between brands. Cross-contamination of GF foods by gluten can also occur during preparation, storage and transport, adding difficulty for patients adhering to this diet.

It is essential that food labels be consulted and checked against listings for GF foods. Coeliac UK (or equivalent association) publishes annual updated food lists that should be used. Some supermarkets and food manufacturers may have their own symbol/flag labelling foods 'suitable for coeliacs' or 'gluten free'. Coeliac UK licenses their Crossed Grain symbol to many food manufacturers who produce GF foods and drinks. Patients should always be encouraged to read labels and check product information to ensure the foods are suitable.

Alternative gluten-free foods

Most foods that have not been processed, such as fresh meats, fish, eggs, cheese, milk, fruit and vegetables can be included safely in the diet. Various manufacturers produce a range of GF substitute products, such as breads, pizza bases, biscuits and flours, although GF foods are generally more expensive to purchase than conventional foods. In some countries financial assistance to compensate for the additional costs is available. In the UK, GF products are available on prescription labelled ACBS (Advisory Committee on Borderline Substances). Published guidance (Gluten-free foods: A prescribing guide www. coeliac.org.uk) is available on the minimum monthly prescription of GF foods on the basis of approximately 15% of energy intake derived from these products. However, in some countries GF foods are tax deductible, and in many European countries monthly financial assistance is available. Regional coeliac associations can provide further information in relation to availability of products and financial assistance, for example in the USA (csaceliacs.org; celiac.org; gluten.net; celiac.com).

GF products are based on GF wheat or other cereals that are safe, such as maize, rice, and oats. GF wheat is wheat starch separated from wheat flour and can be an alternative used in cooking and baking to improve the texture and taste. Evidence suggests that GF wheat starch is tolerated by the majority of people with coeliac disease [32]. Codex wheat starch is specially manufactured wheat starch that has been processed to remove the gluten to a trace level within the Codex Standard. However, very small amounts of gluten can remain that may be sufficient to cause intestinal injury in sensitive patients [33]. Certain sufficiently sensitive individuals may require a wheat and GFD that entails avoiding any products that are manufactured from wheat starch.

9.3.6 Diet in diabetes

People with diabetes are encouraged to adhere to a healthy balanced diet based on adequate energy and carbohydrate to achieve satisfactory glycaemic control (Diabetes UK). The exact proportion of macronutrients (carbohydrate, protein and fat) in the diabetic diet should be consistent with the general population [34] as an ideal percentage of energy from macronutrients in people with diabetes is not supported by evidence [35].

Saturated and trans-fatty acids should be limited and those with diabetes should be encouraged to adhere to a cardioprotective diet that is high in monounsaturated fats and low in saturated fats [36].

Carbohydrate should be consistently distributed throughout the day and incorporated into each meal and snack to improve glycaemic control [35] in all those with diabetes. Lowering the glycaemic index (GI) of the diet is an effective method in improving glycaemic control in those with diabetes [37] as evidence suggests that there is an inverse correlation between the GI of carbohydrates and glycaemic control in those with type 1 diabetes [38]. Foods with a low GI are digested and absorbed more slowly than foods with a high GI. Evidence suggests that dietary fibre is associated with lower HbA1c levels with additional benefit of reduced risk of severe ketoacidosis [39].

Adjusting insulin to the amount of carbohydrate consumed is believed to be an important strategy in achieving good glycaemic control [40]. Structured education programmes that offer education in relation to carbohydrate counting and insulin dose adjustment are recommended for those treated by multiple daily injections or by insulin pump therapy (continuous subcutaneous insulin infusion).

Gluten-free diet for people with diabetes

Carbohydrate is the main nutritional consideration for glycaemic control in those with type 1 diabetes and often is a primary source of gluten requiring the use of substitute GF foods. Many GF foods are made with rice flour and other concentrated, low fibre, highly refined starches (potato, corn starches). Therefore adherence to a GFD may result in a diet higher in GI and reduced fibre.

There is limited information on the GI of GF foods and available evidence is conflicting as to the GI of GF breads and pasta. Saadah et al. [41] suggests that GF foods have a much higher GI than those gluten-containing equivalents however, Packer et al. [42] showed the GI to be similar in both GF and gluten-containing foods.

Naturally GF foods which are high in fibre and have low GI should also be encouraged, for example pulses, legumes, seeds, nuts, buckwheat, rice, millet, sweet potato, sweet corn, fruit and vegetables. Therefore patients with type 1 diabetes and coeliac disease should be encouraged to choose less refined higher fibre GF flours and foods that should not compromise glycaemic control and may improve blood glucose control.

Adherence to a gluten-free diet

Adherence to a GFD varies among those with CD (with and without diabetes) with rates ranging from 24–81% who admitted either occasional or prolonged lapses [43]. Lapses are more likely to occur in those who are asymptomatic [5]. Factors reported to affect the likelihood of compliance include unavailability of GF foods, inconvenient, restrictive, unpalatable, lack of available nutritional information, psychological factors and cost [5]. The clinical impact of adherence to a GFD in those with diabetes is unclear as studies are inconclusive, showing varying results in relation to improvements in hypoglycaemia, weight and glycaemic control [43].

Monitoring

Blood glucose levels should be monitored closely following diagnosis of CD and introduction of a GFD as insulin levels often need to be adjusted due to the increased absorption of carbohydrate.

Those who experienced weight loss prior to diagnosis of diabetes and/or CD may gain weight as absorption of food increases with intestinal recovery. Therefore patients should be educated about weight management.

Complications of coeliac disease

CD requires ongoing review and management. People with undiagnosed CD or those with CD who are not adhering to a strict GFD are at higher risk of complications. CD is associated with reduced bone mineral density, which increases the risk of osteoporosis and osteopenia that is present in 20–50% of people with newly diagnosed CD [5]. This is likely to be due to a delay in diagnosis of coeliac disease with a significant latent period of calcium malabsorption [5]. Establishing a GFD will optimise calcium absorption and improve bone mineral density, although it may not restore it to the level found in comparable non-coeliac people [44]. It is recommended that a daily intake of 1500 mg calcium provides maximal benefit [5]. If dietary intake is likely to be insufficient then supplementation is recommended [5].

People with CD have modest increases in overall risks of malignancy and mortality [45] although the overall number of cases of malignancy and absolute risk remains low [30]. Evidence suggests that the relative risk of all types of malignancy in those with CD has been historically overestimated [30] and is not as significant as was initially estimated. Most of this excess risk occurs in the year of follow-up after diagnosis [45]. The most common association is an increased incidence of intestinal lymphoma, however, the risk is low and this is still a rare condition [5]. Evidence suggests that adherence to a strict GFD may be protective and reduce the risk of malignancy to that of the general population (after at least 5 years on a GFD) [46,47].

CD has been associated with reproductive problems at various stages in adulthood. However, there is a lack of evidence on the impact of CD on reproduction in those with type 1 diabetes [43]. CD is associated with infertility in both men and women and poorer outcomes in pregnancy. Evidence does suggest that for women with CD there is a shortened fertility period and also a greater risk of low-birth-weight babies [43].

Key points

- Coeliac disease is an autoimmune condition associated with type 1 diabetes.
- Coeliac disease is treated by a gluten-free diet.
- Gluten-free diets have a higher glycaemic load and tend to be lower in dietary fibre, which may impact on glycaemic control.
- Structured education including carbohydrate counting, insulin adjustment and frequent blood glucose monitoring are recommended.

References

1. American Gastroenterological Association. Medical position statement? Celiac Sprue. *Gastroenterology* 2001; **120**: 1522–1525.
2. Garcia-Manzanares A, Lucendo AJ. Nutritional and dietary aspects of celiac disease. *Nutr Clin Pract* 2001; **26**: 163–173.
3. Trier JS. Coeliac Sprue. *N Engl J Med* 1991; **325**: 1709–1719.
4. Marsh MN. Gluten major histocompatability complex and the small intestine; a molecular and immunobiologic approach to the spectrum of gluten sensitivity. *Gastroenterology* 1992; **102**: 330–354.
5. British Society of Gastroenterology. The management of adults with coeliac disease. London: BSG, 2010.
6. National Institute for Health and Clinical Excellence. Recognition and assessment of coeliac disease. London: NICE, 2009.
7. Page SR, Lloyd CA, Hill PG, Peacock J, Holmes GK. The prevalence of coeliac disease in adult diabetes mellitus. *Q J Med* 1994; **87**: 631–637.
8. Savilahti E, Simell O, Koskimies S, Rilva A, Akerblom HK. Coeliac disease in insulin dependent diabetes mellitus. *J Pediatr* 1986; **108**: 690–693.
9. Koletzko S, Burgin-Wolff A, Koletzko BT, Knapp M, Burger W, Gruneklee D, et al. Prevalence of celiac disease in diabetic children and adolescents. A multi centre study. *Eur J Pediatr* 1988; **148**: 113–117.
10. Barera G, Bianchi C, Calisti L, Cerutti F, Dammacco F, Frezza E, et al. Screening of children for celiac disease with antigliadin antibodies and HLA typing. *Arch Dis Child* 1991; **66**: 491–494.
11. Saukkonen T, Savilahti E, Reijonen H, Ilonen J, Tuomilehto-Wolf E, Aberblom HK. Coeliac disease: frequent occurrence after clinical onset of insulin-dependent diabetes mellitus. Childhood Diabetes in Finland Study Group. *Diabet Med* 1996; **13**: 464–470.
12. Lorini R, Scaramuzza A, Vitali L, d'Annunzio G, Avanzini MA, De Giacomo, et al. Clinical aspects of celiac disease in children with insulin-dependent diabetes mellitus. *J Pediatr Endocrinol Metab* 1996; **9**: 101–111.
13. Mohn A, Cerruto M, Iafusco D, Prisco F, Tumini S, Stoppoloni O, et al. Coeliac disease in children and adolescents with type 1 diabetes; importance of hypoglycaemia. *J Pediatr Gastroenterol Nutr* 2001; **32**: 37–40.
14. Ravikumara M, Tuthill DP, Jenkins HR. The changing clinical presentation of celiac disease. *Arch Dis Child* 2006; **91**: 969–971.
15. Cronin CC, Shanahan F. Insulin-dependent diabetes mellitus and coeliac disease. *Lancet* 1997; **349**: 1096–1097.

16. Gregory C, Ashworth M, Eade OE, Holdstock G, Smith CL, Wright R. Delay in diagnosis of adult celiac disease. *Digestion* 1983; **28**: 201–204.

17. Collin P, Kaukinen K, Valimaki M, Salmi J. Endocrinological disorders and celiac disease. *Endocr Rev* 2002; **23**: 464–483.

18. Valerio G, Maiuri L, Troncone R, Buono P, Lombardi F, Palmiere R, et al. Severe clinical onset of diabetes and increased prevalence of other autoimmune diseases in children with coeliac diabetes diagnosed before diabetes mellitus. *Diabetologia* 2002; **45**: 1719–1722.

19. Cronin CC, Feighery A, Ferriss JB, Liddy C, Shanahan F, Feighery C. High prevalence of coeliac disease among patients with insulin-dependent (type 1) diabetes mellitus. *Am J Gastroenterol* 1997; **92**: 2210–2212.

20. Sigurs N, Johansson C, Elfstrand PO, Viander M, Lanner A. Prevalence of coeliac disease in diabetic children and adolescents in Sweden. *Acta Paediatr* 1993; **82**: 748–751.

21. Pocecco M, Ventura A. Coeliac disease and insulin dependent diabetes: a causal association. *Acta Paediatr* 1995; **84**: 1432–1433.

22. Westman E, Ambler GR, Royle M, Peat J, Chan A. Children with celiac disease and insulin dependant diabetes mellitus-growth, diabetes control and dietary intake. *J Pediatr Endocrinol Metab* 1999; **12**: 433–442.

23. Rossi TM, Albini CH, Kumar V. Incidence of celiac disease identified by the presence of serum endomysial antibodies in children with chronic diarrhoea, short stature or insulin-dependent diabetes mellitus. *J Pediatr* 1993; **123**: 262–264.

24. Iafusco D, Rea F, Chiarelli F, Mohn A, Prisco F. Effect of a gluten free diet on the metabolic control of Type 1 patients with diabetes and celiac disease. *Diabetes Care* 2000; **23**: 712–713.

25. Acerini CL, Ahmed ML, Ross KM, Sullivan PB, Bird G, Dunger DB. Coeliac disease in children and adolescents with IDDM ; clinical characteristics and response to gluten-free diet. *Diabet Med* 1998; **15**: 38–44.

26. Iafusco D, Rea F, Prisco F. Hypoglycaemia and reduction of insulin requirements as a sign of coeliac disease in children with IDDM. *Diabetes Care* 1998; **21**: 1379–1381.

27. Kaukinen K, Salmi J, Lahtela J Siljamaki-Ojansuu U, Koivisto A-M, Oksa H, et al. No effect of gluten free diet on the metabolic control of type 1 diabetes in patients with diabetes and celiac disease. Retrospective and controlled prospective survey. *Diabetes Care* 1999; **22**: 1747–1748.

28. Korponay-Szabo IR, Dahlbom I, Laurila K, Koskinen S, Woolley N, Partanen J, et al. Elevation of IgG antibodies against tissue transglutaminase as a diagnostic tool for coeliac disease in selective IgA deficiency. *Gut* 2003; **52**: 1567–1571.

29. Picarelli A, Sabbatella L, Di Tola M, Vetrano S, Casale C, Anania MC, et al. Anti-endomysial antibody IgG1 isotype detection strongly increases the prevalence of celiac disease in patients affected by Type 1 diabetes mellitus. *Clin Exp Immunol* 2005; **142**: 1111–1115.

30. Leeds JS, Hopper AD, Sanders DS. Coeliac Disease. *Br Med Bull* 2008; **88**: 157–170.

31. Biagi F, Campanella J, Martucci S, Pezzimenti D, Ciclitira P, Ellis HJ, et al. A milligram of gluten a day keeps the mucosal recovery away: a case report. *Nutr Rev* 2004; **62**: 360–363.

32. Kaukinen K, Collin P, Holm K, Rantala I, Vuolteenaho N, Reunala T, et al. Wheat starch containing gluten free flour products in the treatment of Coeliac Disease and Dermatitis Herpetiformis. A long term follow up study. *Scand J Gastroenterol* 1999; **34**: 163–169

33. Chartrand LJ, Russo PA, Duhaime AG, Seidman EG. Wheat starch intolerance in patients with coeliac disease. *J Am Diet Assoc* 1997; **97**: 612–618.

34. COMA. Report of the Panel on DRVs of the Committee on Medical Aspects of Food Policy (COMA) Report on Health and Social Subjects 41 Dietary Reference Values (DRVs) for Food Energy and Nutrients for the UK. London: The Stationary Office, 1991.

35. Franz MJ, Powers MA, Leontos C, Holzmeister LA, Kulkarni K, Monk A. The evidence for medical nutrition therapy for type 1 and type 2 diabetes in adults. *J Am Diet Assoc* 2010; **110**: 1852–1889.

36. Bantle JP, Wylie-Rosett J, Albright AL, Apovian CM, Clark NG, Franz MJ, et al. Nutrition recommendations and interventions for diabetes: a position statement of the America Diabetes Association. *Diabetes Care* 2008; **31**: S61–S78.

37. Thomas DE, Elliott EJ. The use of low-glycaemic index diets in diabetes control; meta-analysis. *Br J Nutr* 2010; **104**: 797–802.

38. Buyken AE, Toeller M, Heitkamp G, Karamanos B, Rottiers R, Muggeo M; EURODIAB IDDM complications study Group. Glycaemic index in the diet of European outpatients with type 1 diabetes; relations to glycated haemoglobin and serum lipids *Am J Clin Nutr* 2001; **73**: 574–581.

39. Buyken AE, Toeller M, Heitkamp G, Vitelli F, Stehle P, Scherbaum WA, et al. Relation of fibre intake to HbA1c and the prevalence of severe ketoacidosis and severe hypoglycaemia. *Diabetologia* 1998; **41**: 882–890.

40. Sheard NF, Clark NG, Brand-Miller JC, Franz MJ, Pi-Sunyer FX, Mayer-Davis E. Dietary carbohydrate (amount and type) in the prevention and management of diabetes: a Statement by the American Diabetes Association. *Diabetes Care* 2004; **27**: 2266–2271.

41. Saadah OI, Zacharin M, O'Callaghan A, Oliver MR, Catto-Smith AG. Effects of gluten free diet and adherence on growth and diabetic control in diabetics with celiac disease. *Arch Dis Child* 2004; **89**: 871–876.

42. Packer SC, Dornhorst A, Frost GS. The glycaemic index of a range of gluten free foods. *Diabet Med* 2000; **17**: 657–660.

43. Sud S, Marcon M, Assor E, Palmert MR, Daneman D, Mahmud FH. Coeliac disease and paediatric type 1 diabetes: Diagnostic and treatment dilemmas. *Int J Pediatr Endocrinol* 2010; 161285.

44. Pazianas M, Butcher GP, Subhani JM, Finch PJ, Ang L, Collins C, et al. Calcium absorption and bone mineral density in coeliacs after long term treatment with gluten-free diet and adequate calcium absorption. *Osteoporosis Int* 2005; **16**: 56–63.

45. West J, Logan RF, Smith CJ, Hubbard RB, Card TR. Malignancy and mortality in people with celiac disease: population based cohort study. *BMJ* 2004; **329**(7468): 716–719.

46. Holmes GK, Prior P, Lane MR, Pope D, Allan RN. Malignancy in coeliac disease-effect of a gluten free diet. *Gut* 1989; **30**: 333–338.

47. Askling J, Linet M, Grindley G, Halstensen TS, Ekstrom K, Ekbom A. Cancer incidence in a population based cohort of individuals hospitalized with Coeliac Disease or Dermatitis Herpetiformis. *Gastroenterology* 2002; **123**: 1428–1435.

Chapter 9.4

Disorders associated with insulin resistance

Alastair Duncan[1] and Suzanne Barr[2]
[1]Guy's and St Thomas' NHS Foundation Trust, London, UK
[2]Imperial College London, London, UK

9.4.1 Introduction

As part of the developing pandemic of type 2 diabetes many individuals are experiencing increased risk of developing insulin resistance and progression to diabetes [1]. This chapter focuses on three conditions associated with insulin resistance: polycystic ovary syndrome, non-alcoholic fatty liver disease and human immunodeficiency virus (HIV) infection. Insulin resistance refers to an impaired ability of insulin action, principally a reduced glucose-lowering effect, but also a reduction in uptake of circulating triglycerides and increased hydrolysis of fat stores. Peripheral insulin resistance reduces glucose uptake in muscle and fat cells. Insulin resistance in liver cells leads to both reduced glycogen synthesis and storage, and reduced suppression of gluconeogenesis. Together these contribute to elevated blood glucose levels, leading to metabolic syndrome and type 2 diabetes.

Several diseases and conditions are associated with insulin resistance and its aetiology within these conditions may be inherent or extrinsic. In polycystic ovary syndrome, an inherent factor associated with the condition is currently thought to lead to the development of insulin resistance. In liver disease, localised insulin resistance may be extrinsic secondary to obesity or infection. The aetiology of HIV-associated insulin resistance is complex, but may be inherent secondary to inflammation and/or extrinsic secondary to antiretroviral therapy or obesity.

9.4.2 Polycystic ovary syndrome

Disease pathogenesis and consequences

Polycystic ovary syndrome (PCOS) is a heterogeneous condition, with a prevalence of 5 to 20% depending on diagnostic criteria and population investigated [2]. Clinical presentation is heterogeneous, women present with a combination of symptoms including menstrual dysfunction, infertility or increased pregnancy complications, hirsutism (excess hair) or alopecia, acne, central adiposity and insulin resistance [3]. The current diagnostic criteria for PCOS involve the presence of two of the following three features with the exclusion of other endocrine disorders [4]:

(1) Oligo-ovulation leading to oligomenorrhoea (defined as less than nine menses per year) or anovulation leading to amenorrhoea.
(2) Hyperandrogenism defined clinically (hirsutism, male pattern alopecia, acne) and/or biochemically.
(3) Polycystic ovaries (identified on ultrasound).

Although insulin resistance is not included in the current diagnostic criteria, the majority of women with PCOS present with some degree of insulin resistance, which is suggested to be an intrinsic, rather than typical obesity-related

Advanced Nutrition and Dietetics in Diabetes, First Edition. Edited by Louise Goff and Pamela Dyson.
© 2016 John Wiley & Sons, Ltd. Published 2016 by John Wiley & Sons, Ltd.

extrinsic insulin resistance [5]. The inherent factor is largely unknown, however, a post insulin receptor defect has been proposed as *in vitro* studies on adipocytes from women with PCOS show a significant reduction in the number of GLUT-4 transporter molecules, in the absence of abnormalities in insulin receptor number or affinity [6]. Studies are also ongoing in relation to genetic susceptibility of PCOS and insulin resistance. Some studies have suggested an autosomal dominant inheritance, however, others propose an oligogenic basis, due to the heterogeneous nature of PCOS [7], and may be the consequence of the interaction of several genes (in addition to environmental factors). Insulin resistance and compensatory hyperinsulinemia promotes ovarian hyperandrogenism and in turn reduces hepatic production of sex hormone binding globulin (SHBG) thereby increasing free testosterone levels, leading to disrupted follicular growth, menstrual irregularity and anovulatory sub-fertility [8].

Increased risk of type 2 diabetes is common as a result of intrinsic insulin resistance, with up to 50% of women with PCOS developing impaired glucose tolerance or type 2 diabetes by the age of 40 years, and a similar proportion also exhibit features of the metabolic syndrome [9]. Further studies also demonstrate that women with PCOS have greater prevalence of cardiovascular disease risk factors, including hypertriglyceridaemia, low high-density lipoprotein (HDL) cholesterol, hypertension and endothelial dysfunction [10].

Obesity and abdominal obesity are more prevalent in PCOS [11], estimated to affect 30–70% of women [12, 13] and worsen the reproductive and metabolic features including insulin resistance [14]. Weight gain exacerbates symptoms, with obese women generally more symptomatic and at increased health risk compared with lean women with PCOS; however, lean women with PCOS are also at increased disease risk compared with matched controls [14].

Genetic heritability

The exact pathophysiology of PCOS is complex and remains largely unclear, however, it is thought there is a genetic heritability that is enhanced by environmental factors such as obesity or lifestyle [15]. PCOS prevalence also varies by ethnic background, being more prevalent in South Asian and Black women than in Caucasians [3]; yet there is relatively little research in this area.

Patient-centred consequences

The psychological effects of PCOS should also not be neglected, as increased levels of anxiety, depression and reduced quality of life have been described in women with PCOS [16]. This has been attributed to presenting features, such as oligomenorrhoea, hirsutism, acne and obesity [17]. There is some additional evidence that a higher prevalence of eating disorders exists in women with PCOS [18], however, further research is needed in this area.

Nutritional assessment

In addition to standard nutritional assessment, some additional factors should be considered for women with PCOS, as detailed in Box 9.4.1. Clinical (acne, hirsutism), psychological (anxiety and depression), economic and social factors should be considered in the context of dietary and lifestyle recommendations, which should also include behavioural change techniques such as motivational interviewing where appropriate.

Clinical and nutritional management

Clinical management of PCOS focuses on the treatment of presenting symptoms [19] as presently there is no cure for PCOS. Despite this, lifestyle management is widely advocated as the primary therapy in overweight and obese women with PCOS. Clinical management includes suppression of androgen secretion by systemic treatment (such as oral contraceptive pill or antibiotics) or by topical treatment of excess hair growth or acne [19]. Clomiphene citrate is widely used for the induction of ovulation and metformin is commonly prescribed to insulin-resistant individuals [20].

Box 9.4.1 Nutritional assessment for PCOS

- **BMI and waist circumference**. Anthropometric measurements can be used to inform risk of comorbidities and dietary management.
- **Oral glucose tolerance test (OGTT)**. Due to the increased prevalence of impaired glucose tolerance and type 2 diabetes, OGTT should be undertaken in women with PCOS with a BMI >30 kg/m², aged >40 years, a personal history of gestational diabetes or a family history of type 2 diabetes. Where an OGTT is not possible, fasting blood glucose levels may be of value.
- **Blood pressure, plasma total, LDL and HDL cholesterol and triglycerides**. Due to the increased prevalence of cardiovascular risk factors, measurements of these are recommended.
- **Hormone levels** may be considered, however these may not be measured routinely*.
- A **dietary assessment** to determine habitual dietary habits should be undertaken, which should also include details relating to eating behaviours due to increased possibility of eating disorders in this population.

*Typical biochemical features of women with PCOS are elevated testosterone. However, free androgen index (FAI) measurements are generally recommended: FAI = 100 × (total testosterone/SHBG) as direct measurement of biochemical androgens lacks accuracy in women. Women with PCOS also have a raised LH:FSH ratio (raised luteinising hormone (LH) and normal follicle stimulating hormone (FSH)), however these hormones are not routinely measured.

Weight and nutritional management

Weight loss achieved through dietary restriction and increased physical activity remain the key management strategy for overweight and obese women with PCOS. Modest weight loss of just 5–10%, without medical intervention, has been shown to improve many of the symptoms associated with PCOS by lowering fasting insulin levels, increasing SHBG, reducing free testosterone, improving reproductive function, improving symptoms of hirsutism and improving risk factors for diabetes and CVD [21,22]. The optimal method of achieving sustainable weight loss is under debate and, as with the general population, a range of weight loss strategies appropriate to the individual are available.

The optimal dietary composition remains unknown, with proposed modifications to diets including lowering glycaemic index or load, increasing monounsaturated or polyunsaturated fat intake, lowering carbohydrate or increasing protein intake. Studies have demonstrated varying clinical and biochemical benefits to these modifications [22,23] with no conclusive optimum diet advocated to manage PCOS.

There remains a limited body of literature investigating dietary strategies for PCOS, with existing studies comprising small sample sizes, being of short to medium duration, and focused predominantly on Caucasian women, indicating the lack of generalisability of results and contributing to the lack of consensus on the optimum dietary recommendations for this population.

It has been proposed that dietary modification to improve insulin resistance may produce benefits greater than those achieved by weight loss alone and would also be suitable for lean women with PCOS [24], yet few studies have included lean women with PCOS. One small study, which included lean women, demonstrated an improvement in insulin sensitivity through an isocaloric diet with a reduction in dietary glycaemic index [25]. Additional research is warranted to investigate the effects of dietary modification on metabolic and reproductive factors in lean women with PCOS, many of whom are symptomatic and insulin resistant. Clinical guidelines have been recently published in Australia [26], and include comprehensive information on lifestyle strategies and weight management; however, there is a clear need for further clinical guidelines to be developed worldwide.

9.4.3 Non-alcoholic fatty liver disease

Disease pathogenesis and consequences

Non-alcoholic fatty liver disease (NAFLD) is characterised by a spectrum of liver disease, from the relatively benign hepatic steatosis where lipid accumulation within hepatocytes accounts for more than 5% of liver weight, to non-alcoholic steatohepatitis (NASH) where fibrosis and cirrhosis can lead to end-stage liver failure [27]. NAFLD occurs in up to 24% of all adults, 53% of obese children and 74% of obese adults. Insulin resistance is central to the development of NAFLD through influx of free fatty acids, and NAFLD itself can accelerate the onset of type 2 diabetes, as well as being caused by it [28]. In addition to insulin resistance, a range of factors are associated with onset of NAFLD, including rapid weight gain, central (visceral) obesity, dyslipidaemia, hypertension, sleep apnoea, inflammation, excessive dietary fat intake and a sedentary lifestyle [27]. It is important to recognise NAFLD at an early stage and intervene to prevent progression.

Clinical and nutritional management

Primary management of NAFLD is through treatment of insulin resistance and weight loss [29]. A systematic review [29] suggests that weight loss through diet and exercise is safe in NAFLD, improving cardio-metabolic risk. The review suggests that a weight loss ≥7% improves a wide range of measures of NAFLD histological disease. However, less than 50% of patients were able to achieve this goal, but weight loss of 5% is also associated with a reduction in steatosis in isolation. The review also suggests a beneficial role for treatment with metformin, statins and thiazolidinediones, and a potential for treatment with vitamin E supplements.

More recently, diet and exercise without weight loss have been shown to be of benefit in the treatment of NAFLD. After only 7 days of an aerobic exercise programme a significant impact was seen in markers of progression of NAFLD, including insulin resistance [30]. In adults, a 4-week low glycaemic index diet, with a reduced intake of saturated and overall fats resulted in reduced liver steatosis [31]. In children and adolescents with NAFLD, modest reductions in fructose intake and a reduced glycaemic index had a positive impact on markers of NAFLD progression [32].

Bariatric surgery has been observed to have a profoundly beneficial effect on NAFLD, with a rapid reduction in insulin resistance and liver fat following surgery [33]. Observations from a study

> **Box 9.4.2** Lifestyle treatments in NAFLD
>
> - Weight loss of 5% improves hepatic steatosis, but ≥7% has a significant impact on wider measures of improvement in NAFLD.
> - Reduced fructose and fat intakes, and a lower glycaemic index have benefits.
> - The beneficial effect of exercise is almost immediate.
> - Rapid weight loss is not harmful as long as nutritional intake is adequate.
> - In advanced NAFLD with decompensated cirrhosis, it is essential that protein requirements are met when restricting energy intake.

published in 1991 [34] that rapid weight loss may worsen fibrosis in NAFLD have since been disproven, as long as adequate dietetic treatment and support is provided [33].

Finally, advanced NAFLD requires careful nutritional assessment and management. Obese NAFLD patients with decompensated cirrhosis may experience significant protein malnutrition, necessitating care to meet protein requirements when restricting overall energy intake [35].

Lifestyle treatments in NAFLD are summarised in Box 9.4.2.

9.4.4 HIV

Disease pathogenesis and consequences

The HIV pandemic

More than 25 million people have died from HIV since the first cases were reported in 1981. Today there are 35.3 million people in the world living with HIV, two-thirds of whom live in sub-Saharan Africa. In South Africa the prevalence of HIV is 17.3%, with almost 6 million people HIV positive. This compares to the United Kingdom (UK) where 78 000 people are HIV positive – a prevalence of 0.01%. The advent of effective anti-HIV medicines used in combination – highly active antiretroviral therapy (HAART) – has dramatically improved morbidity and mortality for the 9.7 million HIV positive people with access to treatment. In the UK, where HIV treatment is universal and free, people newly diagnosed with HIV are told to expect a near-normal life expectancy. In low and middle income countries access to HAART is more variable and the United Nations has published a short-term aim that half of the world's HIV positive people should have access to HAART [36]. Taken as a whole, people with HIV are ageing, and in both the UK and the United States (US), 50% of people with HIV will be aged 50 or over by 2015. Conditions associated with normal ageing, including cardiovascular disease, cancer, cognitive decline, osteoporosis and type 2 diabetes are occurring more frequently and earlier than expected in HIV, attributed to infection and antiviral therapies [37]. These conditions are now the major cause of morbidity and mortality in HIV amongst those with access to HAART.

The phenotype of insulin resistance in HIV

The mechanism of development of insulin resistance in HIV is not fully understood [38]. There is a high prevalence of impaired fasting glycaemia amongst people newly diagnosed with HIV and not yet prescribed HAART [39]. In treated patients, studies report the estimated risk of development of type 2 diabetes to be up to four times higher than in matched HIV negative controls, although the estimated relative risk varies between populations studied [40–42]. This increased risk may include components directly attributable to certain antiretroviral medicines, chronic inflammation, alterations in fat metabolism with resulting body shape changes, and surprisingly high levels of obesity in this cohort [43]. In the US, 12 months after initiation of HAART, patients experience an average 4.5 kg weight gain, with rates of overweight and obesity increasing from 52 to 66%. This compares to rates in matched HIV negative controls of 91%. Women, those with a lower CD4 count, and those initiating onto protease-inhibitor-containing HAART regimens are more likely to gain excess weight [44]. Factors associated with the development of type 2 diabetes in HIV include increasing age [39–42], higher BMI [39–42], higher waist to hip ratio [40], lower nadir CD4 count (lowest ever surrogate marker of strength of the immune system) [39] and the presence of HIV-associated body shape changes [40, 41].

The consequences of insulin resistance in HIV

Type 2 diabetes is more difficult to treat in HIV patients, with a significantly poorer response to anti-diabetic medicines when compared to matched HIV negative controls [44]. There is growing evidence that diabetes is associated with accelerated cognitive decline in HIV, and is particularly associated with neurocognitive impairment in older participants [45]. In the large international D:A:D study, type 2 diabetes was independently associated with a 2.4-fold increased rate of incident coronary heart disease. With the risk of developing type 2 diabetes up to four times higher, unless prevention can be achieved, in the UK alone, by 2020 as many as 15 000 new HIV-associated diabetes diagnoses will present, with an annual financial burden exceeding £30 million [46,47].

Nutritional assessment

In addition to a standard nutritional assessment, there are several factors to include for people with HIV, at risk of or with type 2 diabetes, as outlined in Box 9.4.3.

Box 9.4.3 Nutritional assessment considering insulin resistance in HIV

- A wide range of anthropometric measures should be used to assess for presence of HAART-associated body shape changes:
  ○ BMI
  ○ Circumferences: mid-arm, chest, waist, hips, mid-thigh
  ○ Skin folds: biceps, triceps, subscapular, suprailiac, mid-thigh
  ○ Patient-reported facial wasting.
- Given the association of type 2 diabetes with higher BMIs, higher waist to hip ratios, lower nadir CD4 counts, and presence of body shape changes, if any of these are present screen for impaired fasting glucose, ideally using an oral glucose tolerance test.
- The potential for the presence of cognitive impairment should be borne in mind when carrying out a nutritional assessment.
- An assessment of dietary intake should be performed, and extended to enquire about timing of and adherence to HAART.
- The dietary assessment should refer to cardiovascular risk as well as diet for insulin resistance.

Clinical and nutritional management

Clinical management of insulin resistance in HIV

In addition to considering the HIV-specific risks for developing insulin resistance and type 2 diabetes mentioned in Box 9.4.3, 10-year diabetes risk can be calculated by a range of online tools. Those at higher risk should be regularly screened, ideally with an OGTT. For those with type 2 diabetes, an assessment of cognitive function should be routinely carried out. Current European HIV guidelines state that management of diabetes should follow general principles, with lifestyle management being a primary treatment [48]. However the following factors should be considered:

- HbA1c values may be slightly changed in those on HAART: underestimated in regimens containing non-nucleoside reverse transcriptase inhibitors and abacavir, and overestimated in regimens containing protease inhibitors, although a value of ≥48 mmol/mol (6.5%) is highly specific in diagnosing type 2 diabetes in HIV [49]
- Metformin should be used as a first line agent if lifestyle interventions prove insufficient, but care must be taken as its use can exacerbate lipoatrophy
- Pioglitazone is of limited use in people with HIV due to side effects.

Nutritional management of insulin resistance in HIV

There are few published studies investigating lifestyle interventions for insulin resistance in HIV and so international guidelines recommend the following general principles [46]. These include: achieving and maintaining weight and waist size within the normal range, with caloric intake balanced with energy expenditure; moderating fat intake to provide <30% of caloric intake; increasing intake of fruits and vegetables to between 5 and 7 portions per day, and wholegrains to comprise more than 50% of carbohydrate intake; consuming less than 40 mmol sodium daily; consuming 2 portions of oily fish weekly; and limiting foods and drinks containing added sugar. A review of lifestyle interventions for insulin resistance in HIV [46] contrasts two small studies showing no statistical effect of diet and exercise interventions on measures of insulin resistance in HIV with three small studies that show limited effects. The strongest evidence is presented in a Danish study ($n = 20$) showing that intensive strength and endurance exercise has a positive effect on HIV-related peripheral insulin resistance [50]. There are no published studies investigating prevention of type 2 diabetes in HIV, however, a Brazilian study ($n = 83$) demonstrated that HIV patients receiving dietetic advice prior to and for 12 months following commencement of HAART, did not experience the weight gain seen when starting treatment [51]. Further research is needed for both the prevention and treatment of insulin resistance in HIV.

Key points

- Insulin resistance is associated with an increased risk of type 2 diabetes.
- Polycystic ovary syndrome, non-alcoholic fatty liver disease and HIV infection are all associated with insulin resistance and type 2 diabetes.
- Weight loss improves both PCOS and NAFLD.
- Insulin resistance and type 2 diabetes are more challenging to treat in those who are HIV positive, where weight gain and weight maintenance, rather than weight loss, is the aim.

References

1. Goff L, Duncan A. Diet and lifestyle in the prevention of the rising diabetes pandemic. *J Hum Nutr Diet* 2010; **23**(4): 333–335.
2. March W, Moore VM, Willson KJ, Phillips DI, Norman RJ, Davies MJ. The prevalence of polycystic ovary syndrome in a community sample assessed under contrasting diagnostic criteria. *Hum Reprod* 2010; **25**(2): 544–551.
3. Azziz R, Carmina E, Dewailly D, Diamanti-Kandarakis E, Escobar-Morreale HF, Futterweit W, et al. Androgen Excess Society. Position statement:

criteria for defining polycystic ovary syndrome as a predominantly hyperandrogenic syndrome: an Androgen Excess Society guideline. *J Clin Endocrinol Metab* 2006; **91**(11): 4237–4245.

4. European Society of Human Reproduction and Embryology (ESHRE/ASRM). Revised 2003 consensus on diagnostic criteria and long term health risks related to polycystic ovary syndrome. *Fertil Steril* 2004; **81**(1): 19–25.

5. Teede H, Hutchison SK, Zoungas S. The management of insulin resistance in polycystic ovary syndrome. *Trends Endocrinol Metab* 2007; **18**(7): 273–279.

6. Rice S, Christoforidis N, Gadd C, Nikolaou D, Seyani L, Donaldson A, et al. Impaired insulin-dependent glucose metabolism in granulosa-lutein cells from anovulatory women with polycystic ovaries. *Hum Reprod* 2005; **20**: 373–381.

7. Prapas N, Karkanaki A, Prapas I, Kalogiannidis I, Katsikis I, Panidis D. Genetics of Polycystic Ovary Syndrome. *Hippokratia* 2009; **13**: 216–223.

8. Goodarzi M, Dumesic DA, Chazenbalk G, Azziz R. Polycystic ovary syndrome: etiology, pathogenesis and diagnosis. *Nat Rev Endocrinol* 2011; **7**(4): 219–231.

9. Ehrmann DA, Kasza K, Azziz R, Legro RS, Ghazzi MN; PCOS/Troglitazone Study Group. Prevalence and predictors of the metabolic syndrome in women with polycystic ovary syndrome. *J Clin Endocrinol Metab* 2006; **91**(1): 48–53.

10. Wild R, Carmina E, Diamanti-Kandarakis E, Dokras A, Escobar-Morreale HF, Futterweit W, et al. Assessment of cardiovascular risk and prevention of cardiovascular disease in women with the polycystic ovary syndrome: a consensus statement by the Androgen Excess and Polycystic Ovary Syndrome (AE-PCOS) Society. *J Clin Endocrinol Metab* 2010; **95**(5): 2038–2049.

11. Escobar-Morreale H, San Millan JL. Abdominal adiposity and the polycystic ovary syndrome. *Trends Endocrinol Metab* 2007; **18**(7): 266–272.

12. Balen AH, Glass MR. What's new in polycystic ovary syndrome? in *Recent Advances in Obstetrics and Gynaecology*, ed. J. Bonnar, London: RSM Press. 2005, pp. 147–158.

13. Yucel A, Noyan V, Sagsoz N. The association of serum androgens and insulin resistance with fat distribution in polycystic ovary syndrome. *Eur J Obstet Gynecol Reprod Biol* 2005; **126**: 81–89.

14. Kaya C, Onalan G, Cengiz SD. An increase in systolic blood pressure and abnormal circadian blood pressure regulation in lean women with polycystic ovary syndrome. *Eur J Obstet Gynecol Reprod Biol* 2010; **150**: 217–218.

15. Pasquali R, Gambineri A, Cavazza C, Gasparini DI, Ciampaglia W, Cognigni GE. Heterogeneity in the responsiveness to long-term lifestyle intervention and predictability in obese women with polycystic ovary syndrome. *Eur J Endocrinol* 2011; **164**(1): 53–60.

16. Dokras A, Clifton S, Futterweit W, Wild R. Increased risk for abnormal depression scores in women with polycystic ovary syndrome: a systematic review and meta-analysis. *Obste Gynecol* 2011; **117**(1): 145–152.

17. Coffey S, Bano G, Mason HD. Health-related quality of life in women with polycystic ovary syndrome: a comparison with the general population using the Polycystic Ovary Syndrome Questionnaire (PCOSQ) and the short form-36 (SF-36). *Gynecol Endocrinol* 2006; **22**: 80–86.

18. Kerchner A, Lester W, Stuart SP, Dokras A. Risk of depression and other mental health disorders in women with polycystic ovary syndrome: a longitudinal study. *Fertil Steril* 2009; **91**: 207–212.

19. Badawy A, Elnashar A. Treatment options for polycystic ovary syndrome. *Int J Womens Health* 2011; **3**: 25–35.

20. Diamanti-Kandarakis E, Christakou C, Kandaraki E, Economou F. Metformin: An old medication of new fashion in PCOS. *Eur J Endocrinol* 2010; **162**: 193.

21. Moran LJ, Hutchison SK, Norman RJ, Teede HJ. Lifestyle changes in women with polycystic ovary syndrome. *Cochrane Database Syst Rev* 2011, Issue 7, Art. No.: CD007506. doi: 10.1002/14651858. CD007506.pub3.

22. Moran L, Ko H, Misso M, Marsh K, Noakes M, Talbot M, et al. Dietary composition in the treatment of polycystic ovary syndrome: a systematic review to inform evidence-based guidelines. *J Acad Nutr Diet* 2013; **113**(4): 520–545.

23. Mehrabani H, Salehpour S, Amiri Z, Farahani SJ, Meyer BJ, Tahbaz F. Beneficial effects of a high-protein, low-glycemic-load hypocaloric diet in overweight and obese women with polycystic ovary syndrome: a randomized controlled intervention study. *J Am Coll Nutr* 2012; **31**(2): 117–125.

24. Marsh K, Brand-Miller J. The optimal diet for women with polycystic ovary syndrome? *Br J Nutr* 2005; **94**(2): 154–165.

25. Barr S, Reeves S, Sharp K, Jeanes Y. An isocaloric low glycemic index diet improves insulin sensitivity in women with polycystic ovary syndrome. *J Acad Nutr Diet* 2013; **113**(11): 1523–1531.

26. PCOS Australia Alliance. Evidence-based guideline for the assessment and management of polycystic ovary syndrome. Jean Hailes Foundation for Women's Health on behalf of the PCOS Australian Alliance; Melbourne, 2011.

27. Ahmed M, Byrne C. Non-alcoholic fatty liver disease. In CD Byrne and SH Wild (eds) *The Metabolic Syndrome*, 2nd edn, Oxford: Wiley-Blackwell, 2011, pp. 245–277.

28. Williams K, Shackel N, Gorrell M, McLennan S, Twigg S. Diabetes and nonalcoholic fatty liver disease: A pathogenic duo. *Endocr Rev* 2013; **34**: 84–129.

29. Musso G, Cassader M, Rosina F, Gambino R. Impact of current treatments on liver disease, glucose metabolism and cardiovascular risk in non-alcoholic fatty liver disease (NAFLD): a systematic review and meta-analysis of randomised trials. *Diabetologia* 2012; **55**: 885–904.

30. Haus J, Solomon P, Kelly K, Fealy C, Kullman E, Scelsi A, et al. Improved hepatic lipid composition following short-term exercise in non-alcoholic fatty liver disease. *J Clin Endocrinol Metab* 2013; **98** (7): 1181–1188.

31. Utzschneider K, Bayer-Carter J, Arbuckle M, Tidwell J, Richards T, Craft S. Beneficial effect of a weight stable, low fat / low saturated fat / low glycaemic index diet to reduce liver fat in older subjects. *Br J Nutr* 2013; **109**: 1096–1104.

32. Mager D, Rivera Iñiguez I, Gilmour S, Yap J. The effect of a low fructose and low glycemic index/load (FRAGILE) dietary intervention on indices of liver function, cardiometabolic risk factors, and body composition in children and adolescents with nonalcoholic fatty liver disease (NAFLD). *JPEN* 2013; doi: 10.1177/0148607113501201.

33. Hafeez S. Ahmed M. Bariatric surgery as potential treatment for nonalcoholic fatty liver disease: A future treatment by choice or by chance? *J Obes* 2013; **2013**, article ID 839275.

34. Andersen T, Gluud C, Franzmann M, Christoffersen P. Hepatic effects of dietary weight loss in morbidly obese subjects. *J Hepatol* 1991; **12**(2): 224–229.

35. Johnson T, Overgard E, Cohen A, DiBaise J. Nutrition assessment and management in advanced liver disease. *Nutr Clin Pract* 2013; **28**(1): 15–29.

36. The UNAIDS Report on the Global Aids Epidemic 2013. www.unaids.org/en/resources/documents/2013/name,85053,en.asp (accessed 21 November 2013).

37. Smith R, de Boer R, Brul S, Budovskaya Y, van der Spek H. Premature and accelerated aging: HIV or HAART? *Front Genet* 2012; **3**: 328. doi: 10.3389/fgene.2012.00328

38. Samaras K. The burden of diabetes and hyperlipidemia in treated HIV infection and approaches for cardiometabolic care. *Curr HIV/AIDS Rep* 2012; **9**(3): 206–217.

39. Shen Y, Wang Z, Liu L, Zhang R, Zheng Y, Lu H. Prevalence of hyperglycemia among adults with newly diagnosed HIV/AIDS in China. *BMC Infect Dis* 2013; **13**: 79. http://www.biomedcentral.com/1471-2334/13/79

40. Brown T, Cole S, Li X, Kingsley L, Palella F, Riddler S, et al. Antiretroviral therapy and the prevalence and incidence of diabetes mellitus in the multicenter AIDS cohort study. *Arch Intern Med* 2005; **165**(10): 1179–1184.

41. Capeau J, Bouteloup V, Katlama C, Bastard J-P, Guiyedi V, Salmon-Ceron D, et al. Ten-year diabetes incidence in 1046 HIV-infected patients started on a combination antiretroviral treatment. *AIDS* 2012; **26**(3): 303–314.

42. Rasmussen L, Mathiesen E, Kronborg G, Pedersen C, Gerstoft J, Obel N. Risk of diabetes mellitus in persons with and without HIV: a Danish nationwide population-based cohort study. *PLoS ONE* 2012; **7**(9): e44575.

43. Lakey W, Yang L, Yancy W, Chow S-C, Hicks C. Short communication: from wasting to obesity: initial antiretroviral therapy and weight gain in HIV-infected persons. *AIDS Res Hum Retroviruses* 2013; **29**(3): 435–440.

44. Han J, Crane H, Bellamy S, Frank I, Cardillo S, Bisson G, et al. HIV infection and glycemic response to newly initiated diabetic medical therapy. *AIDS* 2012; **26**: 2087–2095.

45. McCutchan J, Marquie-Beck J, FitzSimons C, Letendre S, Ellis K, Heaton K, et al. Role of obesity, metabolic variables, and diabetes in HIV-associated neurocognitive disorder. *Neurology* 2012; **78**: 485–492.

46. Dyson P, Kelly T, Deakin T, Duncan A, Frost G, Harrison Z, et al. Diabetes UK evidence-based nutrition guidelines for the prevention and management of diabetes. *Diabet Med* 2011; **28**(11): 1282–1288.

47. Health Protection Agency. HIV in the United Kingdom: 2012 Report. http://www.hpa.org.uk/webc/HPAwebFile/HPAweb_C/1317137200016 (accessed 23/11/2013).

48. The European Aids Clinical Society HIV Guidelines 2013. http://www.eacsociety.org/Portals/0/Guidelines_Online_131014.pdf (accessed 22/11/2013).

49. Eckhardt B, Holzman R, Kwan C, Baghdadi J, Aberg J. Glycated Hemoglobin A1c as Screening for Diabetes Mellitus in HIV-Infected Individuals. *AIDS Patient CareSTDs* 2012; **26**(4): 197–201.

50. Lindegaard B, Hansen T, Hvid T, van Hall G, Plomgaard P, Ditlevsen S, et al. The effect of strength and endurance training on insulin sensitivity and fat distribution in HIV-infected patients with

lipodystrophy. *J Clin Endocrinol Metab* 2008; **93**(10): 3860–3869.

51. Lazzaretti R, Kuhmmer R, Sprinz E, Polanczyk C, Ribeiro J. Dietary intervention prevents dyslipidemia associated with highly active antiretroviral therapy in HIV. *J Am Coll Cardiol* 2012; **59**(11): 979–988.

Recommended website

PCOS Australia Alliance 2011. Evidence-based guidelines for the assessment and management of polycystic ovary syndrome. https://jeanhailes.org.au/contents/documents/Resources/Tools/PCOS_evidence-based_guideline_for_assessment_and_management_pcos.pdf

Chapter 9.5

Cystic fibrosis-related diabetes

Kerry-Lee Watson
King's College Hospital NHS Foundation Trust, London, UK

9.5.1 Introduction

Cystic fibrosis (CF) is the most common autosomal recessively inherited genetic condition in Caucasians, affecting 1 in 2500–3000 births and causing premature death. Mutations of the cystic fibrosis transmembrane regulator (CFTR) gene lead to thick viscous secretions, causing obstruction and fibrosis in the lungs and pancreatic tissue. The most important clinical manifestations are pulmonary disease, leading to respiratory failure and mortality, and pancreatic insufficiency (PI). The median age of survival has dramatically improved due to advances in medical therapies; patients born in the 1990s are expected to live into their 40s [1–3]. Currently median life expectancy is 34.4 years and 37.4 years in the United Kingdom (UK) and the United States (US), respectively [4,5].

As the age of survival increases, long term comorbidities will occur, requiring screening, diagnosis and appropriate management.

Cystic fibrosis-related diabetes (CFRD) is the most common comorbidity in CF, currently diagnosed at median age of 18–21 years [6,7]. CFRD is associated with deterioration in clinical status and contributes to poor nutritional status, decreased lung function, more frequent hospital admissions and increased mortality, particularly in women in their 30s [3,8,9]. CFRD is a distinct entity which shares features of type 1 and type 2 diabetes as shown in Table 9.5.1.

9.5.2 Epidemiology of CFRD

The prevalence of CFRD progressively increases with age, 20% of adolescents and 40–50 % of patients over the age of 30 are affected [3]. Women are diagnosed on average 5–7 years earlier than men; the reasons for this are not completely understood. Marshall et al. suggest that female hormones, a lack of anabolic male hormones and oral contraception are possible reasons [10]. Historically, mortality rates in CFRD were higher than in CF patients without diabetes, along with a higher rate of mortality in women with CFRD than men; one paper indicated that only 25% of patients with CFRD reached the age of 30 compared to 60% of CF patients without diabetes [3]. However, recent studies show a narrowing of these differences [3]. Mortality in CFRD is due to respiratory failure and not macrovascular complications. Incidence of CFRD increases with age, however, reports have been made in patients as young as 3 months [5].

9.5.3 Pathophysiology of CFRD

Understanding the pathogenesis of CFRD supports optimization of treatment and ensures appropriate management. The aetiology of CFRD is complex and not completely understood;

Advanced Nutrition and Dietetics in Diabetes, First Edition. Edited by Louise Goff and Pamela Dyson.
© 2016 John Wiley & Sons, Ltd. Published 2016 by John Wiley & Sons, Ltd.

Table 9.5.1 Characteristics of cystic fibrosis-related diabetes, type 1 and type 2 diabetes

	CFRD	Type 1 diabetes	Type 2 diabetes
Average age of onset (y)	+/- 20	<40	>40
Body weight	Thin/ malnourished	Average	Obese
Insulin secretion	Reduced	Absent	Reduced
Insulin sensitivity	Normal or reduced	N/A	Reduced
Autoimmune Aetiology	No	Yes	No
Ketoacidosis	Rare	Yes	No
Microvascular complications	Yes	Yes	Yes
Macrovascular complications	Unseen (survival in years with CFRD)	Yes	Yes
Treatment	Insulin	Insulin	Diet and lifestyle modifications/ oral hypoglycaemic agents and insulin.

it is likely a combination of insulin deficiency, varying insulin resistance and possibly has a genetic predisposition. Adler et al. showed that CFTR mutation classes, female gender, poor hepatic or pulmonary function, pancreatic insufficiency, and steroids increased the risk of developing CFRD [11].

CFRD mainly occurs in patients with more severe CFTR mutations and PI. Insulin deficiency is believed to be the primary cause of CFRD; however, insulin resistance also occurs in the CF patients without diabetes [1,8]. Insulin deficiency is due to the progressive fatty infiltration and fibrosis of the pancreatic tissue, which causes disruption and progressive destruction of the islet cell architecture leading to the loss of endocrine, beta, alpha and pancreatic polypeptide cells. Beta-cell loss and dysfunction is not related to autoimmune disease in CF, although there are a few reported cases of type 1 diabetes in CF [12]. Autopsy studies in CF patients with and without CFRD showed that the diabetes patients had a decreased number of Islets of Langerhans, with approximately 50% reduction in beta-cell mass and islet amyloidosis [5]. Insulin deficiency is severe in CFRD but not complete. Almost all CF patients with PI have some evidence of beta-cell dysfunction, whether they have diabetes or not. Fasting c-peptide and insulin levels are normal; however, there is a delay in peak insulin secretion, which becomes more noticeable as glucose tolerance worsens

and is caused by a loss of first phase insulin response, which is present in CF patients with normal glucose tolerance [13]. Impaired islet hormones include a loss of glucagon responses, thus reducing the likelihood of diabetic ketoacidosis (DKA) [13,14]. Insulin sensitivity in CF patients is variable. Clinically stable, patients with or without CFRD are insulin sensitive, however, as clinical status worsens insulin resistance occurs. Reduced lung function, infection, inflammation and corticosteroid therapy are linked to increased cytokine production and counter regulatory hormones, which cause insulin resistance [15].

All patients with severe CFTR mutations are pancreatic insufficient and need enzyme replacement therapy but only 50% develop diabetes; the reason for this is unclear. The less severe mutations are less likely to develop CFRD, possibly due to less likelihood of pancreatic dysfunction [16]. Laguna queries whether there are genetic factors related to the severity of CFTR mutation which may predispose a patient with CF to CFRD [5]. Research continues to look for a genetic link between types 1 and 2 diabetes and CFRD.

9.5.4 Screening

CFRD is usually insidious and asymptomatic. Studies showed weight loss, protein catabolism, deteriorating lung function and increased mortality

2–4 years prior to diagnosis of CFRD [7,16], and thus regular screening is warranted. Currently, an oral glucose tolerance test (OGTT) appears to be the most specific and sensitive tool for screening of CFRD; and should be performed annually in clinically stable patients over the age of 10 (US) and 12 (UK) [8,17].

Screening should be considered if weight loss, unexplained decline in lung function, or hyperglycaemic symptoms occurs. Monitoring of blood glucose concentrations is recommended during an infective exacerbation, gluocorticoid therapy and overnight enteral feeding. Screening in pregnancy is essential due to increased insulin resistance. An OGTT should be performed pre-conception, or when pregnancy is confirmed. CF patients are at increased risk of gestational diabetes and therefore OGTT should be completed at the end of the first and second trimester. Patients with gestational diabetes should have an OGTT 6–12 weeks post partum [17]. It is recommended that glycated haemoglobin (HbA1c), continuous glucose monitoring (CGM), fasting plasma glucose and self-monitoring of blood glucose are not used as screening tools [17–19]. Transplant patients often require insulin postoperatively and many require it long term. Screening should occur pre-operatively and close blood glucose monitoring post-operatively. CFRD prior to transplant must be managed aggressively due to the negative impact on survival, especially post procedure [17].

9.5.5 Diagnosis

CFRD is part of a continuum of glucose tolerance abnormalities, with only a few CF patients having completely normal glucose tolerance. Glucose metabolism is affected by unique features in CF; see Box 9.5.1, which may lead to fluctuations in glucose tolerance. Patients move along the glucose tolerance spectrum depending on their clinical status. Normal glucose tolerance patients may have impaired fasting glucose (IFG 5.6–6.9 mmol/l) and they may have increased levels midway through the OGTT categorized as indeterminate glucose tolerance

> **Box 9.5.1** Factors affecting glucose metabolism in cystic fibrosis
>
> - Respiratory infection
> - Inflammation
> - Malnutrition
> - Increased energy expenditure
> - Glucagon deficiency
> - Malabsorption/maldigestion
> - Delayed gastric emptying
> - Slow transit time
> - Liver disease

(INDET), however, the clinical significance of these is unknown. Ode et al. have shown that impaired glucose tolerance (IGT) and INDET are associated with an increased risk of CFRD in children [20]. The spectrum of glucose tolerance abnormalities as per OGTT is seen in Table 9.5.2.

Clinical care guidelines have provided diagnostic criteria for different conditions.

In clinically stable patients, criteria for CFRD can be made using standard American Diabetes Association (ADA) diagnostic criteria or Diabetes UK recommendations (i.e. WHO classification) [8,21]. The tests should be repeated on 2 separate occasions to eliminate error. An HbA1c of ≥48 mmol/mol (6.5%) and fasting plasma glucose >7 mmol/l can be used as confirmatory tests together with the positive OGTT. However, HbA1c is spuriously low in CF, therefore levels < 48 mmol/mol (6.5%) should not exclude CFRD. CFRD is diagnosed in the presence of a random glucose ≥11.1 mmol/l inclusive of hyperglycaemic symptoms (polydipsia and polyuria).

Patients may be diagnosed during an acute illness, continuous enteral feeding and pregnancy where the beta-cell stress is heightened. It is recommended that blood glucose monitoring occurs during the first 48 hours of an exacerbation or steroid use. If fasting hyperglycaemia (≥7 mmol/l) or recurrent post prandial hyperglycaemia (≥11.1 mmol/l) occurs in a previously NGT patient, CFRD is diagnosed and insulin should be commenced. This status can be intermittent and may resolve within 2 days to 6 weeks by which time insulin treatment may be discontinued [17,21].

Table 9.5.2 Classification of glucose tolerance abnormalities in cystic fibrosis

Glucose tolerance	Fasting plasma glucose mmol/l	2 hour OGTT glucose mmol/l
Normal glucose tolerance (NGT)	<7.0	<7.8
Impaired glucose tolerance (IGT)	<7.0	>7.9–11.1
Indeterminate glucose tolerance (INDET)	<7.0 Mid OGTT >11.1 mmol	<7.8
CFRD FH- [a]	<7.0	≥11.1
CFRD FH + [a]	≥7.0	≥11.1
Impaired fasting glucose (IFG)	5.6–6.9	N/A

[a] These groups can now be regarded as similar Moran et al., 2010 [17].

There is controversy around the use of the OGTT as a diagnostic tool due to its sensitivity. Some studies have shown abnormal glucose tolerance between baseline and 2-hour post-glucose load levels using CGM and 30, 60 and 90 min blood levels. CGM is validated in CFRD and can detect abnormalities earlier than the OGTT but clinical significance needs to be ascertained and therefore it cannot be used as a diagnostic tool [22]. Early diagnosis and aggressive treatment have recently been associated with a decline in mortality rates in CFRD [3].

9.5.6 Clinical consequences of CFRD

CFRD is associated with worsening clinical outcomes, poor nutritional status and decline in lung function, more frequent hospital admissions and a higher prevalence of liver disease, increased morbidity and mortality [3,7,10,16].

Acute clinical complications

Mild hypoglycaemia (ability to treat oneself, blood glucose concentrations <3.9 mmol/l) is common in CF, even in patients without diabetes [23]. Fasting hypoglycaemia reflects malnutrition or increased energy requirements due to inflammation and infection. Post-prandial hypoglycaemia (reactive hypoglycaemia) is thought to be due to dysfunctional endogenous insulin secretion, usually occurring before the development of IGT [23]. Severe hypoglycaemia (inability to treat oneself) may be less frequent in CFRD. Patients have a delayed glucagon response to hypoglycaemia, however, they do have a brief catecholamine response and normal hypoglycaemic awareness, unless altered by poor glycaemic control [24]. DKA is rare in CFRD due to endogenous insulin and impaired glucagon secretion, and if reported in a CF patient, assessment of T1 diabetes should be considered.

Chronic complications

Microvascular complications, such as retinopathy, nephropathy and neuropathy, do exist in CFRD and are related to the duration of CFRD and poor glycaemic control, as in diabetes generally [25,26]. Microvascular complications are apparent 5 years post diagnosis and therefore retinal screening, albumin/creatinine ratio and a full neurological assessment are recommended annually. Currently there is no evidence of macrovascular complications in CFRD patients [26]. However, this does not exclude macrovascular complications occurring as age of survival and duration of CFRD increases. Annual monitoring of blood pressure and lipid profile is suggested in CFRD patients, although they are less likely to have an abnormal lipid profile [27].

9.5.7 Management of CFRD

A collaborative multidisciplinary approach between CF specialists and a diabetes team that is familiar with CFRD and its unique features is advised [8,17]. Successful diabetes management is facilitated by excellent communication between the teams and the patient, along with self-management tools and dietary and treatment education. It is noted that the additional diagnosis of CFRD is a significant burden on the CF patients, which needs to be managed by the MDT. Quarterly joint CFRD clinics are advised [8]. Optimal glycaemic control is essential, as it has been shown that insulin intervention and optimizing glycaemic control improves nutritional status and pulmonary function, and reduces mortality [28].

Medical management

CFRD is primarily due to insulin insufficiency and, therefore, insulin is the only form of treatment that is recommended. A few studies, discussed in a review article by Laguna, have compared the use of oral hypoglycaemic agents, showing that they are less effective at improving nutritional status and HbA1c outcomes [5] Concerns were raised about gastrointestinal side-effects, and fatal lactic acidosis in hypoxic patients, associated with metformin. Sulfonylureas are known to bind and inhibit CFTR and therefore are not appropriate in CF [28,29]. Insulin treatment in CFRD patients with and without fasting hyperglycaemia (CFRD FH+) (CFRD FH-) showed improved clinical status and a reduced number of exacerbations. Moran et al. report a reversal in weight loss when patients with CFRD FH- were treated with insulin thus suggesting no difference between the two groups [28].

Varying insulin regimens are used in the treatment of CFRD but there is limited evidence to recommend one regimen over another. Individualized treatment plans based on clinical judgement should be provided. A basal bolus regimen or multiple injections of rapid acting insulin matched to carbohydrate intake are most frequently recommended, due to flexibility. It is important to remember that CFRD patients have some endogenous insulin available and therefore may need lower doses of basal insulin than patients with type 1 diabetes. Alternatively, a positive impact has been seen with the use of insulin pumps [30]. Twice daily isophane insulin with or without rapid-acting insulin is an alternative which is often used in adolescents. However, this may be problematic in patients with nausea or anorexia. In acute illness or glucocorticosteroid use, where there is an increased insulin resistance, insulin requirements can increase 2–4-fold and may take up to 4–6 weeks to gradually reduce back to baseline levels. Treatment of IGT and INDET glucose abnormalities which do not meet the criteria of CFRD is not known and therefore close monitoring is suggested.

Nutritional management

Optimizing nutritional status

The main treatment goal for CFRD patients is optimizing nutritional status which is associated with increased longevity [31]. Nutritional requirements in CF are well established but malnutrition is common due to numerous factors, including maldigestion/malabsorption, declining lung function, increased resting metabolic rate, anorexia and gastro-oesophageal reflux which leads to vomiting. CFRD profoundly affects nutritional status and weight, resulting in greater morbidity and mortality than that of non-diabetic CF patients [7]. CFRD-associated poor weight gain may be related to insulin deficiency, anabolic effects of insulin as a hormone and the effect of hyperglycaemia on protein catabolism [29,32]. Adequate calorie intake is required to achieve and maintain an optimal BMI, which is critical to health and survival; therefore no dietary restrictions are recommended. A high fat, high energy, high salt diet is advised. However, as CF survival increases, it may be that we need to review and alter these recommendations. See Table 9.5.3 for the differences in nutritional advice between type1 and type 2 diabetes and CFRD. All patients should be provided with an individually tailored nutrition treatment plan.

Table 9.5.3 Nutritional management of cystic fibrosis-related diabetes, type 1 and type 2 diabetes [34]

	CFRD	Type 1 diabetes	Type 2 diabetes
Energy	120–150% RDA for age	100% RDA/restriction for weight loss	100% RDA/restriction for weight loss
Advice	Weight gain	Weight maintenance/ weight loss	Weight loss/ weight maintenance
Fat	40%	30–35%	30–35%
Refined sugar	Nil restriction	10% TE	10% TE
Carbohydrate	45–50%	Flexible	Flexible
Fibre	Encouraged, without compromising high energy intake	Encouraged	Encouraged
Protein	20%	10–15%	10–15%
Salt	Increased	Restricted <6 g/day	Restricted <6 g/day
	High energy, high fat, high salt	Flexible, according to lifestyle	Low fat, healthy, well-balanced meals

Optimizing glycaemic control is imperative to reduce the risk of long-term complications along with normalizing metabolism and optimizing nutritional status.

Optimal body mass index (BMI) goals are recommended, as per the CFF guidelines: BMI centile of ≥ 50th in 2–20 years age group, BMI ≥ 22 in adult CF females and BMI ≥ 23 in adult CF males is recommended to achieve optimal lung function and longevity [33].

Nutrition support in CFRD

Oral nutritional supplements and/or overnight enteral feeding are often necessary to meet the CF patient's high nutritional requirements. Close monitoring of blood glucose levels before, during and after-feeds is needed to provide an optimal insulin regimen and glycaemic control.

Carbohydrate counting

Carbohydrate counting and insulin dose adjustment enables patients to maintain their CF diet and manage their diabetes optimally. Whilst considered the most flexible approach to CFRD treatment, it does involve multiple injections, which may be difficult for some patients to manage. Insulin pumps can also be advised and have been shown to improve outcomes in CFRD [30].

Insulin doses are prescribed by the doctors and are matched to either 15 g carbohydrate in the US or 10 g carbohydrate in the UK, a recommendation of 0.5–2 units of insulin to 15 g carbohydrate [33]. Twice daily isophane insulin regimens are managed by encouraging patients to consume similar amounts of carbohydrate at each meal and spread intake throughout the day. Education tools and support are vital for CFRD patients and therefore regular dietetic input along with support from the diabetes specialist nurses with CFRD knowledge is advised.

Exercise

Exercise is recommended in all CF patients. CFRD patients are advised to monitor blood glucose levels pre- and post-exercise and to keep high glycaemic index carbohydrate with them. The insulin regimen may need to be altered depending on the intensity, type and duration of the exercise.

Alcohol in CFRD

Patients are advised to discuss alcohol intake with the CF team due to possible drug interactions. They are advised to adhere to guidelines for alcohol consumption and drink sensibly. However, education on the hypoglycaemic effects of alcohol must be provided and patients are advised to consume alcohol with meals and to monitor blood glucose levels regularly [8].

Pregnancy in CFRD/gestational diabetes

Pregnancy has become a more common occurrence in CF and is safe if planned and monitored closely by the CF specialist team. Adequate weight gain is very important for optimal outcomes. Strict blood glucose goals are set for CFRD patients as they are for the general diabetes population in pregnancy, and therefore aggressive treatment is maintained. Gestational diabetes has been shown to have a high incidence in CF, due to the association with insulin deficiency [35]. No calorie restrictions are recommended in CFRD pregnancy to ensure weight gain.

Treatment goals

Glycaemic goals are the same as for the general diabetes population according to ADA, Diabetes UK and WHO guidance [8, 22]. These are based on the need to reduce the risk of microvascular complications. However, due to the negative impact of CFRD on clinical outcomes it may be that more stringent goals need to be followed in CFRD. Currently there is no evidence to support this [18].

Recommendations

Achieve optimal glycaemic control, blood glucose target levels as per general diabetes targets. Self-monitoring of blood glucose at home is essential to achieve optimal glycaemic control and should be done at least 3 times daily.

HbA1c target recommendation is ≤ 53 mmol/ mol (7%) due to microvascular complications occurring in patients with HbA1c of 53 mmol/ mol (7%) [25].

9.5.8 Conclusion

As survival increases due to advances in therapies, so the prevalence of CFRD and glucose tolerance abnormalities will increase. CFRD is mainly caused by insulin deficiency with varying insulin

resistance, along with possible genetic links. CFRD is a distinct clinical entity which shares features with type 1 and type 2 diabetes. Annual OGTT over the age of 10 is recommended, and if CFRD is diagnosed early intervention is advised. Insulin is the only treatment for CFRD. The overall management goal for CFRD is to improve and maintain optimal clinical status, optimize glycaemic control and limit the risk of microvascular complications. Early detection, diagnosis and treatment is advised, due to increased morbidity and mortality associated with CFRD.

9.5.9 Unanswered questions

- Should target goals for glucose and HbA1c in CFRD be lower than those recommended by the ADA?
- Would CF patients with abnormal glucose tolerance benefit from insulin and, if so, what method of treatment would provide the greatest impact on clinical status?

Key points

- CFRD is the most common comorbidity in cystic fibrosis, affecting approximately 40–50% over the age of 30 years.
- CFRD is associated with worsening clinical outcomes, poor nutritional status and increased morbidity and mortality.
- A multi disciplinary approach is recommended for management.
- Malnutrition is common, and an energy dense diet is recommended, supplemented with enteral feeding if necessary.
- Insulin is the medical treatment for CFRD, although there is no evidence for the most effective regime.

References

1. Moran A, Hardin D, Rodman D, Allen HF, Beall RJ, Borowitz D, et al. Diagnosis screening and management of cystic fibrosis related diabetes: a consensus conference report. *Diabetes Res Clin Pract* 1999; **45**: 61–73.

2. Elborn JS, Shale DJ, Britton JR. Cystic Fibrosis: current survival and population estimates to year 2000. *Thorax* 1991; **46**: 881–885.

3. Moran A, Dunitz J, Nathan B, Saeed A, Holme B, Thomas W. Cystic fibrosis-related diabetes: current trends in prevalence, incidence, and mortality. *Diabetes Care* 2009; **32**:1626–1631.

4. UK CF Registry. Annual Data Report 2009. Bromley, UK: Cystic Fibrosis Trust, 2011.

5. Laguna TA, Nathan BM, Moran A. Managing diabetes in cystic fibrosis: review article. *J Diab Obes Metabol* 2010; **12**: 858–864.

6. Rosenecker J, Eichler I, Kuhn L, Harms HK, von der Hardt J. Genetic determination of diabetes mellitus in patients with cystic fibrosis. *J Pediatr* 1995; **127**: 441–443.

7. Finkelstein SM, Wielinski CL, Elliott GR, Warwick WJ, Barbosa J, Wu SC, et al. Diabetes mellitus associated with cystic fibrosis. *J Pediatr.* 1988; **112**: 373–377.

8. UK Cystic Fibrosis Trust Working Group. Management of cystic fibrosis related diabetes mellitus 2004. Bromley, UK: Cystic Fibrosis Trust, 2004.

9. Milla CE, Billings J, Moran A. Diabetes is associated with dramatically decreased survival in female but not male subjects with cystic fibrosis. *Diabetes Care* 2005; **28**: 2141–2144.

10. Marshall BC, Butler SM, Stoddard M, Moran AM, Liou TG, Morgan WJ. Epidemiology of cystic fibrosis-related diabetes. *J Pediatr* 2005; **146**: 681–687.

11. Adler AI, Shine BSF, Chamnan P, Haworth CS, Bilton D. Genetic determinants and epidemiology of cystic fibrosis-related diabetes: Results from a British cohort of children and adults. *Diabetes Care* 2008; **31**: 1789–1794.

12. O' Riordan SMP, Robinson PD, Donaghue KC, Moran A. Management of cystic fibrosis-related diabetes. *Pediatr Diabetes* 2008; **9**(1): 338–344.

13. Moran A, Diem P, Klein DJ, Levitt MD, Robertson RP. Pancreatic endocrine function in cystic fibrosis. *J Pediatr* 1991; **118**: 715–723.

14. Lanng S, Thorsteinsson B, Roder ME, Orskov C, Holst J, Nerup J, et al. Pancreas and gut hormone responses to oral glucose and intravenous glucagon in cystic fibrosis patients with normal, impaired, and diabetic glucose tolerance. *Acta Endocrinol* 1993; **128**: 207–214.

15. Hardin DS, LeBlanc A, Lukenbough S, Seilheimer DK. Insulin resistance is associated with decreased clinical status in cystic fibrosis. *J Pediatr* 1997; **130**: 948–956.

16. Koch C, Cuppens H, Rainisio M, Maddessani U, Harms H, Hodson M, et al. European Epidemiologic Registry of Cystic Fibrosis (ERCF): comparison of major disease manifestations between patients with different classes of mutations. *Pediatr Pulmonol* 2001; **31**: 1–12.

17. Moran A, Brunzell C, Cohen RC, Katz M, Marshall BC, Onady G, et al. Clinical care guidelines for cystic fibrosis related diabetes: A position statement of the American Diabetes Association and a clinical practice guideline for the Cystic Fibrosis Foundation, endorsed by the Pediatric Endocrine Society. *Diabetes Care* 2010; **33**: 2697–2708.

18. Hardin DS, Moran A. Diabetes mellitus in cystic fibrosis. *Endocrinol Metab Clin North Am* 1999; **28**: 787–800.

19. Lanng S, Hansen A, Thorsteinsson B, Nerup J, Koch C. Glucose tolerance in cystic fibrosis: a five year prospective study. *BMJ* 1995; **311**: 655–659.

20. Ode KL, Frohnert B, Laguna T, Philips J, Holme B, Regelmann W, et al. Oral glucose tolerance testing in children with cystic fibrosis. *Pediatr Diabetes* 2010; **11**(7) : 487–492.

21. American Diabetes Association. Clinical Practice Recommendations – 2010. *Diabetes Care* 2010; **33**(Suppl. 1): S1–S100.

22. Lek N, Acerini CL. Cystic fibrosis related diabetes: Diagnostic and management challenges. *Curr Diabetes Rev* 2010; **6**: 9–16.

23. Battezzati A, Battezzati PM, Costantini D, Seia M, Zazzeron L, Russo MC, et al. Spontaneous hypoglycemia in patients with cystic fibrosis. *Eur J Endocrinol* 2007; **156**: 369–376.

24. Moran A, Diem P, Klein DJ, Levitt MD, Robertson RP. Pancreatic endocrine function in cystic fibrosis. *J Pediatr* 1991; **118**: 715–723.

25. Van den Berg JM, Morton AM, Kok SW, Pijl H, Conway SP, Heijerman HG. Microvascular complications in patients with cystic fibrosis related diabetes (CFRD). *J Cyst Fibros* 2008; **7**: 515–519.

26. Schwarzenberg SJ, Thomas W, Olsen TW, Grover T, Walk D, Milla C, et al. Microvascular complications in cystic fibrosis-related diabetes. *Diabetes Care* 2007; **30**(5): 1056–1061.

27. Figueroa V, Milla C, Parks EJ, Schwarzenberg SJ, Moran A. Abnormal lipid concentrations in cystic fibrosis. *Am J Clin Nutr* 2002; **75**: 1005–1011.

28. Moran A, Pekow P, Grover P, Zorn M, Slovis B, Pilewski J, et al. Insulin therapy to improve BMI in cystic fibrosis-related diabetes without fasting hyperglycaemia: Results of the cystic fibrosis-related diabetes therapy trial. *Diabetes Care* 2009; **32**: 1783–1788.

29. Moran A, Phillips J, Milla C. Insulin and glucose excursion following premeal insulin lispro or repaglinide in cystic fibrosis-related diabetes. *Diabetes Care* 2001; **24**(10): 1706–1710.

30. Hardin DS, Rice J, Rice M, Rosenblatt R. Use of the insulin pump in treat cystic fibrosis-related diabetes. *J Cyst Fibros* 2009; **8**(3): 174–178.

31. Corey M, McLaughlin FJ, Williams M, Levison H. A comparison of survival, growth and pulmonary function in patients with cystic fibrosis in Boston and Toronto. *J Clin Epidemiol* 1988; **41**: 583–591.

32. Moran A, Milla C, Ducret R, Nair KS. Protein metabolism in clinically stable adult cystic fibrosis patients with abnormal glucose tolerance. *Diabetes* 2001; **50**: 1336–1343.

33. Stallings VA, Stark LJ, Robinson KA, Feranchak AP, Quinton H. Clinical Practice Guidelines on Growth and Nutrition Subcommittee, Ad Hoc Working Group, for the Clinical Practice Guidelines on Growth and Nutrition Subcommittee. Evidence-based practice recommendations for nutrition-related management of children and adults with cystic fibrosis and pancreatic insufficiency: results of a systemic review. *J Am Diet Assoc* 2008; **108**: 832–839.

34. Brunzell C, Schwarzenberg SJ. CFRD and abnormal glucose tolerance: overview and medical nutrition therapy. *Diabetes Spectrum* 2002; **15**: 124–127.

35. Giljam M, Antoniou M, Shin J, Dupuis A, Corey M, Tullis DE. Pregnancy in cystic fibrosis. Fetal and maternal outcome. *Chest* 2000; **118**: 85–91.

Chapter 9.6

Diabetic gastroparesis

Pamela Dyson

University of Oxford, Oxford Centre for Diabetes, Endocrinology and Metabolism, Churchill Hospital, Oxford, UK

9.6.1 Introduction

Diabetic gastroparesis (DGP) is a well-established complication of diabetes and is defined as a clinical syndrome characterised by delayed gastric emptying in the absence of mechanical obstruction of the stomach, together with specific symptoms [1]. Stomach emptying is normally under the control of complex interactions between muscles and autonomic nerves (vagal and splenic) and DGP appears to be associated with a degree of central neuropathy causing vagal autonomic dysfunction. The symptoms of DGP are similar to those of idiopathic gastroparesis; early satiety, nausea, vomiting, abdominal bloating, upper abdominal pain, heartburn, gastro-oesophageal reflux (GORD), but also include diabetes-specific symptoms of erratic blood glucose control and post-prandial hypoglycaemia in those treated by insulin [2].

9.6.2 Prevalence

The true prevalence of DGP is unknown, with estimates ranging from 1% among those in the community with type 2 diabetes, to 50% in people with long-standing type 1 diabetes. Prevalence in community studies in the United States estimate that 5% of people with type 1 and 1% of people with type 2 diabetes have DGP [3]. Studies from tertiary centres in people with long-standing diabetes suggest higher rates, with reports of delayed gastric emptying in 30% of people with type 2 diabetes [4], and DGP prevalence rates of 30–50% in people with type 1 diabetes [5]. There is recent evidence of increasing prevalence, with reports of a three-fold increase over the past ten years, and indication of a gender difference, with women having a four-fold increased risk of gastroparesis [1].

9.6.3 Risk factors for DGP

The risk factors for DGP include those that are non-modifiable – female gender, age and duration of diabetes – and modifiable ones including erratic blood glucose control and use of pharmaceutical agents that delay gastric emptying (narcotic pain medication, calcium channel blockers, some antidepressants, aluminium-containing antacids and GLP-1 receptor agonists) [2]. Some have suggested that the presence of the so-called 'triopathy' of retinopathy, nephropathy and neuropathy indicate that DGP is also likely to be present.

9.6.4 Diagnosis

Diagnosis of DGP is made on the basis of symptomology together with an assessment of delay in gastric emptying. The gold standard

Advanced Nutrition and Dietetics in Diabetes, First Edition. Edited by Louise Goff and Pamela Dyson.
© 2016 John Wiley & Sons, Ltd. Published 2016 by John Wiley & Sons, Ltd.

Table 9.6.1 Grades of severity of gastroparesis

Grade	Severity	Retention at 4 hours (%)
1	Mild	11–20
2	Moderate	21–35
3	Severe	36–50
4	Very severe	>50

Source: Abell et al. [6].

for the assessment of gastric emptying is scintigraphy (gastric emptying scintigraphy, GES), where a standard radiolabelled meal is administered after an overnight fast, and images of the stomach are taken at 5–30 minute intervals over 4 hours [1]. General preparation for GES includes an overnight fast and cessation of all agents, including prokinetics and narcotics, that affect gastric emptying for 48 hours before the test. In addition, tobacco should be avoided for 12 hours before testing. There are additional preparations for people with diabetes and they include stopping GLP-1 receptor agonists for 48 hours before the test, reducing pre-test insulin dose by 50% and aiming for blood glucose levels of >11.1 mmol/l [6]. Blood glucose control is of importance in testing for the presence of gastroparesis, as hyperglycaemia delays stomach emptying and will directly affect the results.

Gastroparesis is diagnosed if more that 10% of the stomach contents are retained at 4 hours [6]. The severity of gastroparesis is graded from 1–4 depending on the amount of retention, see Table 9.6.1.

9.6.5 Effects of DGP

DGP has far-reaching effects on people with diabetes, including a negative effect on glycaemic control. Unpredictable duodenal food delivery increases the risk of post-prandial hypoglycaemia in those treated with insulin or insulin sectretagogues [7]. Historically, gastroparesis has been associated with an increase in both mortality and morbidity [8], although more recent evidence suggests that DGP is not associated

with increased mortality [9]. DGP increases the risk of phytobezoars leading to intestinal obstruction and has a negative impact on quality of life [10].

9.6.6 Treatment of DPG

There are a variety of options available for the treatment of DGP including:

Maintaining blood glucose levels as near to the normal range as possible
Avoiding pharmaceutical agents that delay gastric emptying, including GLP-1 agonist therapy
Dietary modification
Prokinetic therapy
Gastric pacing, also known as gastric electrical stimulation
Surgical treatment (partial or total gastrectomy)
Acupuncture.

These options are discussed fully in the first book in this series: *Advanced Nutrition and Dietetics in Gastroenterology* [21] and only diabetes-specific strategies are explored here.

9.6.7 Glycaemic control

The inter-relationship between blood glucose levels and gastric emptying is extremely complex and is only now being understood [11]. Post-prandial blood glucose levels both influence and are influenced by the rate of gastric emptying, highlighting the challenges of determining cause and effect, although evidence shows that blood glucose control is fundamental to successful management of DGP [12]. There is no evidence-base for guidelines for blood glucose management in DGP, although recommendations include frequent blood glucose testing to assess post-prandial fluctuations, transferring from oral medication to insulin therapy in those with type 2 diabetes, adopting a basal prandial insulin regime, taking smaller and more frequent insulin doses and taking short-acting insulin after meals in order to minimise post-prandial hypoglycaemia [13].

9.6.8 Dietary treatment

Dietary interventions are the first-line treatment for DGP [14] and are an effective sole therapy in mild to moderate cases. Dietary advice is based on consensus recommendations [1,2,5,13] and can be summarised as follows:

Small, regular meals
Food should be chewed well before swallowing
Liquid intake should be increased, and liquid-based meals may be necessary
Carbonated drinks, high fat foods, high fibre foods and alcohol should be avoided.

Small, regular meals are recommended as large amounts of food delay gastric emptying and exacerbate GORD [15]. In people treated with insulin, doses of short-acting insulin should be matched to food intake, resulting in more frequent injections, and insulin doses may need to be delayed until after eating [13]. The consistency of meals may need manipulation as large food particles delay gastric emptying [16] and liquid-based meals may be necessary, as gastric emptying of liquids is frequently maintained where there is a delay for solid foods [17]. In practice, this translates to advice to the patient to chew foods thoroughly before swallowing, increasing the liquid component of a meal and, in moderate to severe cases, a soft or liquidised diet may be instigated.

A low fat, low dietary fibre diet is recommended for people with DGP as both fat and fibre delay gastric emptying [2]. Alcohol is also contraindicated [18], as are carbonated drinks as they may promote gastric distension [19].

In mild and moderate cases of DGP, maintaining good oral intake is the goal, but in more advanced cases of DGP, nutrition may be compromised and deficiencies in energy, vitamins and minerals are common [20]. In patients who are unable to maintain adequate nutrition through oral intake, enteral or, in extreme cases, parenteral nutrition may be required [2]. It is recommended that enteral feeding by-passes the stomach, and jejunal feeding has been shown to improve nutritional status and relieve symptoms in people with gastroparesis [2].

In summary, DGP is a widely over-looked complication of diabetes that is more common in women, those who have had diabetes for more than 10 years and who have evidence of other complications. DGP causes erratic blood glucose control and post-prandial hypoglycaemia and, although there is no cure, it can be managed by a combination of diet and medication.

Key points

- Diabetic gastroparesis (DGP) is a complication of diabetes.
- The true prevalence is unknown, with estimates ranging from 1–50%.
- Diagnosis is made by means of symptomology and assessment of gastric emptying.
- DGP can cause erratic blood glucose control and post-prandial hypoglycaemia.
- Medical management includes prokinetic agents, gastric pacing or surgery.
- Dietary management is based on consensus recommendations.

References

1. Camilleri M, Parkman HP, Shafi MA, Abell TL, Gerson L. Clinical guideline: management of gastroparesis. *Am J Gastroenterol* 2013; **108**(1): 18–37.
2. Camilleri M, Bharucha AE, Farrugia G. Epidemiology, mechanisms, and management of diabetic gastroparesis. *Clin Gastroenterol Hepatol* 2011; **9**(1): 5–12.
3. Choung RS, Locke GR 3rd, Schleck CD, Zinsmeister AR, Melton LJ 3rd, Talley NJ. Risk of gastroparesis in subjects with type 1 and 2 diabetes in the general population. *Am J Gastroenterol* 2012; **107**(1): 82–88.
4. Horowitz M, Harding PE, Maddox AF, Wishart JM, Akkermans LM, Chatterton BE, et al. Gastric and oesophageal emptying in patients with type 2 (non-insulin-dependent) diabetes mellitus. *Diabetologia* 1989; **32**(3): 151–159.
5. Parkman HP, Fass R, Foxx-Orenstein AE. Treatment of patients with diabetic gastroparesis. *Gastroenterol Hepatol (N Y)* 2010; **6**(6): 1–16.
6. Abell TL, Camilleri M, Donohoe K, Hasler WL, Lin HC, Maurer AH, et al. American Neurogastroenterology and Motility Society and the Society of Nuclear Medicine. Consensus recommendations for gastric emptying

scintigraphy: a joint report of the American Neurogastroenterology and Motility Society and the Society of Nuclear Medicine. *Am J Gastroenterol* 2008; **103**(3): 753–763.

7. Lysy J, Israeli E, Strauss-Liviatan N, Goldin E. Relationships between hypoglycaemia and gastric emptying abnormalities in insulin-treated diabetic patients. *J Neurogastroenterol Motil* 2006; **18**(6): 433–440.

8. Jung HK. The incidence, prevalence, and survival of gastroparesis in olmsted county, Minnesota, 1996–2006. *J Neurogastroenterol Motil* 2010; **16**(1): 99–100.

9. Chang J, Rayner CK, Jones KL, Horowitz M. Prognosis of diabetic gastroparesis - a 25-year evaluation. *Diabet Med* 2013; **30**(5): e185–8.

10. Talley NJ, Bytzer P, Hammer J, Young L, Jones M, Horowitz M. Psychological distress is linked to gastrointestinal symptoms in diabetes mellitus. *Am J Gastroenterol* 2001; **96**: 1033–1038.

11. Chang J, Rayner CK, Jones KL, Horowitz M. Diabetic gastroparesis-backwards and forwards. *J Gastroenterol Hepatol* 2011; **26**(Suppl. 1): 46–57.

12. Chang J, Rayner CK, Jones KL, Horowitz M. Diabetic gastroparesis and its impact on glycemia. *Endocrinol Metab Clin North Am* 2010; **39**(4): 745–762.

13. Sadiya A. Nutritional therapy for the management of diabetic gastropareis: a clinical review. *Diabetes Metab Syndr Obes* 2012; **5**: 329–335.

14. Vanormelingen C, Tack J, Andrews CN. Diabetic gastroparesis. *Br Med Bull* 2013; **105**: 213–230.

15. Camilleri M. Integrated upper gastrointestinal response to food intake. *Gastroenterology* 2006; **131**: 640–658.

16. Olausson EA, Alpsten M, Larsson A, Mattsson H, Andersson H, Attvall S. Particle size of a solid meal increases gastric emptying and late postprandial glycaemic response in diabetic subjects with gastroparesis. *Diabetes Res Clin Pract* 2008; **80**: 231–237.

17. Abell TL, Bernstein VK, Cutts T, Farrugia G, Forster J, Hasler WL, et al. Treatment of gastroparesis: a multidisciplinary clinical review. *Neurogastroenterol Motil* 2006; **18**: 263–283.

18. Bujanda L. The effects of alcohol consumption upon the gastrointestinal tract. *Am J Gastroenterol* 2000; **95**(12): 3374–3382.

19. Parkman HP, Hasler WL, Fisher RS; American Gastroenterological Association. American Gastroenterological Association technical review on the diagnosis and treatment of gastroparesis. *Gastroenterology* 2004; **127**(5): 1592–1622.

20. Parkman HP, Yates KP, Hasler WL, Nguyan L, Pasricha PJ, Snape WJ, et al; NIDDK Gastroparesis Clinical Research Consortium. Dietary intake and nutritional deficiencies in patients with diabetic or idiopathic gastroparesis. *Gastroenterology* 2011; **141**(2): 486–498.

21. Lomer M. (ed.) Advanced Nutrition and Dietetics in Gastroenterology, Oxford: Wiley-Blackwell, 2014.

Nutrition support in diabetes

Hilary McCoubrey
Birmingham Children's Hospital, Birmingham, UK

9.7.1 Introduction

People with diabetes make up a disproportionately high percentage of hospital inpatients in the United States (US) and the United
Kingdom (UK) [1,2]. This is unsurprising as
people with diabetes have an increased risk of
disorders such as coronary artery disease,
stroke, peripheral artery disease, chronic kidney disease, neuropathy, lower extremity
infection, ulceration and amputations. The
causes of emergency admissions in diabetes
patients include diabetic ketoacidosis (DKA),
hyperosmotic hyperglycaemic state (HHS) and
hypoglycaemia, however, the UK National
Diabetes Inpatient Audit (NaDIA) [3] report
suggests that the majority of admissions in
people with diabetes are not directly diabetes-
related and are for other medical or surgical reasons [3]. The NaDIA established that diabetes
patients have a longer length of hospital stay than
other patients, an average of 8 nights compared
with 5 nights for all patients. Hyperglycaemia is
associated with an increased risk of adverse
clinical outcomes, for example delayed surgical
healing and healing of foot ulcers and pressure
sores [4]. Furthermore, patients with unstable blood
glucose levels are likely to experience delayed
discharges as it takes time to ensure safety at
home in this potentially vulnerable population.

Dietetic management is an essential component of inpatient blood glucose management and in the coordination of appropriate
insulin therapy [5–7]. Nutritional needs often
differ in the hospital setting and are affected
by hospital routines, such as investigations
and procedures and strict meal delivery times,
which can make optimising glucose management challenging [4]; this chapter explores
the role of the dietitian in providing advice
about food or artificial feeding during the
inpatient stay and the impact of this on glycaemic management.

It is well established that inadequate intake
of energy and protein in hospital patients
results in slower recovery rates, increased
length of admission and increased rates of
readmission, morbidity and mortality [8]. In
addition, it has been shown that optimising
blood glucose concentrations can speed up
recovery times in hospitalised patients [9].
Appropriate and adequate nutrition is, therefore, vitally important for diabetes patients
receiving any kind of nutrition support.

In the UK, national initiatives such as 'Think
Glucose' have highlighted the importance of
improving the management of patients with diabetes, and offer a structured programme with
resources to improve the hospital experience and
quality of care for these patients [10].

9.7.2 Standards of care

Blood glucose targets

There is controversy surrounding optimal blood
glucose targets. The Leuvan study [11] cited in the
ESPEN guidelines [12] reported that maintaining

blood glucose concentrations below 6.7 mmol/l (110 mg/dl) in patients with diabetes reduced hospital mortality by 34%. However, a review of the evidence by Sawin et al. [9] suggests that hospitalised patients do not benefit from very tight blood glucose control and that levels should be maintained only at random levels of less than 10 mmol/l (180 mg/dl). The Joint British Diabetes Society (JBDS) guidelines state that evidence for target ranges is weak but the expert opinion of the authors is that blood glucose concentrations should be kept above 6 mmol/l and below 12 mmol/l during enteral nutrition in stroke patients with diabetes [13]. The NaDIA defined acceptable control as blood glucose concentrations above 4 mmol/l but below 11 mmol/l [3]. A Cochrane review of glycaemic control for prevention of surgical site infections recommended blood glucose concentrations below 11 mmol/l (<200 mg/dL), concluding that there was insufficient evidence for strict glycaemic control when compared with conventional management [14]. Although there is no consensus on exact targets, it is agreed that a strategy to avoid extremely high or low blood glucose concentrations is important, and blood glucose targets should be individualised.

Dietetic review

The aims of inpatient dietetic care for patients with diabetes are to optimise glycaemic control, provide adequate nutrition to meet needs, address individual needs and preferences, and provide a discharge plan for ongoing care [15–17]. Individualised dietetic care, alongside intensive medical management, is usually required for patients with diabetes to achieve optimal blood glucose control [18]. 69% of diabetes patients interviewed in the latest NaDIA had not been seen by a member of the diabetes team [3]. A draft report by the Diabetes Management and Education Group (DMEG) of the British Dietetic Association recommended that diabetes patients who are enterally fed, or who have gastroparesis, should be seen within 48 hours of admission by a diabetes specialist dietitian [19]. The recommendation by Diabetes UK is that there be four dietitians specialising in diabetes for every 250 000

members of the population [20], but unfortunately this is not always the case in UK hospitals and diabetes services concentrate heavily on outpatients, where longer-term education and goals to improve glycaemic control are agreed. This usually means that diabetes healthcare professionals have the opportunity to form relationships with people with diabetes, and visiting them during a hospital admission may provide reassurance for patients and improve continuity of care.

Treatment changes

Infection and physical trauma, including burns, surgery or stroke, initiate a stress response and an increase in the production of pro-inflammatory cytokines and counter-regulatory hormones, which raise blood glucose concentrations by increasing glucose production and decreasing glucose uptake [21]. The introduction of new medications, such as corticosteroids (which inhibit glucose uptake and thus significantly affect post-prandial glycaemia), also increases blood glucose concentrations in a hospital setting [9]. This is often frustrating for patients who usually have good glycaemic control and they are likely to need more frequent monitoring and advice about dietary and medication changes. The dietitian needs to have a good understanding of the mechanisms by which diabetes medications work in order to advise patients on relevant food changes that complement revised drug regimes.

In patients with gastroparesis, dietitians may need to incorporate advice on delaying insulin injections in line with reduced gastric emptying. Reduced fat and fibre content of meals may be relevant in some patients to reduce symptoms, however, it may be more appropriate, in patients who are under-nourished, to maximise the use of regular prokinetic medications and relax food restrictions to ensure adequate energy and protein intake [22]. It is important to check renal function in hospitalised diabetes patients and note decreases in medications as a result of decreasing eGFR and enhanced circulation of oral agents and insulin. It is also worth noting that raised blood glucose concentrations may also be responsible for raised serum potassium levels in renal patients and dietary advice to limit potassium intake should be given cautiously to prevent an excessively restricted diet once glycaemia is normalised.

The American Association of Clinical Endocrinologists (AACE) guidelines for optimal glucose goals in hospitalised patients [23] recommend a consistent carbohydrate intake for patients, which would need liaison with catering services and information provision to patients on the carbohydrate content of meals and snacks. This should always be available at ward level but is frequently an underutilised resource.

9.7.3 Oral nutrition support

The hospital meal service

There is no consensus on a diabetes meal plan that is ideal for hospitalised patients. Bantle et al. suggested that a consistent carbohydrate load in which the daily carbohydrate content of the main meals and snacks is kept consistent may be beneficial, however, there is a lack of controlled trial evidence to demonstrate clinical benefit of such an approach [6, 24].

The NaDIA was designed to look at a number of questions, including how patients rated their stay in hospital in various areas, such as the provision of meals and snacks [3]. 27 and 23%, respectively, reported that choice and timing of meals were only sometimes or rarely suitable. Those reporting poor meal timing or choice were more likely to have had a severe hypoglycaemic episode during admission.

Food choices and flexibility for hospitalised patients are frequently limited because food preparation is often off-site, with 34% of hospitals buying in ready-made meals in the UK [24]. Current meal provision planning usually aims to ensure adequate energy through a combination of main meal, dessert and, frequently, sweet snacks such as biscuits and cakes. Food choices will not necessarily match advice given in an outpatient setting, where the bulk of dietary education takes place. Increased energy requirements relating to illness, in addition to frequent taste preferences for sweet foods (e.g. in uraemic patients), mean that there is a reliance on desserts and sweet

snacks for energy provision. Readily available fats such as butter and cream are very useful for fortification. Diabetes patients should not be denied foods that many would not think of as suitable if they were well. Working with the multidisciplinary team (MDT) and the patient to re-educate on dietary recommendations in an inpatient setting is crucial to ensure food choices are not restricted and that medication changes are made when necessary to accommodate (sometimes limited) hospital food choices.

Complaints about meal choice and timings are among the most common patient concerns but have not, as yet, been addressed in most hospitals. The Diabetes Inpatient Treatment Satisfaction (DIPSat) study also investigated this area, and although their findings were similar, they did not gather any qualitative information useful for shaping change in hospital food provision [25]. Further research in this area is needed.

Oral nutritional supplements

The majority of oral nutritional supplements (ONS) contain carbohydrate in varying forms and quantities, which is fairly rapidly absorbed since it is in liquid form. Drinks that are higher in protein or fibre, in theory, should increase blood glucose levels more gradually. There are not, however, any readily available data about the glycaemic index (GI) of ONS. In order to minimise impact on appetite for meals, ONS are usually prescribed between meals, potentially resulting in extended periods when blood glucose concentrations maybe elevated. Low carbohydrate ONS drinks are available, although not globally, and provide carbohydrate in the form of isomaltulose, which has a lower GI than other carbohydrates used in ONS. Additionally, there are various fat and fat and protein-only supplements available in liquid and powder forms, which can be prescribed in combination with a multivitamin and mineral tablet to reduce the intake of carbohydrates.

Many of the neutral flavour ONS contain hydrolysed starch, which is likely to have the same impact on raising blood glucose concentrations as the sugars in some of the flavoured supplements, which needs to be considered when prescribing.

It is generally accepted that carbohydrate is absorbed more slowly when it is accompanied by fibre, protein and fat, due to delayed gastric emptying [26]. Those ONS with particularly high total carbohydrate content but low fibre, protein and fat, such as some of the juice-based drinks will probably have the greatest impact on glycaemia and should ideally be used in diabetes patients only as a last resort, or as suitable treatment for hypoglycaemia. If milk-based ONS are disliked, they may be advised for consumption in medicinal doses or fat and fat/protein supplements may be prescribed to add to food or again to be taken in medicinal 'shot' form.

9.7.4 Enteral nutrition

Exclusive enteral nutrition induces a more pronounced insulin and glucose response than solid, oral nutrition. It is important to consider, therefore, whether the type of formulas used in enteral nutrition plays a part in managing glycaemia in diabetes patients. The guidelines considered below investigated the effect of specialist enteral formulas on blood glucose control.

Specialist enteral formulas

ESPEN guidelines have reviewed the evidence for the use of different enteral formulas in diabetes [12]. Traditionally, formulas used in diabetes have been rich in complex carbohydrate (55–60%) with low lipid content (30%), whilst newer formulas have replaced some of the carbohydrate with monounsaturated fatty acids (MUFAs), and may include dietary fibre [27, 28]. Although there is no consensus on the most relevant markers to measure, studies of high MUFA formulas report lower mean fasting and/or post-prandial glucose levels and trends towards lower HbA1c or fructosamine and lower insulin requirements [29–34]. Some studies have also shown improved lipid profiles on

such formulae [29, 31]. Further reported benefits include a trend towards fewer pressure ulcers and infections [30] and reduced length of hospital stay compared with higher carbohydrate formulas [32]. These formulas may be of more importance outside the intensive care setting where less stringent monitoring is carried out. Whilst there is a general acceptance of the benefits of these specialised formulas [27, 35] ESPEN concludes that more evidence demonstrating clinical outcome benefits is needed, particularly to justify the additional expenditure on specialised formulas [12].

The JBDS report for inpatient care of stroke patients with diabetes was published in 2012 [13]. Athough diabetes patients are at increased risk of stroke and myocardial infarction and also have increased risk of death or poor functional recovery with hyperglycaemia [36, 37], the report does not consider there to be sufficient evidence or clinical experience in the UK to recommend the use of diabetes-specific enteral formulas. The use of standard enteral formulas is advised [37].

A US review in 2005 suggests that enteral formulae with reduced carbohydrate and modified fat content have been shown to result in lower blood glucose concentrations and should be used, if possible, in hyperglycaemic patients, but persistent hyperglycaemia should be treated with scheduled insulin doses [35].

Fluid requirements

Dehydration is a common complication in enteral nutrition and is an often-overlooked cause of hyperglycaemia. The risk of dehydration should be routinely checked and either highlighted to nursing staff, patient and family to encourage increased oral fluids or changes made to flushes on the enteral regimen.

The role of the dietitian in a multi-disciplinary approach

The JBDS report [13] makes a wide range of recommendations, many of which are aimed at nursing care, for the management of this patient group. It is an important reference document outlining the roles and responsibilities of the MDT in ensuring that standards of care are being met at ward level during enteral nutrition. Blood glucose monitoring, for example, should take place every 4–6 hours during feeding or hourly if feeding is unexpectedly switched off. Dietetic reviews represent an ideal opportunity to monitor these standards.

This report highlights the risk of hypoglycaemia if insulin has been administered and feeding stopped and recommends intravenous (IV) glucose substitute feed, if there is no alternative to stopping enteral nutrition. Treatment of hypoglycaemia in patients with impaired swallow involves administration of glucose-based liquids via the feeding tube or glucogel and a water flush, to provide 15–20 g of rapidly absorbed carbohydrate followed by 15–20 g of carbohydrate from the enteral formula.

The overall recommendation to dietitians starting enteral nutrition in diabetes patients is to:

- Be clear on the dietetic rationale for the enteral regime and rest periods proposed and assess the amount of carbohydrate provided per hour.
- Involve the diabetes specialist team before starting any enteral regime and subsequently if blood glucose concentrations are outside target levels. Provide rationale and information on the formula (as above), previous blood glucose monitoring, HbA1c and existing mediation/insulin regime and weight of patient.
- Advise the MDT on aspects of care such as hypo treatment and frequency of blood glucose monitoring in accordance with guidelines or refer to the diabetes specialist team as appropriate.

9.7.5 Medication changes

Dietitians should be aware of appropriate insulin and medication regimes suited to different feeding rates and timings. Factors to be considered when planning nutritional support include individual nutritional requirements, gut absorption, suitability and tolerance of night-time enteral nutrition and the need for breaks for procedures or other events. Metformin powder is highlighted in the JBDS guidelines as being suitable for nasogastric administration, whereas

other forms of oral medications in a crushed form are not recommended. Different insulin regimens are detailed with a biphasic regimen of mixed insulin being used with continuous feeding, or basal bolus insulin regimes with short-acting insulin given at 6 hourly intervals. It suggests that rapid-acting insulin be administered as part of a basal bolus regime, 20 minutes prior to administration of a bolus feed (due to the rapid digestion and absorption of enteral formulas). Some guidance on insulin to carbohydrate ratios is provided depending on insulin sensitivity levels and usual total daily doses.

The AACE guidelines recommend that oral agents be discontinued during acute illness and that glycaemia be managed with insulin only, partly due to the slow onset of action and dissipation of oral medications and partly due to unsuitability in a number of acutely unwell patient groups [38].

Principles recommended in these guidelines are very similar to those used in the DAFNE course (dose adjustment for normal eating), which is widely utilised in Europe and Australia for those with type I diabetes. It recommends glucose monitoring before meals and at bedtime and suggests the calculation of a sensitivity or correction factor. This can be calculated by the formula: 100/total daily dose of insulin and calculates the predicted mmol/l decrease in blood glucose concentration from administering one unit of insulin.

The guidelines make recommendations for those patients who are newly started on insulin and suggest that many patients will not need to continue with insulin post hospital discharge.

Basal bolus insulin regimens

A review by Umpierrez suggests that basal bolus insulin regimens (rapid-acting and background insulin) are superior to sliding scale regimens for patients on oral intake, in terms of numbers of patients reaching target blood glucose concentrations [39]. They are also generally preferred to IV insulin for patients who are consuming food orally or via enteral nutrition support, as it lessens the risk of hypoglycaemia. It has been recommended that basal bolus regimens based on

0.4–0.5 units of background insulin/kg/day, combined with rapid-acting insulin with meals may provide improved blood glucose control compared with a sliding scale approach [9].

In the NaDIA, insulin was reported to have been given at inappropriate times, with 6.7% of those patients on insulin prescribed or given insulin at the wrong time [3]. Dietitians are well placed to support the MDT in providing correct information about insulin administration with appropriate carbohydrate. Information about the type and quantity of carbohydrate in food should be available from hospital food services and nutritional data about ONS and enteral or parenteral nutrition are available from the manufacturers.

Variable rate intravenous insulin infusion – previously known as sliding scale

The protocol for using variable rate intravenous insulin infusion (VRIII) will vary between hospitals but is generally used perioperatively for patients on insulin and sometimes for those on oral medications. It is also used in patients who are unable to manage a normal diet and may occasionally be used in patients admitted with DKA or HHS for ongoing glycaemic control.

VRIII requires regular blood glucose monitoring and adjusting of insulin given intravenously via a dedicated cannula, usually together with a glucose infusion. Insulin doses are calculated based on patients' usual requirements or on guidelines based on units of insulin per kg (patient weight) and an hourly infusion rate is calculated, which is adjusted also according to blood glucose concentrations. Protocols that consider the rate of change of blood glucose in addition to current values are more effective than those that look at current values only [23].

Frequency of monitoring is usually 2–4 hourly. Discontinuation of VRII needs cautious management. There may be decreased requirements of basal insulin associated with reductions in illness or surgery-related stress, and increases in appetite and food intake will require increased rapid-acting insulin. Initially, IV insulin should be continued when basal bolus is re-started, to prevent ketoacidosis in patients with type 1 diabetes.

9.7.6 Total parenteral nutrition

Current guidelines do not make full recommendation for management of patients requiring total parenteral nutrition (TPN). It is known that patients receiving exclusive TPN have substantially higher insulin requirements to achieve the same blood glucose targets compared with those receiving enteral nutrition [40]. Nutrients enter the systemic circulation directly, thus bypassing the splanchnic circulation and the insulinotrophic effect of incretins. TPN commonly leads to hyperglycaemia, even in the absence of diabetes. 75% of patients with type 2 diabetes not previously treated with insulin will require insulin with TPN. In patients in intensive care units, strict glycaemic control is relatively easily achieved, probably because more frequent monitoring and adjustment of insulin takes place [40].

Studies have shown that TPN-associated hyperglycaemia is a risk factor for development of infection, cardiac, and renal dysfunction and increased mortality in critically ill and non-critically ill patients [41].

In TPN patients, blood glucose concentrations of over 10 mmol/l have been shown to be associated with an increased risk of pneumonia and acute renal failure. Pre-TPN blood glucose concentrations between 8.3 mmol/l and 10 mmol/l independently predicted mortality as well as a blood glucose>10 mmol/l within 24 hours of TPN when compared with normoglycaemia. It is hypothesised that immune function and inflammatory response may be the underlying mechanisms for this result. Any hyperglycaemia (>8.3 mmol/l) was an indicator of increased hospital stay and risk of complications [40].

The AACE guidelines recommend 0.1 units of insulin for every gram of carbohydrate administered, with daily increases of 80% of the previous day's correctional insulin. IV insulin can be used to correct hyperglycaemia more rapidly [23]. This is a typical approach that would be outlined in individual hospital guidelines on TPN. It has been considered that cyclical rather than continuous nutrition allows insulin concentrations to drop, helping to prevent further insulin resistance. In addition it may be possible to manipulate proportions of fat, protein and carbohydrate in TPN in order to reduce the impact on BG concentrations. Since there is some evidence that if fat provides more than 50% of the required energy it impacts on clearance by the reticuloendothelial system, it is usually restricted to 30% of total energy [42].

9.7.7 Discharge from hospital

DMEG have made recommendations regarding those patients who should be followed up by a dietitian post hospital discharge as a priority, including those with newly diagnosed type I, those started on insulin for the first time in hospital, and those with pancreatitis/pancreas surgery and hypoglycaemia linked to undernutrition. It also provides guidance on which patients should have routine follow up by dietitians and is a useful guide for General Practitioners, since many of these patients will not be routinely reviewed by ward dietitians and will not, therefore, always be referred into appropriate outpatient clinics.

9.7.8 Conclusion

Increasing numbers of diabetes inpatients across all hospital wards and specialities means that dietitians working in all areas need to have a good understanding of the guidelines for diabetes inpatients and how these apply to their particular patients' needs. They should liaise closely with their hospital's diabetes team to ensure the optimal glycaemic management while patients are in hospital, especially if they are receiving nutrition support during their stay. Optimising glycaemic management during the delivery of appropriate nutrition support is beneficial in terms of a wide range of patient outcomes.

References

1. Jiang HJ, Stryer D, Friedman B, Andrews R. Multiple hospitalisations for patients with diabetes. *Diabetes Care* 2003; **26**(5): 1421–1426.
2. Donnan PT, Leese GP, Morris AD. Hospitalisation for people with type 1 and type 2 diabetes compared with the nondiabetic population of Tayside, Scotland: a retrospective cohort study of resource use. *Diabetes Care* 2000; **23**(3): 1774–1779.
3. National Diabetes Audit 2010-2011 Report 1: Care Processes and Treatment Targets. Internet: http://www.hqip.org.uk/assets/NCAPOP-Library/NCAPOP-2012-13/Diabetes-Audit-Report-2010-11-Care-Process-and-Treatment-Targets-published-2012.pdf (accessed 29 June 2015).
4. Gosmanov AR, Umpierrez GE. Medical nutrition therapy in hospitalised patients with diabetes. *Curr Diab Rep* 2012; **12**(1): 93–100.
5. Ziegler TR. Parenteral nutrition in the critically ill patient. *N Engl J Med* 2009; **361**: 1088–1097.
6. Curll M, Dinardo M, Noschese M, Korytkowski MT. Menu selection, glycaemic control and satisfaction with standard and patient-controlled consistent carbohydrate menu plans in hospitalised patients with diabetes. *Qual Saf Health Care* 2010; **19**: 355–359.
7. Inzucchi SE. Clinical practice. Management of hyperglycaemia in the hospital setting. *N Engl J Med* 2006; **355**: 190311.
8. Stratton RJ, Green CJ, Elia M. *Disease-related Malnutrition: An evidence-based Approach to Treatment.* Wallingford, Oxon.: CAB International, 2003.
9. Sawin G, Shaughnessy AF. Glucose control in hospitalized patients. *Am Fam Physician* 2010; **81**(9): 1078–1080.
10. NHS Institution for Innovation and Improvement. Think Glucose (Improving care for people with diabetes). http://www.institute.nhs.uk/quality_and_value/think_glucose/issues_that_thinkglucose_addresses.html. Accessed Oct 2012.
11. Van den Berghe G, Wouters P, Weekers F, Verwaest C, Bruyninckx F, Schetz M, et al. Intensive insulin therapy in the critically ill patient. *N Engl J Med* 2001; **345**(19): 1359–1367.
12. Lochs H, Allison SP, Meier R, Pirlich M, Kondrup J, Schneider S, et al. Introductory to the ESPEN Guidelines on Enteral Nutrition: Terminology, Definitions and General Topics. *Clin Nutr* 2006; **25**: 180–186.
13. Joint British Diabetes Societies (JBDS) for inpatient care. NHS Diabetes. Glycaemic management during the inpatient enteral feeding of stroke patients with diabetes. June 2012.
14. Kao LS, Meeks D, Moyer VA, Lally KP. Cochrane Summary. Strict control compared with conventional glycaemic control for preventing surgical site infections in adults. *Cochrane Database Syst Rev* 2009 Jul 8; (3): CD006806. doi: 10.1002/14651858.CD006806.pub2.
15. American Diabetes Association. Standards of medical care in diabetes – 2011. *Diabetes Care* 2011; **34**(Suppl. 1): S11–S61.
16. Clement S, Braithwaite SS, Magee MF, Ahmann A, Smith EP, Schafer RG, et al. Management of diabetes and hyperglycaemia in hospitals. *Diabetes Care* 2004; **27**: 553–591.

17. Schafer RG, Bohannon B, Franz MJ, Freeman J, Holmes A, McLaughlin S, et al. Diabetes nutrition recommendations for health care institutions. *Diabetes Care* 2004; **27**(Suppl. 1): S55–S57.

18. Swift CS, Boucher JL. Nutrition therapy for the hospitalised patient with diabetes. *Endocr Pract* 2006; **12**(Suppl. 3): 61–67.

19. DMEG. Draft DMEG Position Statement. The Role of the Diabetes Specialist Dietitian (DSD) in Inpatient Diabetes Management. 2010 for the 2010 Dietitian Workforce Survey. March 2012. Internet: http://www.dmeg.org.uk/news.html (accessed Sept 2012).

20. Diabetes UK. Commissioning Specialist Diabetes Services for Adults with Diabetes. A Diabetes UK Task and Finish Group Report. October 2010. Internet: http://www.diabetes.org.uk/Professionals/Publications-reports-and-resources/Reports-statistics-and-case-studies/Reports/Commissioning-Specialist-Diabetes-Services-for-Adults-with-Diabetes---Defining-A-Specialist-Diabetes-UK-Task-and-Finish-Group-Report-October-2010 (accessed Oct 2012).

21. McDonnell ME, Umpierrez MD. Insulin therapy for the management of hyperglycaemia in hospitalised patients. *Endocrinol Metab Clin North Am* 2012; **41**(1): 175–201.

22. Camilleri M, Bharucha AE, Farrugia G. Epidemiology, mechanisms, and management of diabetic gastroparesis. *Clin Gastroenterol Hepatol* 2011; **9**(1): 5–12.

23. Magaji V, Johnston J. Inpatient management of hyperglycemia and diabetes. *Clin Diabetes* 2011; **29** (1): 4–9.

24. Bantle JP, Wylie-Rosett J, Albright AL, Apovian CM, Clark NG, Franz MJ, et al. Nutrition recommendations and interventions for diabetes: a position statement of the American Diabetes Association. *Diabetes Care* 2008; **31** (Suppl. 1): S61–S78.

25. Rutter CL, Jones C, Dhatariya KK, James J, Irvine L, Wilson EC, et al. Determining in-patient diabetes treatment satisfaction in the UK–the DIPSat study. *Diabet Med* 2013; **30**(6): 731–738.

26. Diabetes UK. Glycaemic Index. http://www.diabetes.org.uk/Guide-to-diabetes/Food_and_recipes/The-Glycaemic-Index/. Accessed Oct 2012.

27. Kreymann KG, Berger MM, Deutz NE, Hiesmayr M, Jolliet P, Kazandjiev G, et al. ESPEN Guidelines on Enteral Nutrition: Intensive care. *Clin Nutr* 2006; **25**: 210–223.

28. Via MA, Mechanick JI. Inpatient enteral and parenteral nutrition for patients with diabetes. *Curr Diab Rep* 2010; **11**: 99–105.

29. Garg A, Grundy SM, Koffler M. Effect of high carbohydrate intake on hyperglycemia, islet function, and plasma lipoproteins in NIDDM. *Diabetes Care* 1992; **15**: 1572–1580.

30. Craig LD, Nicholson S, Silverstone FA, Kennedy RD. Use of a reduced-carbohydrate, modified-fat enteral formula for improving metabolic control and clinical outcomes in longterm care residents with type 2 diabetes: results of a pilot trial. *Nutrition* 1998; **14**: 529–534.

31. Gumbiner B, Low CC, Reaven PD. Effects of a monounsaturated fatty acid-enriched hypocaloric diet on cardiovascular risk factors in obese patients with type 2 diabetes. *Diabetes Care* 1998; **21**: 9–15.

32. Leon-Sanz M, Garcia-Luna PP, Sanz-Paris A, Gómez-Candela C, Casimiro C, Chamorro J, et al. Glycemic and lipid control in hospitalized type 2 diabetic patients: evaluation of 2 enteral nutrition formulas (low carbohydrate- high monounsaturated fat vs high carbohydrate). *J Parenter Enteral Nutr* 2005; **29**: 21–29.

33. Low CC, Grossman EB, Gumbiner B. Potentiation of effects of weight loss by monounsaturated fatty acids in obese NIDDM patients. *Diabetes* 1996; **45**: 569–575.

34. McCargar LJ, Innis SM, Bowron E, Leichter J, Dawson K, Toth E, et al. Effect of enteral nutritional products differing in carbohydrate and fat on indices of carbohydrate and lipid metabolism in patients with NIDDM. *Mol Cell Biochem* 1998; **188**: 81–89.

35. Elia M, Ceriello A, Laube H, Sinclair AJ, Engfer M, Stratton RJ. et al. Enteral nutrition support and use of diabetes-specific formulas for patients with diabetes: a systematic review and meta-analysis. *Diabetes Care* 2005; **28**: 2267–2279.

36. Capes SE, Hunt D, Malmberg K, Gerstein HC. Stress hyperglycaemia and increased risk of death after myocardial infarction in patients with and without diabetes: a systematic overview. *Lancet* 2000; **355**(9206): 773–778.

37. Fowler M. Inpatient Diabetes Management. *Clin Diabetes* 2009; **27**(3): 119–122.

38. American Association of Clinical Endocrinologists and American Diabetes Association: Consensus statement on inpatient glucose control. *Endocr Pract* 2009; **15**: 353–369.

39. Umpierrez GE, Palacio A, Smiley D. Sliding scale insulin use: myth or insanity? *Am J Med* 2007; **120**(7): 563–567.

40. Pasquel FJ, Spiegelman R, McCauley M, Smiley D, Umpierrez D, Johnson R, et al. Hyperglycemia during total parenteral nutrition. An important marker of poor outcome and mortality in hospitalized patients. *Diabetes Care* 2010; **3**(4): 739–741.

41. McMahon M, Manji N, Driscoll D, Bistrian B. Parenteral Nutrition in Patients with Diabetes Mellitus: Theoretical and Practical Considerations. *J Parenter Enteral Nutr* 1989; **13**(5): 461–464.

42. Kumar P R, Crotty P, Raman M. Hyperglycemia in hospitalized patients receiving parental nutrition is associated with increased morbidity and mortality: A review. *Gastroenterol Res Pract* 2011; 2001, Article ID 760720.

Further reading

Diabetes UK. Commissioning Specialist Diabetes Services for Adults with Diabetes. A Diabetes UK Task and Finish Group Report. Oct 2010.

Diabetes UK. Evidence-based nutrition guidelines for the prevention and management of diabetes. May 2011.

Diabetes UK. State of the Nation 2012 England. Care Connect Campaign. 2012.

Donelan A(Chair), Bowen L, Gimson A, Hanazawa S, Saied S, Slee C, et al.; BDA. Delivering Nutritional Care through Food and Beverage Services. A Toolkit for Dietitians. http://www.scribd.com/doc/68226530/Delivering-Nutritional-Care-Through-Food-Beverage-Services#scribd

Durao MS, Marra AR, Moura DF, Almeida SM, Fernandes CJ, Akamine N, et al. Tight glucose control versus intermediate glucose control: a quasi-experimental study. *Anaesth Intensive Care* 2010; **38**(3): 467–473.

Liu Z, Liu J, Jahn LA, Fowler DE, Barrett EJ. Infusing lipid raises plasma free fatty acids and induces insulin resistance in muscle microvasculature. *J Clin Endocrinol Metab* 2009; **94**(9): 3543–3549.

McKnight KA, Carter L. From trays to tube feedings: Overcoming the challenges of hospital nutrition and glycemic control. *Diabetes Spectr* 2008; **21**(4): 233–240.

Parrish CR. The effect of diabetes-specific enteral formulae on clinical and glycemic indicators. *Pract Gastroenterol* 2009; **74**: 20–36.

Preiser JC, Devos P. Clinical experience with tight glucose control by intensive insulin therapy. *Crit Care Med* 2007; **35**(9): S503–S507.

Index

Note: Page numbers in *italics* refer to Figures; those in **bold** to Tables.

Advanced Nutrition and Dietetics in Diabetes, First Edition. Edited by Louise Goff and Pamela Dyson.
© 2016 John Wiley & Sons, Ltd. Published 2016 by John Wiley & Sons, Ltd.

Printed and bound by CPI Group (UK) Ltd, Croydon, CR0 4YY

27/10/2024

14580289-0002

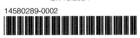